Nurses' Guide to Clinical Procedures

Jean Smith-Temple, DNS, RN

Associate Professor of Nursing
University of South Alabama
Mobile, Alabama

Joyce Young Johnson, PhD, RN, CCRN

Dean and Professor, College of Health Professions
Department of Nursing
Albany State University
Albany, Georgia

EDITION

5

LIPPINCOTT WILLIAMS & WILKINS
A **Wolters Kluwer** Company
Philadelphia · Baltimore · New York · London
Buenos Aires · Hong Kong · Sydney · Tokyo

Acquisitions Editor: Quincy McDonald
Developmental Editors: Megan Klim, Mackenzie Lawrence
Director of Nursing Production: Helen Ewan
Managing Editor / Production: Erika Kors
Senior Production Editor: Tom Gibbons
Design Coordinator: Brett MacNaughton
Senior Manufacturing Manager: William Alberti
Indexer: Nancy Newman
Compositor: Circle Graphics
Printer: R. R. Donnelley

9 8 7 6 5 4 3 2 1

Library of Congress Cataloging-in-Publication Data

Smith-Temple, Jean.
  Nurses' guide to clinical procedures / Jean Smith-Temple, Joyce Young Johnson.—5th ed.
    p. ; cm.
  Includes bibliographical references and index.
  ISBN 0-7817-5379-1 (pbk. : alk. paper)
 1. Nursing—Handbooks, manuals, etc. I. Johnson, Joyce Young. II. Title.
    [DNLM: 1. Nursing Process—Handbooks. 2. Home Care Services—Handbooks. 3. Nursing Care—Handbooks. 4. Patient Care Planning—Handbooks.]
  RT51.S655 2005
  610.73—dc22
                                        2004023826

To my husband, Richard, and son, Benjamin . . . for your encouragement, support, sacrifice, and love in the midst of many life transitions.

To my mother, Louise ("Sunshine"), who is the silent wind beneath my wings.

Jean

To my husband, Larry, and my children, Virginia and Larry, Jr., for your hugs, love, and patience.

To my mother, Dorothy, and in memory of my father, Riley Young Sr., who taught me perseverance, and are a source of encouragement in everything I do.

Joyce

To our students and colleagues for contributing to our professional growth and development.

To our Lord and Savior, through whom we can do all things.

Jean and Joyce

Contributors

Linda W. Alford, RN MEd, MSN, APRN, FNP
Department of Nursing
College of Health Professions
Albany State University
Albany, Georgia

Peggy Boullier, RN, MSN
Clinical Assistant Professor
College of Nursing
University of South Alabama
Mobile, Alabama

Phyllis Prather Hicks, RN, BSN
Nursing Instructor
Harrisburg Community College
Harrisburg, Pennsylvania

Michael Jacobs, RN, MSN, CCRN, CEN
Clinical Assistant Professor
University of South Alabama
Mobile, Alabama

Debra Lett, MSN, MPA, RN
Instructor, School of Nursing
Auburn University
Montgomery, Alabama

Julie Sanford, DNS, RN
Assistant Professor
Spring Hill College
Mobile, Alabama

Kathleen A. Schachman, RN, FNP-C, PhD
Assistant Professor
Director, Family Nurse Practitioner Track
Albany State University
Albany, Georgia

Annette Smith, RN, MSN
Assistant Professor
Coordinator, Undergraduate Nursing Program
Albany State University
Albany, Georgia

Betty J. Tinson-Jenkins, RN
Clinical Skills Lab Coordinator
Department of Nursing
College of Health Professions
Albany State University
Albany, Georgia

Janet Wills, APRN, MEd, MSN, FNP-C
Assistant Professor
Department of Nursing
College of Health Professions
Albany State University
Albany, Georgia

Reviewers

Harrison Applin, RN, BSN, MEd
Nursing Instructor, Course Leader
Grant MacEwan College
Edmonton, Alberta, Canada

Kay Barrington, RN, MEd
Coordinator
Centre for Nursing Studies
St. John's, Newfoundland, Canada

Madeline Buck, BSN, MSN
BSN Nursing Program Coordinator
McGill University
Montreal, Canada

Cheryl Conces, MSN, RN
Assistant Professor, ASN Program Director
University of Indianapolis
Indianapolis, Indiana

Shelba Durston, RN, ADN, BSN, MSN, CCRN
Nursing Instructor
San Joaquin College
Stockton, California

M. Victoria Greensdale, RN, BN, Med, PhD
Nurse Educator
Centre for Nursing Studies
St. John's, Newfoundland, Canada

Pamela Gwin, RNC
Vocational Nursing Program Director
Brazosport College
Lake Jackson, Texas

Karen Hoffman, RN, BSN, MSN
Assistant Professor
Indiana Wesleyan University
Marion, Indiana

Lynda Jackson, RN, BSN, IBCLC
Nursing Instructor
Douglas College
New Westminster, British Columbia, Canada

Caroline Ostand, BC, MSN, RN
Clinical Instructor
University of Charleston
Charleston, West Virginia

Stacey Zampogna-Douglas, BSN
Nursing Learning Resource Coordinator
University of San Francisco
San Francisco, California

Nurses' Guide to Clinical Procedures, Fifth Edition, is a quick-reference clinical-support tool designed to serve students in all types of educational programs and practicing nurses in any clinical setting. The book explains the key steps necessary to perform nursing skills and provides cues to the critical thinking needed for client care.

A detailed Table of Contents and Index are provided for easy reference to procedures. This guide contains information on over 200 skills and now is reorganized to emphasize procedures basic to nurse and client safety and communication by placing them in the first two chapters. The procedures within the 13 chapters of *Nurses' Guide to Clinical Procedures* are organized in a nursing process format, with procedures listed at the beginning of each chapter for convenience. Chapter overviews review basic principles and concepts, including general delegation guidelines. A list of potential nursing diagnoses accompanies each procedure. Nursing procedures are organized as follows:

Purpose(s)
Equipment
Assessment
Nursing Diagnoses
Outcome Identification and Planning
    - Desired outcomes
    - Special considerations
        General
        Pediatric
        Geriatric
        End-of-life care
        Home health
        Transcultural
        Cost-cutting tips
        Delegation guidelines, when appropriate
Implementation (actions with rationales)
Evaluation
Documentation (includes examples of charting)

Actions are presented concisely, with clear illustrations to assist the user. Standard precautions are considered whenever applicable. An icon next to the procedure title indicates that gloves should be worn.

Nursing procedures have been organized to facilitate safe, expedient performance. *Nurses' Guide to Clinical Procedures* should be used as a clinical reference; it is not intended for initial instruction of nursing procedures. The user should review principles in the chapter overview before proceeding to the nursing procedures. Procedures should be read in their entirety to ensure that all relevant health-care matters are considered during performance. Narrative documentation format will be used for charting examples, although many other forms of documentation may be used in the clinical setting. Illustrations, tables, and appendices provide further support. Users should refer to these aids as well as to related nursing procedures, as needed.

Jean Smith-Temple, DNS, RN
Joyce Young Johnson, PHD, RN, CCRN

Acknowledgments

We would like to thank our contributors for their contributions of excellence.

We would like to thank Quincy McDonald and Megan Klim for their insight, support, guidance and patience.

We would also like to thank Troycia Webb, Shondra Green, and Markeeta Williams for their invaluable assistance.

We would also like to thank the many nurse colleagues and colleagues from other disciplines who provided us direction in the preparation of this guidebook.

Contents

1

Safety, Asepsis, and Infection Control

OVERVIEW

- Knowledge of principles of body mechanics and proper body alignment is essential to injury prevention. Improper usage of body mechanics when moving a client could result in injury to client and nurse.
- Proper body mechanics, with prevention of injury, conserves time and energy expenditure, as well as preventing financial expense resulting from injury.
- The occupational group documented as most frequently absent from work with back injury for more than 3 days is nurses.
- Some major nursing diagnostic labels related to body mechanics in association with activity and mobility include impaired physical mobility, risk of physical injury, and activity intolerance.
- Unlicensed assistive personnel should receive training on how to move or transfer clients correctly and monitor for signs of complications; however, routine monitoring remains the responsibility of the nurse. Some techniques should be delegated only to assistive personnel specifically trained or certified in physical rehabilitation maneuvers.
- The chain of infection requires that six links be present:
  - Infectious agent in sufficient amount to cause an infection
  - Place for the agent to multiply and grow (reservoir)
  - Point at which the agent can exit the growth area (portal of exit)
  - Method of transportation from the growth area to other sites (transmission)

- Available access or entrance to another site (portal of entry)
- Susceptible host or medium for agent growth (client)
- The aim of all precaution procedures (standard precautions as well as expanded precautions—contact precautions, droplet precautions, airborne infection isolation, and protective environment) is to decrease exposure to and the spread of microorganisms and disease; all actions are aimed at breaking the chain of infection by eliminating the links, thus maintaining biologic safety (safety from infection).
- Protective devices, particularly gloves, should be worn whenever exposure to body secretions is likely. ALWAYS WEAR GLOVES WHEN EMPTYING DRAINAGE CONTAINERS. Gowns, masks, and goggles should be worn when splashing of secretions is likely.
- Biohazardous waste must be properly discarded and disposed of to prevent exposure to other clients, visitors, or agency personnel. Use biohazard labels and proper containers for specified materials for maximum protection.
- Some major nursing diagnostic labels related to infection control and biologic safety include risk for infection, impaired tissue integrity, knowledge deficit, and anxiety.
- Unlicensed assistive personnel should be trained in safety protocols that prevent exposure to microorganisms such as application of gowns and gloves, use of precaution (isolation) protocols, and disposal of biohazardous wastes.

● Nursing Procedure 1.1

Using Principles of Body Mechanics

Purpose

Prevents physical injury of caregiver and client
Promotes correct body alignment
Facilitates coordinated, efficient muscle use when moving clients
Conserves energy of caregiver for accomplishment of other tasks

Equipment

- Equipment needed to move client or lift object (e.g., Hoyer lift, sling scales, trapeze bar)
- Turn sheets
- Chair, stretcher, or bed for client
- Adequate lighting

- Positioning equipment (e.g., trochanter rolls, pillows, foot-boards)
- Nonsterile gloves
- Visual and hearing aids needed by client

Assessment

Assessment should focus on the following:
- Presence of deformities or abnormalities of vertebrae or limbs
- Physical characteristics of client and caregiver that will influence techniques used (e.g., weight, size, height, age, physical limitations and abilities, condition of target muscles to be used in moving client, problems related to equilibrium)
- Characteristics of object to be moved during client care (e.g., weight, height, shape)
- Immediate environment (e.g., amount of space available to work in; distance to be traveled; presence of obstructions in pathway; condition of floor; placement of chairs, stretchers, and other equipment being used; lighting)
- Adequacy of function and stability of all equipment to be used
- Extent of knowledge of assistive personnel, client, and family regarding proper use of body mechanics and body alignment
- Equipment attached to client that must be moved (e.g., IV machines, tubes, drains)

Nursing Diagnoses

Nursing diagnoses may include the following:
- Risk of physical injury related to improper use of body mechanics
- Deficient knowledge about proper use of body mechanics related to lack of exposure to information

Outcome Identification and Planning

Desired Outcomes

Sample desired outcomes include the following:
- Client displays no evidence of physical injury, such as new bruises, tears, or skeletal trauma after moving.
- Before discharge, client demonstrates proper use of body mechanics to be used in performing major lifting and moving tasks at home.

Special Considerations in Planning and Implementation

General

Secure as much additional assistance as is needed for safe moves. As a general rule, if equipment is available that will make lifting, turning, pulling, or positioning easier, use it. NEVER BECOME SO IMPATIENT THAT SAFETY BECOMES JEOPARDIZED WITH ANY TYPE OF MOVE. Check all equip-

ment to be used, including chairs, for adequate function and stability. *If physical injury of personnel is sustained because of performance of any work-related activity, follow agency policies regarding
follow-up medical attention and completion of incident report forms.
This provides for proper care and ensures financial assistance as
needed.* Avoid excessive pressure and shearing on skin when
moving the client by lifting and not dragging the client.

Pediatric

If child is restless, agitated, or confused, secure assistance to
prevent injury during the moving process.

Geriatric

If client is restless, agitated, or confused or has a condition that
causes loss of muscle control, secure assistance to prevent injury
during the moving process.

Home Health

Assess the home environment to determine the need to rearrange furniture and other items and to secure mechanical
equipment to ensure the safety of client and family as they move
client and perform care.

Delegation

If special precautions are to be used when moving a client,
reinforce the precautions with assistive personnel to make they
understand the client's care needs.

Implementation

Action	Rationale
1. Perform hand hygiene (see Procedure 1.2).	*Reduces microorganism transfer*
2. Determine factors indicating need for additional personnel, such as: • Is there equipment attached to client? • Does the move require persons of approximately the same height?	*Promotes efficiency and enhances safety of client and caregiver*
3. Apply client's glasses and hearing aids if client is able to assist.	*Enables client to assist in making a safe move*
4. Explain required movement techniques to assistive personnel, family, and client; instruct and allow client to do as much as possible.	*Facilitates coordinated movement and prevents physical injury; promotes independence*

Action	Rationale
5. Don gloves if contact with body fluids is likely.	*Prevents exposure to body secretions*
6. Organize equipment so that it is within easy reach, stabilized, and in proper position: • If moving client to chair, place chair so back of chair is in same direction as head of bed. • If placing client on stretcher, align stretcher with side of bed.	*Avoids risks once movement begins; minimizes number of actions needed for the move*
7. Raise or lower bed and other equipment to a comfortable and suitable height.	*Prevents unnecessary use of back muscles when performing tasks*
8. Maintain proper body alignment by using the following principles when handling equipment and when moving, lifting, turning, and positioning client: • Stand with back, neck, shoulders, pelvis, and feet in as straight a line as possible; knees should be slightly flexed and toes pointed forward (Fig. 1.1).	*Maintains proper body alignment*
• Keep feet apart to establish broad support base; keep feet flat on floor (Fig. 1.2).	*Provides greater stability*
• Flex knees and hips to lower center of gravity (heaviest area of body) close to object to be moved (Fig. 1.3).	*Establishes more stable position; prevents pulling on spine*
• Move close to object to be moved or adjusted; do not lean or bend at waist.	*Promotes use of large muscles of extremities rather than of spine*
• Use smooth, rhythmic motions when using bedcranks or any equipment requiring a pumping motion.	*Prevents improper alignment and inefficient muscle use*
• Use arm muscles for cranking or pumping and arm and leg muscles for lifting	*Avoids use of spine and back muscles*

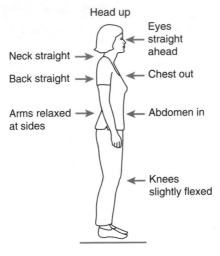

FIGURE 1.1

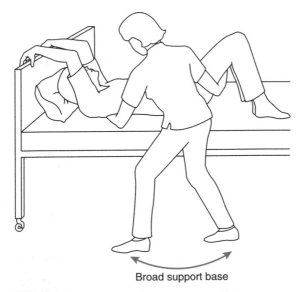

FIGURE 1.2

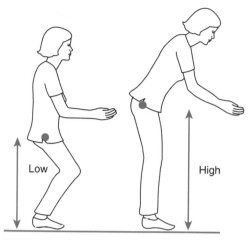

Low

High

FIGURE 1.3

Action	Rationale
9. Secure tubes, drains, traction, and other equipment by whatever means are needed for proper functioning during moving, lifting, turning, and positioning.	*Prevents dislodgment of tubes and reflux of contaminants into body*
10. Move client close to edge of bed in one unit or move client to side of bed at any time during procedure, moving one unit of the body at a time from top to bottom or vice versa (i.e., head and shoulders first, trunk and hips second, and legs last). Coordinate move so everyone exerts greatest effort on count of three; the person carrying the heaviest load should direct the count.	*Maintains correct alignment; facilitates comfort; prevents physical injury*
11. Use the following principles to move a heavy object or client: • Review each move again before move is made.	*Reinforces original plan*

Action	Rationale
• Face client or object to be moved.	*Allows full use of arm and leg muscles*
• Place hands or arms fully under client or object; lock hands with assistant on opposite side, if necessary.	*Provides extra leverage*
• Prepare for move by taking in a deep breath, tightening abdominal and gluteal muscles, and tucking chin toward chest. (If client cannot provide assistance, instruct client to cross arms on chest.)	*Facilitates use of large muscle groups; prevents injury to arms during move and centers client's weight*
• Allow adequate rest periods, if needed.	*Prevents fatigue and subsequent physical injury*
• When performing move, keep heaviest part of body within base of support.	*Promotes stability*
• Perform pulling motions by leaning backward and pushing motions by leaning forward, maintaining wide base of support with feet, keeping knees flexed and one foot behind the other; push and pull (instead of lifting, whenever possible) using the muscles of the arms and legs, not back.	*Prevents injury to vertebrae and back muscles*
• Always lower head of bed as much as permissible.	*Avoids pulling against gravity*
• When moving from a bending to a standing position, stop momentarily once in standing position before completing next move. When getting client into a chair, stop to allow client and self to stand to establish stability before pivoting into chair.	*Allows time to straighten spine and reestablish stability*

Action	Rationale
• Move in as straight and direct a path as possible, avoiding twisting and turning of spine.	*Avoids vertebral and back injury related to rotating and twisting spine*
• When turning is unavoidable, use a pivoting turn; when positioning client in chair or carrying client to a stretcher, pivot toward chair or stretcher together.	*Avoids twisting of spine and possible muscle strain*
12. Position props and body parts for appropriate body alignment of client after move is completed:	*Maintains body alignment*
• When client is sitting, ensure that hips, shoulders, and neck are in line with trunk and knees, hips, and ankles are flexed at a 90-degree angle with toes pointing forward.	
• When client is in bed, ensure that neck, shoulders, pelvis, and ankles are in line with trunk, with knees and elbows slightly flexed.	
13. After move is completed, provide for comfort and safety of client with the following actions, if applicable:	
• Raise protective rails.	*Prevents falls*
• Apply safety belts on stretchers and wheelchairs.	*Promotes safety*
• Lower height of bed.	*Promotes safety*
• Elevate head properly.	*Supports airway clearance*
• Restore all tubes, drains, and equipment being used by client to proper functioning and placement.	*Reestablishes proper functioning of equipment*
• Place pillows and position equipment properly.	*Promotes proper body alignment and supports airway, if client is intubated*
• Replace covers.	*Provides warmth and privacy*
• Place call light within reach.	*Provides means of communication*

Action	Rationale
• Place frequently used items within client's reach.	*Enhances comfort and general satisfaction*
14. Discard gloves and perform hand hygiene.	*Reduces microorganism transfer*

Evaluation

Were desired outcomes achieved? Examples of evaluation include:
● Desired outcome met: Client displays no evidence of physical injury.
● Desired outcome met: Client demonstrated proper use of body mechanics to be used in performing major lifting and moving tasks at home.

Documentation

The following should be noted on the client's chart:
● Amount of assistance given by client
● Position in which client was placed (e.g., in chair, returned to bed, on stretcher)
● Reports of discomfort, dizziness, or faintness during or after move
● Reestablishment of proper functioning of equipment
● Safety belts applied
● Status of side rails
● Auxiliary equipment used
● Status of equipment being used to maintain alignment

Sample Documentation
Date: 1/19/05
Time: 1030

Assisted client into chair. Client able to provide partial assistance; reported slight dizziness when standing. IV remains intact and infusing at prescribed flow rate. Vest restraint reapplied. Call light within reach.

Using Principles of Medical Asepsis

Purpose

Prevents the growth and spread of pathogenic microorganisms from one individual or the environment to another individual

Equipment

- Soap and warm running water
- Nonsterile gloves
- Clean gown
- Mask
- Waste disposal materials: trash can, bags (precaution bags optional)
- Precaution stickers
- Linen bags
- Specimen bags, as needed

Assessment

Assessment should focus on the following:
- Data from medical history and physical or diagnostic studies indicating susceptibility to or presence of infection (fever, cloudy urine, positive culture, decreased white blood count, history of immunosuppression or steroid intake)
- Doctor's orders or agency policy regarding standard and expanded precaution procedures
- Client's or nurse's allergy to soap or bacteriostatic solutions
- Client's assignment (ward, double or single room)
- Client's knowledge of principles of asepsis
- Ability of client to cooperate and not contaminate sterile field

Nursing Diagnoses

Nursing diagnoses may include the following:
- Risk for impaired skin integrity related to wound drainage
- Risk for infection related to immunosuppressive therapy for renal transplant

Outcome Identification and Planning

Desired Outcomes

Sample desired outcomes include the following:
- Client's skin remains intact and irritation-free around ostomy site.
- Client remains free of signs of infection or of additional infection.

Special Considerations in Planning and Implementation

General

Display 1.1 discusses hand hygiene. Keep your fingernails short and filed. Dirt and secretions that lodge under fingernails contain microorganisms. Long fingernails can scratch client's skin.

Pediatric

If a child is restless or too young to understand the importance of maintaining a sterile field, prevent the child from moving using linen or soft restraints during the medical procedure.

Geriatric

If a client is disoriented and restless, gently prevent him or her from moving during procedures that require maintenance of sterile or clean materials.

Home Health

Bar pets from the room in which a medical procedure is being performed. Remember that procedures are performed with clean rather than sterile technique.

Implementation

Action	Rationale
Performing Hand Hygiene: Handwashing (Medical)	
1. Stand in front of sink, being careful that uniform does not touch the sink during the washing procedure.	*Sinks are considered contaminated; uniforms can carry organisms from place to place*
2. Remove rings (often may retain wedding band) and chipped nail polish; move watch to position high on wrist.	*Removes sources that harbor and promote growth of microorganisms*
3. Wet hands from wrist to fingertips under flowing water.	*Aids in removal of microorganisms from least to most dirty*
4. Keep hands and forearms lower than elbows when washing.	*Water flows from least to most contaminated area; hands are the most contaminated parts to be washed; permits cleaning of the dirtiest areas without risking contamination of other less dirty areas*
5. Place soap, preferably bacteriostatic, on hands and rub vigorously for 15 to 30 seconds, massaging all	*Creates friction to remove organisms; permits cleaning around and under ring*

● Display 1.1 Hand Hygiene

The Centers for Disease Control and Prevention uses specific terminology related to infection prevention. **Hand hygiene** refers to any of the following:
- Handwashing with non-antimicrobial soap and water
- Handwashing with antiseptic soap
- Using an antiseptic handrub (waterless product that is usually alcohol-based)
- Performing surgical hand antisepsis (discussed in Procedure 1.3)

Handwashing is indicated when hands are visibly soiled. Handwashing is also mandatory after contact with bodily fluids or excretions, mucous membranes, non-intact skin, or wound dressings. If hands are not visibly soiled and have not come in contact with the fluids or surfaces listed above, using an antiseptic handrub is permitted.

Action	Rationale
skin areas, joints, finger-nails, between fingers, and so forth; slide ring up and down while rubbing fingers (if unable to remove).	
6. Rinse hands from fingers to wrist under flow of water.	*Washes dirt and organisms from cleanest to least clean area*
7. Dry hands with paper towel, moving from fingers to wrist to forearm.	*Dries hands from cleanest to least clean area*
8. Turn off faucet with paper towel.	*Prevents recontamination of hand*

Performing Hand Hygiene: Using an Antiseptic Handrub

1. Apply amount of product recommended by manufacturer to palm of one hand.	*Ensures that correct amount of handrub is used*
2. Rub hands together, covering all surfaces of the hands from wrists to fingers. Continue rubbing until hands are dry.	*Distributes handrub; decontaminates hands*

Managing Contaminated Materials

1. Don gloves when contact with body fluids or infected area is possible.	*Prevents contamination of hands; prevents contact with secretions*

Action	Rationale
2. Use specimen bags for any specimens collected.	*Prevents exposure to microorganisms found in specimens*
3. Don mask if organism can be transmitted by airborne route through contact with mucous membranes.	*Prevents exposure to airborne microorganisms or projectile body fluids*
4. Don gown if contact with body secretions or contaminated area is likely, if client has highly contagious condition, or if client is immunosuppressed.	*Avoids contact with potentially infectious material; avoids spread of infection; protects client from exposure to microorganisms*
5. Place disposable contaminated materials in bag before leaving bedside; place in dirty utility room or send for waste disposal personnel; or place in precaution (isolation) bag or mark "BIOHAZARD or Precaution (isolation)" on bag; use double bagging, if agency policy.	*Provides added protection against exposure to body fluids or infectious materials; alerts housekeeping department to dispose of materials properly*
6. Bag reusable items, labeled "Precaution (isolation)," and send to central supply unit for sterilization or to appropriate department for cleaning; items too large to bag should be sprayed with disinfectant and sent for thorough cleaning.	*Decreases spread of microorganisms on used medical equipment*
7. Place linens in linen bags before leaving bedside and place in central hamper or linen chute (agency may require double bagging).	*Decreases spread of organisms; clears environment of dirty materials*
8. Clean stethoscope between use for different clients with soap and water and wipe with alcohol swab (if used in an infected area or with an infected client, thorough disassembly and cleaning may be needed). Use a separate stethoscope for a client with an infection, if possible.	*Decreases spread of microorganisms on stethoscope; limits exposure to infection*
9. Spray or wipe sphygmomanometers, thermometers, ECG leads, or similar daily-use items with a bacteriosta-	*Decreases exposure to potentially infectious medium, because these items provide a good medium for organism growth*

Action	Rationale
tic substance between use with different clients.	
10. Place used syringes and needles, scalpels, and other sharp disposables in appropriately marked container. DO NOT REPLACE CAPS ON NEEDLES.	*Prevents accidental stick and contact with client's blood; prevents accidental sticks during attempts to recap needle*
11. Discard gown, gloves, and mask before leaving client's room.	*Prevents spread of infection*

Handling Clients' Personal Items

Action	Rationale
1. Place items in bags and send home with family; if client is discharged and does not want certain items, dispose of these as described.	
2. NEVER SHARE PERSONAL-CARE ITEMS BETWEEN CLIENTS.	*Prevents general spread of infection*
3. If papers, books, or other items become soiled with infectious material, discard items unless sterilization is possible and desired.	*Prevents spread of microorganisms from contaminated materials to client or others*

Determining Room Assignment

Action	Rationale
1. Placement in a private room is preferable but is required only when a highly virulent or infectious microorganism is present, the microorganism is airborne, or the client is highly susceptible to infection.	*Protects client or other clients from cross-contamination*
2. Use a semiprivate room when the microorganism is limited to one body area; however, good medical asepsis must be maintained by staff, client, family, and visitors.	*Prevents spread of infection*

Cleaning Room

Action	Rationale
1. Ensure that room is cleaned with disinfectant daily. If soiled materials spill on floor, clean area	*Reduces microorganisms in the environment*

Action	Rationale
with disinfectant or bactericidal agent specific to organism, if known. 2. When client with known infection is discharged, is transferred, or dies, ensure that room is cleaned and disinfected thoroughly and allowed to remain vacant for 12 to 24 hours. (See Procedure 12.3 for post-mortem care and Procedure 1.4 for additional information on precaution techniques.)	*Promotes thorough removal of microorganisms*

Evaluation

Were desired outcomes achieved? Examples of evaluation include:
● Desired outcome met: Skin around ostomy is clean and intact.
● Desired outcome met: Client shows no signs of infection or reinfection.

Documentation

The following should be noted on the client's chart:
● Status of source of infection/potential infection (wound, dressing, breath sounds, secretions)
● Procedure performed
● Protective garments used
● Client teaching completed

Sample Documentation
Date: 1/2/05
Time: 1200

Abdominal abscess site dressed. Site clean and without redness. Drains intact. Client tolerated procedure without complaint of unusual discomfort. States understands dressing change process and would like to change dressing in morning. Contact precautions maintained.

Using Principles of Surgical Asepsis 🧤

Purpose

Avoids introducing microorganisms onto a designated sterile field

Equipment

- Bactericidal or antimicrobial soap
- Sink with side or foot pedal
- Surgical scrub brush
- Sterile gloves
- Sterile gown
- Mask
- Hair covering and booties (optional)
- Sterile materials (dressing, instruments)
- Sterile sheets or towels (occasionally found in dressing tray)
- Waste disposal materials: trash can, bags (precaution [isolation] bags optional)

Assessment

Assessment should focus on the following:
- Data from medical history and physical or diagnostic studies indicating susceptibility to infection (decreased leukocyte count, history of immunosuppression, or steroid intake)
- Doctor's orders or agency policy regarding dressing changes and precaution procedures
- Client's or nurse's allergy to soap or bacteriostatic solutions
- Client's room assignment (ward, double or single room)
- Date of expiration and sterility indicator on sterile supplies and solutions
- Client's knowledge of principles of asepsis
- Client's ability to cooperate and not contaminate sterile field
- Agency policy regarding surgical scrub procedure

Nursing Diagnoses

Nursing diagnoses may include the following:
- Risk for infection related to central line insertion and total parenteral nutrition (TPN) therapy
- Deficient knowledge related to immunosuppression from renal transplant therapy

Outcome Identification and Planning

Desired Outcomes

Sample desired outcomes include the following:
- Client shows no signs of infection or of additional infection.
- Client verbalizes understanding of need for protective environment.

Special Considerations in Planning and Implementation

General

Variations in sterile technique (e.g., the omission of some protective coverings [hair cover, booties, mask]) may be used in performing some procedures. CONTINUE TO USE ASEPTIC PRINCIPLES TO GOVERN ACTIONS DURING A PROCEDURE. IF UNSURE OF STERILITY OF MATERIAL, GLOVE, OR FIELD, CONSIDER IT CONTAMINATED. Consult appropriate policies and procedures manuals.

Pediatric

If a child is restless or too young to understand the importance of maintaining a sterile field, restrain the child with linen or soft restraints during the procedure. Use a family member to assist in holding the child still and allaying fears, if possible. Provide sedation or pain medication before the procedure to comfort and calm the child.

Geriatric

If a client is disoriented and restless, enlist assistance or use manual protective device(s) to hold client still during procedures requiring maintenance of sterile materials (see Procedure 1.6).

Home Health

Bar pets from the room in which a sterile or clean procedure is being performed. Keep in mind that most procedures are performed with clean rather than sterile technique. Enlist and instruct a family member to serve as an assistant. Remove biohazardous waste from home each visit. See Display 1.2 for various considerations in teaching the client/family about infection control and disposal of biohazardous waste in the home. Disposal requirements for biohazardous waste vary by state and by agency.

● Display 1.2 Infection Control in the Home (Including Teaching Points)

Assessment

Assess the following:

- Client's and family's ability to understand and perform necessary infection control procedures (see "Implementation")
- General environmental cleanliness
- Possibility of insect or rodent infestation
- Number and status of people living in the home
- Specific client conditions requiring special infection control techniques

Planning

Sample desired outcomes:

- No transfer of microorganisms will occur from client to others.
- No contamination of sterile and clean supplies by microorganisms will occur.

Special considerations:

- Basic infection control practices should be a basic part of instruction in healthy lifestyle, particularly in multi-generational families living in one house.
- Handwashing, environmental cleaning, and laundry may have cultural implications. Contact a resource person before proceeding with teaching.
- Be alert for the possibility that poor compliance with infection control practices may be related to insufficient funds; contact social service agencies and other community resources, if necessary. Insect or rodent infestation may be a major obstacle to infection control in the home. If needed, contact the public health department for advice and assistance.
- Prepare to teach. Gather supplies, including nonsterile gloves, gown/apron, masks, goggles, 10% bleach solution, biohazardous waste containers, rigid plastic container (e.g., detergent jug), household disinfectant, and paper towels.
- Remember that the nurse must arrange for pickup of biohazardous waste containers from the home.
- All family members and caregivers must be instructed in standard precautions if they are going to be exposed to blood or body fluids.

Implementation

1. Instruct all family members to perform handwashing before and after doing client care, after using the toilet,

(display continues on page 20)

● Display 1.2 Infection Control in the Home
(Including Teaching Points) (continued)

and whenever handling trash or biohazardous materials, including raw meats. Provide the following instruction about handwashing technique:

a. Turn on water.
b. Apply soap, using vigorous friction to all skin surfaces for at least 10 seconds.
c. Rinse hands under running water and turn off faucet with paper towel.
d. Dry hands with paper towel, not cloth towel used by others.

2. Teach about general environmental cleaning:
a. Use disinfectant and/or bleach solution to clean the bathroom and kitchen.
b. Clean surfaces in client area with disinfectant (avoid strong odors if client has respiratory condition or arrange for client to be out of room until odor dissipates).
c. Vacuum and dust as needed (also remove client from area until completed).
d. Remove heavy carpet and difficult-to-clean furniture from client area, if possible.
e. All family members must use own towel, washcloth, and toothbrush.

3. Instruct family and client regarding avoidance of blood-borne transmission:
a. Wash garments, linens, and towels soiled with blood and body fluids:
   • Wear gloves.
   • Rinse all items in cold water.
   • Wash separately from family laundry in washer with hot water and bleach.
b. To dispose of used dressings soiled with blood or body fluids:
   • Wear gloves.
   • Wear other personal protective equipment if splashing is anticipated.
   • Place soiled dressings in an approved biohazardous waste container.
c. If needles are being used, use sharps container (heavy plastic jug with lid).
   • Place small amount of bleach solution in jug.
   • Place all used sharps in jug and replace lid each time.
   • Discard when two-thirds full.
   Note: If a sharps container exchange program is available in the community, instruct caregivers in how to access this resource.

4. Teach about maintenance of supplies if sterile or clean supplies are to be left in the home for client use:

● Display 1.2 Infection Control in the Home
(Including Teaching Points) (continued)

a. Place supplies in a clean, protected storage area that
   may be used for supplies only.
b. Cover supplies with clean plastic or towel.

Documentation

In the visit note, include the infection control instructions
given and to whom, special circumstances in the home, and
activities taken to address them.

Implementation

Action	Rationale
Determining Room Assignment	
Use a private room (preferable) for performing a sterile procedure; transfer client to treatment room, if necessary.	*Minimizes microorganisms in environment*
Performing Surgical Hand Antisepsis (Surgical Scrub)	
1. Don mask, hair cover, and booties, if required.	*Prevents introduction of contaminants from mouth, hair, or shoes into environment*
2. Perform surgical scrub using counted brush stroke method.	*Reduces organisms on hands; counted brush stroke method places emphasis on specific areas and ensures that all skin surfaces are exposed to sufficient friction*
• Remove rings (often must remove wedding band), chipped nail polish, and watch.	*Removes sources that harbor and promote growth of microorganisms*
• Stand in front of sink, being careful that uniform does not touch sink during washing procedure.	*Avoids sink, which is considered contaminated; prevents uniform, which can carry organisms from place to place, from coming into contact with a contaminated surface*
• Wet hands and arms from elbows to fingertips under flowing	*Cleans from least to most dirty area; aids in removal of microorganisms*

Action	Rationale
water (use sink with side or foot pedal).	
• Place soap, preferably antimicrobial/ bacteriostatic, on hands and rub vigorously for 15 to 30 seconds; use scrub brush gently— do not abrade skin.	*Reduces microorganisms on hands; creates friction to remove organisms*
• Using circular motion, scrub all skin areas, joints, fingernails, between fingers, and so forth (on all sides and 2 inches above elbows); slide ring, if present, up and down while rubbing fingers.	*Works soap thoroughly over skin surface to increase removal of dirt and organisms; permits cleaning around and under ring*
• Continue scrub for 5 to 10 minutes or per agency policy.	
• Rinse hands from fingers to elbows under flow of water.	*Washes dirt and organisms from cleanest to least clean area*
• Repeat soaping, rubbing, and rinsing until hands and arms are clean.	
• Pat hands dry with sterile towel, moving from fingers to wrist.	*Dries hands from clean to least clean area*
• Turn off faucet with side or foot pedal.	*Prevents recontamination of hands*

Managing a Sterile Field

Action	Rationale
1. To create a sterile field:	
• Arrange sterile supplies on overbed table or surgical stand. NEVER USE OPENED ITEMS OR ITEMS OF QUESTIONABLE STERILITY.	*Organization reduces the risk of error and contamination*
• Open packages to reveal supplies, using insides of packages to form sterile field; open package's outer flap away from you, open side flaps next, and then pull inner flap toward you	*Prevents reaching over exposed materials; reduces risk that edges, which are considered unsterile, will contaminate field*

Action	Rationale
(Fig. 1.4); spread edges of package cover over table with fingertips. 2. To add items to sterile field: • Drop sterile items onto field, keeping packaging between items and hands (Fig. 1.5); use sterile forceps or tongs to remove items from package if unable to do so with sterile technique; if unable to remove item from package without contamination, wait until sterile garb is applied, then place items on sterile field.	*Prevents contamination of supplies*
• Use sterile gloves or sterile tongs to remove sterile towels from field, and cover field and supplies if not beginning procedure immediately. DO NOT REACH OVER OPEN STERILE FIELD, AS THIS EXPOSES FIELD TO CONTAMINATION.	*Prevents loss of sterility if field is exposed to air for extended period of time*
• Don sterile gown and sterile gloves (see	*Prevents exposure of sterile field to hands or clothing*

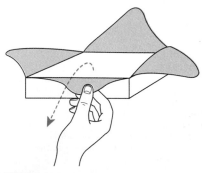

FIGURE 1.4

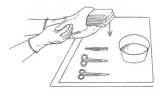

FIGURE 1.5

Action	Rationale
Procedures 11.1 and 11.2).	
• Begin procedure with hands held above waist.	*Maintains area above the waist as sterile; area below waist is considered nonsterile*
3. To maintain a sterile field:	
• Drape sterile sheets or towels over area surrounding site being treated.	*Decreases chance of exposure to nonsterile sites*
• Use tongs or forceps to clean site thoroughly with bactericidal agent.	*Maintains sterility of gloves; reduces microorganisms*
• Discard tongs from sterile field.	*Prevents field contamination*
• Pour liquids into a sterile basin held by an assistant in sterile garb or by holding bottle over 1-inch outer parameter of field; avoid splashing on field. IF FIELD BECOMES WET, CONSIDER IT CONTAMINATED.	*Prevents reaching over sterile field; allows water to conduct microorganisms from nonsterile area to sterile field*

Maintaining Asepsis During Procedure

Action	Rationale
1. Remove soiled equipment from area or sterile field and drop trash in bag or receptacle; avoid touching nonsterile surfaces.	*Prevents introduction of microorganisms onto sterile field*
2. When procedure is complete and dressing is intact, label dressing with date, time, and your initials.	*Indicates when next dressing change is due*

Action	Rationale
Limiting Microorganisms in the Environment	
Maintain a clean protective environment for immuno-suppressed clients or burn clients:	
• Place client in single room.	*Decreases exposure to micro-organisms*
• Use a separate stetho-scope, sphygmomano-meter, and thermome-ter for client, if possible.	*Prevents exposure to micro-organisms*
• Use only hospital gowns, linens, and ma-terials; allow no items from home unless ap-proved and sterilized by hospital.	*Prevents introduction of possible source of contamination*
• When client is severely immunosuppressed, remove papers, books, and other personal items from immediate area unless sterilization is possible.	*Removes items that may be contaminated*
• Use special food trays, disposable or pre-sterilized.	

Evaluation

Were desired outcomes achieved? Examples of evaluation include:
• Desired outcome met: Client showed no signs of infection.
• Desired outcome met: Client verbalized understanding of need for protective environment.

Documentation

The following should be noted on the client's chart:
• Status of wound, dressing, and incision site, with indication of signs of infection, if any
• Procedure performed
• Protective garments used
• Client teaching done regarding maintenance of dressing and sterile protective environment and verbalized understanding by client

Sample Documentation
Date: 12/2/05
Time: 1200

Temporary pacemaker inserted at bedside by Dr. Hope using sterile technique. Chest site clean and without redness. Clean, sterile dressing applied to site. Client tolerated procedure without complaint of unusual discomfort. Client states understanding of dressing change process and need for sterility.

● **Nursing Procedures 1.4, 1.5**

Using Precaution (Isolation) Techniques: Infection Prevention (1.4) 🧤
Disposing of Biohazardous Waste (1.5) 🧤

Purpose

Prevents spread of infection from client to others
Decreases exposure of susceptible client to infection

Equipment

- Precaution (isolation) cart
- Precautions door card indicating that visitors must see nurse before entry, depending on type of precaution (see Appendix F)
- Soap and source of water
- Paper towels
- Approved sharps container
- Approved rigid biohazardous waste container
- Approved biohazardous waste bags
- Spill kit or spill cloth

If a precaution cart is unavailable or not preferred, substitute the following materials:

- Masks
- Gloves (nonsterile or sterile)
- Gowns
- Plastic bags (or cloth linen bags)
- Tape, bag ties, or fasteners

Assessment

Assessment should focus on the following:
- Type of precaution indicated
- Site of infection
- Kind of barrier restrictions needed in addition to standard precautions
- Perceptions of client and family regarding information provided by doctor
- Usual duration of infection
- Adequate ventilation in room (often door is kept closed)
- Associated physical symptoms of client, such as elevated temperature, chills, stiff neck
- Items considered to be biohazardous waste
- Requirements and methods for safe disposal of biohazardous waste (agency and community)

Nursing Diagnoses

Nursing diagnoses may include the following:
- Deficient knowledge related to minimizing exposure to pathogens
- Impaired skin integrity related to burn

Outcome Identification and Planning

Desired Outcomes

Sample desired outcomes include the following:
- Client verbalizes three procedures needed to maintain specified precaution (isolation) by end of day.
- Client shows no signs of additional infection.

Special Considerations in Planning and Implementation

General

Refer to Display 1.3 for discussion of standard and expanded precautions. Hand hygiene is the single most important measure used to prevent the spread of infection. Perform hand hygiene before entering and upon leaving precaution (isolation) rooms, as well as between care procedures for different clients. Often handwashing is the required form of hand hygiene. Most hospital policies require a nurse to obtain a culture from a draining body area and to initiate precaution (isolation) procedures when positive cultures are reported. Consult the agency policy man-

● Display 1.3 Infection Prevention: Standard and Expanded Precautions

Standard Precautions are infection prevention techniques that apply in all health care settings and to all patients, regardless of their infection status. Standard Precautions are rooted in the fact that all blood, body fluids (including secretions and excretions, except sweat), and open skin may have infectious agents.

Expanded Precautions, previously called transmission-based precautions, aims to control transmission of highly infectious agents or epidemiologically important infectious agents. Expanded Precautions include Contact Precautions, Droplet Precautions, Airborne Infection Isolation, and Protective Environment.

ual. A client may become withdrawn, depressed, and feel abandoned due to precaution (isolation). Plan frequent visits with the client and follow through as promised.

Home Health

Provide family members with an information sheet with clear instructions.

Implementation

Action	Rationale
Using Precaution Techniques	
1. Clearly explain to client and family the precaution (isolation) type, reason initiated, how microorganisms are spread, staff and visitor restrictions related to dress and duration of contact (if applicable), and compliance needed; demonstrate procedure for applying sterile mask and gown. THE DOCTOR SHOULD INITIALLY INFORM THE CLIENT OF THE DIAGNOSED INFECTION.	*Increases compliance of client, family, and visitors; decreases anxiety*
2. Ensure that precaution (isolation) cart is complete and that sufficient trash cans and linen bags are in room.	*Promotes organized, efficient, and proper disposal of contaminated materials*

Action	Rationale
3. Keep sufficient linens and towels in room.	*Avoids unnecessary trips into and out of room; decreases spread of microorganisms*
4. Have housekeeping staff check room daily for sufficient soap and paper towels.	*Facilitates compliance with need for frequent handwashing*
5. Perform hand hygiene and organize equipment.	*Reduces microorganism transfer; promotes efficiency*
6. Note doctor's orders or refer to precaution (isolation) guidelines adopted by agency for precautions necessary to establish appropriate type of precaution (isolation) (see Appendix D).	*Provides sufficient protection from microorganisms with minimum stress and restrictions on client, visitors, and staff*
7. Obtain appropriate precaution (isolation) card and place on client's door. (If card must be filled out, include instructions on hand hygiene; use of masks, gloves, and gowns; handling of linen and disposable items; and need for private room, if appropriate.)	*Alerts visitors and staff to follow dress and hand hygiene restrictions*
8. Review disinfectants needed to eliminate specific microorganisms.	*Prepares nurse for environmental and client management*
9. Inform any visitors of necessary precautions.	*Allays fears to prevent withdrawal of friends and family from client; increases compliance*
10. Maintain precaution (isolation) supplies and cart outside door of client's room.	*Facilitates maintenance of precaution (isolation)*
11. Obtain supplies needed for wound care, if required, and keep sufficient supplies in client's room.	*Avoids unnecessary trips into and out of room; decreases spread of microorganisms*

Disposing of Biohazardous Materials

1. Don gloves, maintain asepsis while handling waste.	*Prevents contact with bodily fluids*
2. Keep disposal equipment readily available for use at all times (e.g., if using	*Allows for safe disposal of waste even if not anticipated before care*

Action	Rationale
sharps, take sharps container into client area; replace sharps container when it is two-thirds full to avoid needlesticks when putting additional sharps in a nearly full container).	
3. Dispose of used supplies taken into room or place them inside appropriate precaution (isolation) bag for removal.	*Prevents spread of infection from objects used on or by client*
4. When removing full sharps container, close securely (date and label, if agency policy). If transporting in car, place in second rigid-walled container. Log in sharps container for disposal per agency policy.	*Prevents contamination of supplies in car; adds extra barrier*
5. Use plastic bags for trash and reusable equipment. Use biohazard bags to bag disposable drainage systems and soiled non-sharp biohazardous materials before delivering to agency's disposal unit. If removing to car for disposal, place bags in rigid container in car.	*Prevents spread of infection from contaminated materials; keeps biohazardous waste separate from other supplies*
6. Label reusable equipment.	*Indicates date of use and possible replacement time*
7. Place soiled linens in proper linen bags; double-bag linens if required by agency. Take linen bags to soiled utility room. (Instruct family to wash soiled linen and clothing separate from family wash.)	*Allows for washing without removing from bag*
8. Clean room thoroughly with appropriate anti-microbial agent. If blood or body fluids spill in client's home, use spill kit or spill cloth.	*Kills virulent organisms; prevents exposure of other clients or family members to infection*
9. Leave room unoccupied after client discharge for appropriate time period.	*Minimizes exchange of organisms between clients*
10. Perform hand hygiene.	*Reduces microorganism transfer*

Evaluation

Were desired outcomes achieved? Examples of evaluation include:
- Desired outcome met: Client verbalizes three procedures needed to maintain specified precaution (isolation).
- Desired outcome met: Client shows no signs of additional infection.

Documentation

The following should be noted on the client's chart:
- Status of client's infection (identity of infection and extent of areas involved)
- Client's, family's, and visitors' understanding of and compliance with precaution (isolation) and required precautions
- Staff compliance with precaution (isolation) precautions and biohazardous waste disposal
- Periodic culture reports to establish need for continued precaution (isolation)

Sample Documentation
Date: 2/3/05
Time: 1400

Lab report obtained on culture of sputum specimen; results show pneumococcal pneumonia. Doctor notified. Client and family instructed on precaution (isolation) procedures; understanding voiced. Airborne precautions noted on sign placed on door. Masks and gloves placed outside of room. Visitors instructed on use of mask. Understanding verbalized by visitors and compliance noted.

● **Nursing Procedure 1.6**

Using Protective Devices: Limb and Body Restraints

Purpose

Prevents injury to client from falls, wound contamination, and tube dislodgment

Prevents injury to others from disoriented or hostile client when other methods of control have been ineffective

Equipment

- Restraint appropriate for limb or body area (e.g., wrist, ankle, vest, or waist restraint)
- Washcloths for each limb restraint (if restraints are not padded)
- Lotion and powder (optional)
- Stretch (Kerlix) gauze (3- or 4-inch roll)
- 2-inch tape

Assessment

Assessment should focus on the following:
- Specific client behaviors and circumstances indicating need for protective devices
- Client's orientation and level of consciousness
- Alternative activities attempted to avoid use of restraints (unless part of care standard or protocol)
- Effectiveness of other safety controls and precautions
- Availability of staff or family members to sit with client
- Doctor's order (obtain if not on chart)
- Agency policy regarding use of restraints
- Skin and circulatory status in areas requiring restraint

Nursing Diagnoses

Nursing diagnoses may include the following:
- Risk of injury related to confusion and disorientation
- Risk of impaired skin integrity related to use of restraints

Outcome Identification and Planning

Desired Outcomes

Sample desired outcomes include the following:
- Client experiences no falls or injury while under nurse's care.
- Client demonstrates intact skin and circulation at and below the site of restraint, with capillary refill <3 seconds and warm skin temperature.

Special Considerations in Planning and Implementation

General

Because restraints may actually cause injury instead of preventing it, whenever possible use alternative protective measures specific to the problem resulting in the use of restraints (e.g., minimize use of invasive treatments, disguise tubing or keep out of client's view, wrap infusion sites in stockinette or bandage, and use abdominal binder for dressings to prevent disruption of lines or wounds).

Always obtain a doctor's order before applying restraints, unless an approved protocol or standard is in place. Notify the doctor of the time when restraints were initiated so a face-to-face evaluation can be performed within 1 hour of restraint use as required by the Joint Commission on Accreditation of Healthcare Organizations (JCAHO) and the Health Care Financing Administration (HCFA). Learn standards and protocols and agency policy regarding use of restraints (some agencies require that restraints be used in certain situations, such as presence of an endotracheal tube). Note that JCAHO standards limit restraint use to emergent dangerous client actions; addictive disorders; as an adjunct to planned care; and as a component of an approved protocol, or in some cases as part of standard practice. While a client is in restraints, perform assessments every 15 minutes; in some agencies, one-on-one supervision of the client is required for the entire period.

Pediatric

Use mittens, which may be preferable to wrist restraints because they are less restrictive and permit growth and development activities.

Geriatric

Restrain elderly clients with linen or soft restraints applied loosely because the skin in elderly people is often very sensitive and the blood vessels are easily collapsed. Check the circulation frequently. Remove restraints frequently to check the skin underneath.

Home Health

Suggest using sheets to help secure a client to a bed or chair to prevent falls.

Cost-Cutting Tips

Use socks or other soft pieces of cloth to make wrist restraints; mittens made with socks or gauze restraints may be used to prevent pulling of tubes. However, commercial restraints may be cost-effective due to decreased friction on skin.

Delegation

Train unlicensed assistive personnel before they are allowed to apply restraints. Training focuses on appropriate application and client monitoring. However, monitoring the client's physical status remains the primary responsibility of the nurse.

Implementation

Action	Rationale
1. Perform hand hygiene and organize equipment.	*Prevents microorganism transfer; promotes efficiency*

Action	Rationale
2. Explain procedure to client and state why restraints are needed.	*Promotes cooperation; reduces anxiety*
3. Place client in a comfortable position with good body alignment.	*Promotes client cooperation in remaining in proper position while movement is restricted*
4. Wash and dry area to which restraint will be applied; massage area and apply lotion if skin is dry; apply powder, if desired.	*Facilitates circulation to skin; decreases friction on skin from dirt and dead skin cells*
5. Apply restraint. **To apply wrist or ankle restraints:** • For non-commercial restraint: Use 10-inch strip of stretch (Kerlix) gauze folded to 2-inch width; apply washcloth or cotton padding around wrist. Wrap strip in a figure-eight (Fig. 1.6) and fold the circles of the figure over one another; slip wrist or ankle through loop.	
• For commercial restraint: Wrap padded portion of restraint around wrist or ankle, thread tie through slit in	*Holds restraint intact around wrist/ankle*

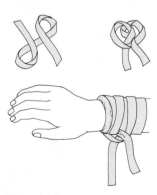

FIGURE 1.6

Action	Rationale
restraint, and fasten to second tie with secure knot, or apply Velcro as indicated on package.	
• Secure ends of ties to bed frame. DO NOT SECURE TO BED RAILS (with some two-part restraints, the wrist section snaps into a separate section that is secured to the bed frame).	*Prevents accidental pulling on limb with movement of bed rail; allows removal of restraint for skin care without removal of portion secured to bed*

To apply a vest restraint (used to prevent client from getting out of bed without restricting arm and hand mobility):

Action	Rationale
• Place vest on client with opening in front.	
• Pull tie on end of vest flap across chest and slip through slit in opposite side of vest.	
• Wrap other end of flap across client and around chair or upper portion of bed.	*Secures vest to client*
• Fasten ends of ties together behind chair or to sides of bed frame.	*Secures vest to chair or bed*
• Check respiratory status for distress related to restriction from vest	*Determines client tolerance of vest or need to loosen or remove due to respiratory compromise*

To apply a waist restraint (used to prevent client from getting out of bed without binding the chest):

Action	Rationale
• Wrap restraint around waist.	
• Slip end of one tie through slit in restraint.	*Secures waist restraint to client*
• Fasten ends of ties to bed frame.	*Secures restraint to bed*
• Monitor for complaints of nausea or abdominal distress.	*Determines client tolerance and need for removal due to restriction on abdomen*

To apply hand mittens (used to prevent client from pulling on tubes):

Action	Rationale
• Wrap stretch (Kerlix) gauze around hand until totally covered.	*Allows mobility of limb*
• Fold hand into fist and continue to wrap fist.	*Decreases client's ability to use fingers to dislodge tubings*
• Put tape around fist to secure gauze; cover with sock or stocking.	*Minimizes pulling of gauze and disruption of mitt*
6. While a client is in restraints:	
• Remove restraint every 2 to 4 hours, as well as when staff or family are at bedside to prevent injury.	*Decreases continuous pressure on skin and allows for movement*
• Massage skin beneath restraint and apply lotion or powder; wrap folded washcloth around limb and place restraint on top of cloth.	*Increases circulation to skin; decreases friction and skin irritation*
• Monitor the extremity distal to the restraint every 15 minutes for color, temperature, and capillary refill.	*Determines adequacy of circulation below restraint; identifies need for restraint removal*
• Check every 15 minutes for skin irritation or added pull on restraints and limb, tangled ties, or pressure points from knots; remove and adjust restraint to eliminate problem.	*Prevents loss of skin integrity due to excessive pressure*
• Offer client fluids and mouth care hourly.	*Promotes hydration and client comfort*
• Assist client with activities of daily living.	*Promotes client comfort and cooperation*
• Offer opportunities for elimination on a regular schedule.	
7. Continually assess client's orientation and continued need for restraints. Remove them as soon as safe to do so.	*Decreases risk of disruption of skin integrity; restores sense of self-control*

Evaluation

Were desired outcomes achieved? Examples of evaluation include:
- Desired outcome met: Client experienced no falls during morning shift.
- Desired outcome partially met: Client exhibits intact skin at and below the site of restraint. Capillary refill takes 5 seconds and skin is cool.

Documentation

The following should be noted on the client's chart:
- Reason for restraint application (per JCAHO standard in overview)
- Activities taken to attempt to avoid use of restraints
- Time physician's order obtained or protocol/standard activated
- Time of restraint and type of restraint applied
- Time doctor notified of restraint application
- Time of doctor's visit
- Client's response to restraints
- Frequency of checks of client and restraint site
- Status of restraint site and distal circulation
- Frequency of removal of restraints
- Skin care performed

Sample Documentation
Date: 1/2/05
Time: 1200

Admission history reveals pulling of tubes and disruption of wound during recent stay at nursing home. Client diagnosed with senile dementia, anorexia, and severe dehydration. IV and feeding tube inserted. Dr. Knowles ordered restraints at 1100. Bilateral wrist restraints applied after use of bandage wrap around IV and use of mitts failed to keep client from pulling out tubes. Client monitored q15 minutes; circulation and skin integrity intact. Dr. Knowles notified and will see client in 30 minutes. No family available at this time.

Documenting and Reporting

OVERVIEW

Effective Communication
- Simple: briefly and comprehensively relates data using commonly known and understood terms
- Clear: states exactly what is meant, covering the who, what, when, where, why, and how of the matter
- Pertinent: contains data that are important to the current situation and ties data to an apparent need to show significance
- Sensitive: considers readiness of the receiver and adapts depth and breadth of data to meet receiver's needs
- Accurate: includes factual information related with confidence and credibility
- Interdisciplinary communication is vital to maintaining continuity of care.

Privacy
- Client privacy must be maintained in all settings and through all reasonable means, whether verbal or written. In addition to the ethical obligation of the nurse to maintain privacy, the client is protected through federal legislation under the Health Insurance Portability and Accountability Act (HIPAA, 1996, 2003). Violations of protection of the client's privacy could result in criminal or civil litigation. Verbal and written communication must be confined to the appropriate settings and appropriate individuals to facilitate client care.

- All conversations about the client should take place in a private setting away from uninvolved parties and should be kept confidential. If a tape or other recording of client information is made, the recording should remain on the nursing unit in the designated place or at the service agency.
- All electronic communication should take place over secure, private channels. Minimal personal client information should be provided over cellular phones or other open channels.

Verbal Communication
- Verbal communication involves a sender, a receiver, a message, and the environment in which the interaction takes place.
- Verbal communication includes the attitude projected—gestures, voice tone, rhythm, volume, and pitch—in addition to words spoken.
- Building effective communication skills requires a constant awareness of oneself as a sender and a receiver of messages.
- Communication approaches should be modified to meet the individual needs of the client (e.g., cultural, age-related, and religious orientation).
- Consider the following factors in the communication process: knowledge level; personal perceptions, values, and beliefs; language; environmental setting; roles in the family and interpersonal relationships; space; and the general status of one's health.
- Often, patterns of client behavior warrant the use of special approaches for client communication. Clients who are anxious, depressed, in denial, angry, and potentially violent present additional considerations for effective communication.
- The home setting may provide unique challenges to verbal communication. Efforts should be made to minimize distractions and to include all family members in communication, as appropriate.

Written Communication
- Written communication involves the process of providing clear descriptions and documentation of client assessment and needs, client care activities, and nursing process activities directed toward meeting the client's needs.
- Written communication is often the major and occasionally the only medium for data exchange between health care team members.
- Communication that is client-oriented and reflects the nursing process is more focused and organized than disjointed, task-oriented communication.
- Written communication often provides proof of practice or malpractice. Legally speaking, if it wasn't documented, it wasn't done. Overall, charting should reflect that standards of care were upheld. Focus charting or charting by exception may be used to minimize lengthy narrative charting through the use of checklists. Clear documentation is the best proof that responsible, well-planned nursing care was given.

- Nurses' notes and plans of care often will be the only proof in future years that clients were monitored and cared for.
- Well-written plans of care, completed flow sheets, and progress notes provide a strong foundation for continuity of client care.
- Standardized plans of care may be used in some settings; however, individualization of the plan of care should be possible, and basic knowledge of plan of care preparation remains beneficial.
- The terms *goals, outcomes,* and *objectives* are often used interchangeably; however, distinctions are made between the terms in some settings. Nurses should be familiar with the use of the terms in the setting in which they work.
- Client outcome or critical path timeline plans may guide patient care. Documentation of client outcomes remains important for evaluation.
- Although nursing diagnoses accepted by the North American Nursing Diagnosis Association (NANDA, 2001) are available as a reference, additional clinically useful diagnoses such as collaborative problems (Carpenito, 2003) may be used if accepted by the institution.

● Nursing Procedure 2.1

Establishing a Nurse–Client Relationship

Purpose

Facilitates client's sense of well-being and control
Promotes beneficial interaction between the nurse and the client/family
Anticipates barriers to communication

Equipment

- Calendars
- Clocks
- Picture or word boards
- Any items needed to add clarity to message

Assessment

Assessment should focus on the following:
- Client's age, developmental level, cultural or ethnic background, educational level
- Physical and mental barriers to communication (e.g., poor sight or hearing, speech impediment, pain level)

- Client's use of nonverbal gesturing
- Client's perceptions of people and situations
- Sources of stress for client
- Client's use of defense and coping mechanisms
- Immediate environment (e.g., noise, lighting, visitors)
- Support systems (e.g., family, friends, community agencies; See Nursing Procedure 13.4, Support System Assessment)

Nursing Diagnoses

Nursing diagnoses may include the following:
- Anxiety related to inability to communicate needs
- Noncompliance related to feeling of lack of control
- Ineffective coping related to multiple stressors

Outcome Identification and Planning

Desired Outcomes

Sample desired outcomes include the following:
- Client shows no signs of anxiety and communicates needs effectively.
- Client complies with dietary, activity, or home health regimen.
- Client discusses current major stressors in life.

Special Considerations in Planning and Implementation

General

Anticipate questions and concerns when explaining factual information to clients. Plan interaction times to ensure privacy and avoid interruptions. When planning interactions, consider the phase of the nurse–client relationship:
- Orientation phase: Initial meeting of client and nurse; verbal contract is made
- Working phase: Basic nurse–client trust established and relationship solidified through meeting of objectives
- Termination phase: Preparation for discharge and ending of relationship

Avoid statements or behaviors that might result in barriers to communication (Display 2.1). When interacting with clients, consider their stage of coping or possible grief: denial, anger, bargaining, depression, and acceptance (Display 2.2). Special considerations are needed in communicating with potentially violent clients (Display 2.3).

Pediatric

Consider the child's developmental stage. Approach the child slowly after informing him or her of your intentions, as children may perceive sudden body movements by an adult as threatening.

● Display 2.1 Barriers to Therapeutic Communication

Giving advice	Stereotyping
Using responses that imply approval or disapproval	Imposing judgment
	Providing false reassurance
Agreeing or disagreeing	Using clichés
Not listening attentively	Questioning with bias
Appearing distracted	Excessive probing
Responding defensively	

● Display 2.2 Considerations for Interactions With Special Clients/Families

*When interacting with an **anxious client:***
- Recognize client's decreased ability to focus on and respond to multiple stimuli.
- Maintain quiet, calm environment.
- Keep messages simple, concrete, and brief.
- Repeat messages often.
- Minimize need for extensive decision making.
- Monitor anxiety level, using verbal and nonverbal cues.

*When interacting with an **angry or potentially violent client:***
- Use careful, unhurried, deliberate body movements.
- Provide an open, nonthreatening environment.
- Clear area of anger-provoking stimuli (persons, objects, etc.).
- Maintain a nonthreatening demeanor, using open body language, soft voice tones, etc.

*When interacting with a **depressed client:***
- Allow additional time for interactions.
- Emphasize use of physical attending.
- Avoid giving client time-limited tasks due to slowed reflexes.
- Monitor closely for cues of self-destructive tendencies.
- Keep messages simple, concrete, and brief.
- Minimize need for extensive decision making.

*When interacting with a **client exhibiting denial:***
- Use direct questions to determine the situation triggering use of coping mechanism.
- Do not avoid the reality of the situation, but allow client to maintain denial defense; it often serves a protective function.
- Recognize that denial may be the first of a series of crisis phases, to be followed by phases of increased tension, disorganization, attempts to reorganize, attempts to escape the problem, local reorganization, general reorganization, and possibly resolution.
- Be alert for cues that the phase is ending (i.e., questions from client regarding the disturbing situation).

● **Display 2.3** Special Considerations in Communication With Potentially Violent Clients

- Maintain a heightened awareness of triggers of increased agitation. *Signs associated with impending violence include:*
  - Verbal expression of anger and frustration
  - Body language, such as threatening gestures
  - Signs of drug or alcohol use
  - Presence of a weapon
- *Violence often occurs during times when high interaction or high client or unit activity takes place,* such as mealtime, personal care, increased physical activity, visiting hours, or client transport.
- Assaults may occur when limits are set relative to eating, drinking, alcohol or tobacco use, when service is denied, or when a client is involuntarily admitted.
- Avoid behavior that could be considered threatening or aggressive: loud talking, moving too quickly and hurriedly, touching, getting too close.
- *Communication is aimed toward avoiding an escalating situation and defusing anger.*
  - Maintain a calm, unhurried approach.
  - Keep messages simple, concrete, and brief.
  - Acknowledge the client's feelings (e.g., "I know you are frustrated").
  - Minimize need for extensive decision making.
  - Don't match threats.
  - Don't give orders.
- *Be alert and remain vigilant* throughout the encounter.
  - Don't isolate yourself with a potentially violent person.
  - Ascertain that others know you are entering the room of a potentially violent client.
  - Keep an open path for exiting. Do not allow the potentially violent person to stand between you and the door/exit.
- *If the situation cannot be defused quickly:*
  - Remove yourself from the situation.
  - Call security for help.
  - Report any violent incidents.

Geriatric

Elderly clients may have one or more communication barriers that may readily be removed once discovered; dentures, hearing aids, and glasses should be acquired, if possible. With increasing age, a client's speech and comprehension may be slowed, requiring more time for communication.

End-of-Life Care

Communication with the dying client is vital, as it is believed that hearing is the last sense to leave the body. When in the room with the client, speak in a normal tone of voice, as whispering causes unnecessary strain. Do not speak as if the client is not in the room. During the final hours of life, the client may become restless, as agitation is common; however, unresolved physiological (including pharmacological), emotional, or spiritual issues should also be considered. Those who have come to terms and are at peace with death tend to become less communicative; therefore, explanations should be provided to family members that this process is common and does not indicate their loved one is rejecting them. Client and family wishes should be granted as much as possible. Family members should be allowed to remain with the client as much as possible and explanations should be provided.

Home Health

Encourage the client and family to prepare a list of questions or concerns during the time between the nurse's visits. Use of a diary or journal may promote communication of the content as well as the context of the client's concerns.

Transcultural

Use of an interpreter for clients whose native language is not English may reduce the chance of miscommunication by client and nurse. Sociocultural differences should be considered when interpreting a client's nonverbal behavior. For example, clients from some cultures may view direct eye contact as offensive and intrusive. It is best to follow the cues of the client in developing rapport.

Delegation

All levels of personnel interacting with clients and families should receive training and education about appropriate client communication, including clients with special needs. When clients have special communication needs, appropriate personnel should be assigned to work with those clients, and the staff should be informed of the communication needs to facilitate appropriate communication. Communication specifically addressing the progress or status of the client should not be delegated, but rather should be done by the nurse or other appropriate and trained personnel as designated by the agency policies. All levels of staff should be informed about potential dangers in communicating with agitated, angry, or potentially violent clients.

Implementation

Action	Rationale
1. Approach the client in a purposeful but unhurried manner.	*Promotes a controlled and non-threatening interaction*

Action	Rationale
2. Identify self and relationship to client.	*Initiates orientation phase of nurse–client relationship*
3. Arrange environment so it is conducive to type of interaction needed (ask client or family permission and assistance if in the home setting).	*Eliminates environmental distractions*
4. Use the following physical attending skills throughout the interaction process:	
• Face directly and lean toward client.	
• Maintain eye contact and an open posture (do not cross legs or arms).	*Exhibits nonverbal body language consistent with verbalizations; conveys interest, attentiveness, sincerity, and lack of defensiveness*
5. Begin interactions using the following therapeutic techniques when eliciting or sharing information or responses:	*Promotes purposeful and mutually beneficial interactions between nurse and client*
• Use open-ended statements and questions.	*Allows client to express feelings and concerns most important to him or her at the time*
• Restate or paraphrase client's statements when indicated.	*Confirms significance of client's comments*
• Clarify unclear comments.	*Ensures that intended message was received*
• Focus the statement when client tends to ramble or is vague.	*Promotes concreteness of message*
• Explore further when additional information is needed.	*Promotes gathering of complete information*
• Provide rationale why more information is needed, when appropriate.	*Maintains professional integrity of interaction*
• Use touch and silence, when appropriate.	*Conveys compassion and allows time for client to gain composure*
6. Use the following active listening techniques:	*Conveys interest, attentiveness, sincerity, and lack of defensiveness*
• Do not interrupt client in the middle of comments.	*Prevents distraction*
• Use verbal indicators of acceptance and understanding (e.g., "um-hmm," "yes").	*Expresses interest*

Action	Rationale
7. When client is speaking, note his or her gestures, facial expressions, and elements of speech (e.g., tone, pitch, emphasis of words).	*Facilitates receipt of complete message*
8. When you are speaking, note client's nonverbal gestures (e.g., grimacing, smiling, crossing arms or legs).	*Allows nurse to detect cues indicating acceptance or non-acceptance of message*
9. Toward the end of the interaction, summarize important aspects of the conversation.	*Avoids abrupt and incomplete close to interaction*

Evaluation

Were desired outcomes achieved? Examples of evaluation include:
- Desired outcome partially met: Client showed signs of anxiety but communicated needs effectively.
- Desired outcome met: Client complied with dietary, activity, or home health regimen.
- Desired outcome met: Client discussed current major stressors in life.

Documentation

The following should be noted on the client's chart:
- Date, time, and place of interaction
- Client's reaction to initial meeting and interaction
- Any adaptations made to the environment
- Nature and significant highlights of the discussion
- Communication barriers (if any) and interventions used
- Client's gestures, facial expressions, and elements of speech while talking
- Client's significant nonverbal gestures while listening

Sample Documentation
Date: 2/29/05
Time: 1400

Client in bed and tearful; upset because husband has not visited in 3 days. States concern about husband's feelings regarding loss of her breast. Reach to Recovery support group discussed. Nurse will contact husband this PM.

Providing Client and Family Education

Purpose

Assists client in learning information necessary for participation in self-care

Assists family in learning information necessary for participation in care of client/family

Facilitates client transition to home and care of client/family in the home setting

Reduces anxiety

Equipment

Selected teaching tools (e.g., booklets, pamphlets, audiovisual materials, games)

Assessment

Assessment should focus on the following:
- Presence of those persons participating in client's care
- Client's or significant others' readiness to learn and ability to comprehend
- Age and education level of learner(s)
- Amount and accuracy of client's and significant others' prior knowledge about content
- Community resources for referral
- Presence of any communication barriers such as visual, hearing, or speech problems
- Presence of any physical or emotional barriers (e.g., conditions or medications that alter mental state or cause pain or stress)
- Environmental distractions (e.g., TV, radio, noise, visitors not involved in client care or education session)

Nursing Diagnoses

Nursing diagnoses may include the following:
- Deficient knowledge related to unfamiliarity with new illness and treatment
- Anxiety related to deficient knowledge

Outcome Identification and Planning

Desired Outcomes

Sample desired outcomes include the following:
- Client demonstrates knowledge of new illness and treatment by:
  - Stating purpose of procedure before beginning procedure
  - Demonstrating procedure correctly with 100% accuracy by time of discharge from facility or agency service
  - Stating solutions to potential complications of procedure by time of discharge
- Client shows no signs of anxiety related to deficient knowledge.

Special Considerations

General

Individuals with similar problems are frequently helpful in facilitating client learning. A list of support or referral groups may be available through an agency or a nursing association website.

Pediatric

Visual aids and demonstrations are often effective when teaching children. Always include parents or other family members (for reinforcement), if available. Same-age-group teaching can be used.

Geriatric

Elderly clients may require more response time during teaching and evaluation due to delayed reaction times that occur with normal aging. Consider response time when planning time frame for teaching.

End-of-Life-Care

Explanations concerning the client or client care should be provided as needed to the client and family/significant others to facilitate a peaceful transition to death. See also Special Considerations in Planning and Implementation under Procedure 2.1, Establishing a Nurse–Client Relationship.

Home Health

In the acute care setting, discharge teaching should begin as soon as is reasonably possible given the client's condition due to shortened hospital stays. A well-planned, concerted effort must be made to be sure the client and family have the information needed to participate in care in the home setting. Incorporate adaptations or modifications of procedures that are likely to occur in the home setting.

 ### Transcultural

Examples used for clarification or explanation of information are sometimes understood more easily if they relate to some aspect of the client's culture. Pictures may be useful if the client speaks a different language. Many facilities have access to interpreters. It is important to find out how the client views health. For example, clients of various cultures may view illness as a curse or bad luck. This may affect the nurse's ability to engage the client in active learning.

Cost-Cutting Tips

Group education is a cost-effective way to teach general principles to a large number of clients. Video/DVD materials may be purchased to teach frequently taught patient information; this may reduce staff teaching time and will allow the client to review material repeatedly as needed or desired. Interdisciplinary teaching plans and documentation should be well coordinated to avoid time-consuming, costly duplication of services.

Delegation

Generally, documentation of teaching is the ultimate responsibility of the registered nurse. The appropriate level of personnel should provide teaching to clients and family. Teaching about early detection and prevention of complications, health maintenance, reporting pertinent observations, medications, treatments, care directed toward problem resolution, and discharge teaching should always be conducted by the registered nurse or licensed vocational nurse, as designated by agency policies within specific guidelines for the roles of each level of nurse. Any teaching by other nursing staff related to procedures to be done by the client/family should be reinforced or directed by the nurse, and the effectiveness of the teaching should be evaluated by the registered nurse, with appropriate documentation.

Implementation

Action	Rationale
1. Establish verbal contract with client regarding teaching plans.	*Provides mutual goals for client and nurse*
2. Eliminate environmental distractions such as excess noise, poor lighting, uncomfortable room temperature, clutter in room, excess visitor and staff traffic, and clinical treatments and procedures.	*Creates optimal environment for communication and learning*
3. Secure a private environment.	*Maintains confidentiality and promotes free exchange of information*
4. During assessment and along with client, determine exactly what infor-	*Provides teaching focus and involves client. Teaching is most effective when it occurs in*

Action	Rationale
mation the client needs and is able to retain.	*response to specific needs expressed by the learner.*
5. Determine nursing diagnoses based on assessment findings.	*Provides focus for goal-setting*
6. Set realistic, measurable goals with client and family/significant others.	*Promotes client participation; provides focus for teaching*
7. Develop a teaching plan (Display 2.4) that specifically addresses the following: • Objectives to be met by the end of the teaching session • Content to be taught • Methods of teaching • Methods of evaluation	*Facilitates optimal learning; guides teaching plan preparation*
8. Obtain all necessary equipment.	*Promotes efficiency*
9. Implement teaching plan.	*Assists client in understanding self-care; reduces anxiety*
10. Evaluate plan and implementation.	*Determines whether further teaching is needed*

● **Display 2.4** Preparation Guide for Development of a Teaching Plan

Objectives to be met by end of session
Content
    What content will be taught to meet objectives?
    Will complex content need to be taught in divided stages?
Teaching methods
    What reading materials are needed?
    What audiovisual aids are needed?
    Will games or role-playing be used?
    Will support groups or group sessions be used?
    What equipment/supplies are needed?
    Will tours or visits to related agencies be helpful?
    How much time is needed to cover each section of
      material?
    Will practice time be needed?
    How much time is realistic for this client?
Evaluation methods
    How much time will be needed to evaluate learning?
    Will evaluation be: Verbal? Written? Return
      demonstration?

Evaluation

Were desired outcomes achieved? Examples of evaluation include:
● Desired outcome met: Client demonstrated knowledge of illness and treatment.
● Desired outcome met: Client showed no signs of anxiety.

Documentation

The following should be noted on the client's chart:
● What information the client needs
● Goals as set by client and nurse
● Teaching plan to be implemented (including objectives, content to be taught, methods of teaching, and methods of evaluation)
● Extent to which each objective was met (fully, partially, not met)
● Nature of material taught
● Persons other than client included in session
● Client's response to teaching
● Client concerns expressed during teaching
● Need for additional teaching or alternate method of teaching
● Need for revision of plans with client input

Sample Documentation
Date: 6/11/04
Time: 0900

Provided client teaching regarding importance of low-sodium diet in relation to managing hypertension. Client demonstrated selection of low-sodium foods from list with 80% accuracy. Participated actively in learning. Denies concerns in relation to topic at this time.

● **Nursing Procedure 2.3**

Preparing a Shift Report (Interdisciplinary Information Exchange)

Purpose

Facilitates continuity of client care through accurate and comprehensive communication of relevant client data among nurses and various care providers (may occur in the form of shift-to-shift updates, interdisciplinary consultation, and client-care conferences)

Equipment

- Client Kardex or plan of care/clinical pathway
- Client summary notes (kept throughout shift or visit)
- Tape recorder, if warranted by facility protocol
- Form to document verbal communication
- Provider or payer phone and fax numbers or e-mail address as indicated

Assessment

Assessment should focus on the following:
- Current status of client (e.g., comfort, medications/fluid infusions) and treatments pending
- Identity and availability of care providers and payer sources involved in client's care
- Information needed by various care providers and payer sources
- Desired method of communication (e.g., phone, fax, computer, e-mail). Determine that method is secure and private.

Outcome Identification and Planning

Desired Outcomes

Sample desired outcomes include the following:
- Appropriate treatments, medications, and other care measures and support consistent with plan of care are received as scheduled or needed.
- All applicable care providers and payer sources will have accurate information concerning the client and any changes in client condition.

Special Considerations in Planning and Implementation

General

Under the Health Insurance Portability and Accountability Act (HIPAA, 1996, 2003), client privacy must be maintained through all reasonable means, whether verbal or written. Verbal and written communication must be confined to the appropriate settings and appropriate individuals as necessary to facilitate client care, as violations of protection of the client's privacy could result in criminal or civil litigation. When "walking rounds" are employed, verbal information about the client should be shared in a more private setting (e.g., in a report room) before going to the client's room for visual verification of or supplemental information on the client's condition. When reporting to caregivers with little previous exposure to the client, more background may be needed or desired. Caregivers with extensive previous exposure to the client may require only a brief update of pertinent changes. Take a few minutes to determine exactly what information is needed (e.g., a medical supply company about to make a delivery will need a correct address; a payer source will need to know client condition, care being received, and expected duration of care). Remember to report data or occurrences from previous shifts, days, or visits, when pertinent. Include concerns of the client, family members, or significant others. Establish with the agency a method for routing information received from the physician's office. In some agencies, the field nurse is called directly by pager or by cellular phone, whereas in others the supervisor is the go-between. All parties involved in the communication must have the same information.

End-of-Life Care

Reports on dying clients should remain focused on providing optimal care to facilitate a peaceful death for the client and provide support to the family/significant others as needed.

Home Health

The assessment and report of a homebound client should include the client's status at the time of the last home health visit, the client's response to interventions, any restrictions present in the environment (e.g., no running water, no electricity), and any adaptations that have been made in client-care procedures (e.g., irrigating a wound while in the bathtub). The visit report should also include the client's address (with directions if the home is difficult to locate), any special supplies or equipment to be taken on the next visit, and client teaching needs. It is rare that the home health nurse will speak directly with the physician during physician office hours. Establish a contact at the office who will reliably transfer information to the physician. Check with the office to determine the best time and method (e.g., fax, voicemail, e-mail) to leave nonemergency messages for the physician.

Transcultural

Pertinent data about the client's sociocultural background should be included if the data are significant to some aspect of the client's care.

Cost-Cutting Tips

Tape-recording reports may be less time-consuming and therefore more cost-effective, but follow agency guidelines to avoid violating client privacy. If interdisciplinary shift reports are not a standard daily routine, a periodic interdisciplinary conference may prevent unnecessary resource utilization due to duplications from various service departments.

Delegation

Direct communication ensures the greatest accuracy of information exchange. However, if information must be relayed to the doctor, another member of the health care team, a payer, or the client through a third party, the nurse should follow up as soon as possible to validate that the correct information was relayed. Reports should never be delegated to unlicensed personnel. As a clinical nursing student, remember that reports should be given only to licensed personnel or the instructor prior to leaving your unit.

Implementation

Action	Rationale
Preparing an Inpatient Report	
1. Gather information and equipment.	*Facilitates organizing report*
2. Report client identification data (name, room number, age, medical diagnosis [primary and secondary], and doctor's name).	*Ensures association of reported data with correct client*
3. Record the following special circumstances of client: • Sight or hearing deficits • Language or cultural barriers • Safety needs (e.g., client at high risk for falls) • Support needs • Family concerns • Religious concerns	*Promotes client safety and psychosocial well-being* *Recognizes ethical and legal concerns; individualizes care*
4. Summarize client's status using nursing diagnoses or outcomes to indicate active emotional and physical problems (Display 2.5). Begin with the diagnoses or outcomes of highest priority and proceed to those of least priority.	*Validates established nursing diagnoses and outcomes and need for continued intervention*
5. For each diagnosis or outcome addressed, record the following: • Nursing diagnosis or outcome • Assessment data (e.g., complaints, wound/dressing status, IVs, drains, oxygen) • Interventions used (e.g., medications, IVs, treatments, monitoring, teaching)	

● **Display 2.5** Report Format—Summary

Client identification data
Special circumstances
Client status—physical/emotional
Priority nursing diagnoses
Assessment data
Interventions (treatments, teaching, monitoring needs)
Evaluation (client response to interventions)
Recent diagnostic test results
New orders medical/nursing
Environmental concerns
Tubes
Infusions (fluid count)
Drains
Immediately pending treatments
Family's or significant others' concerns or considerations

Action	Rationale
• Evaluation (e.g., intake and output, client response to treatments, teaching)	*Summarizes current status of client and treatments*
6. Report recent results of diagnostic procedures and lab tests.	*Provides status update*
7. Report new medical/nursing orders (diagnostic tests, medications, treatments, surgery, dietary or activity restrictions, or discharge planning).	*Provides update on planned medical and nursing interventions*
8. Summarize general environmental concerns (e.g., tubes, drains, infusions with fluid counts, and mechanical supports [include setting]).	*Facilitates maintenance of support equipment*
9. Summarize information required during first hour of oncoming shift (e.g., treatments, fluid replacements, medication needs, tests).	*Facilitates punctuality and continuity in treatment regimen*

Preparing a Report in Outpatient/Home Setting

1. Determine what information is needed before making the phone call.	*Increases the clarity and focus of the communication*

Action	Rationale
2. Have all related information with you at the time of the call, and make the call in as quiet an environment as possible.	*Allows the nurse to answer questions and to hear and understand the other party*
3. Clearly state who you are, the agency you represent, and what the call is about.	*Allows party receiving the call to route you to the proper person*
4. Obtain the name of the person with whom you are speaking.	*Permits the nurse to follow up with the same person, if needed*
5. Give all information in a clear and concise manner. If giving a condition report, know current vital signs, symptoms, medications and doses, and so forth.	*Promotes efficiency and reduces the need for additional calls*
6. If receiving a phone order from a physician, repeat it back to the physician for verification, spell medications for clarity, and put it in writing immediately to be sent out for physician signature.	*Reduces the chance of acting on a misunderstood order*
7. Document all verbal and phone communication concerning any client.	*Provides a clear picture in the client record and reduces the reliance on any individual's memory*

Evaluation

Were desired outcomes achieved? Examples of evaluation include:
- Desired outcome met: Appropriate treatments, medications, and other care measures and support were consistent with plan of care and received as scheduled or needed.
- Desired outcome met: All applicable care providers and payer sources received accurate information concerning the client and any changes in client condition.

Documentation

The following should be noted on the client's chart:

Inpatient

- Client's identification data
- Any special circumstances
- Results of any procedures or lab tests

- Any new nursing orders
- Environmental concerns

Outpatient

- All physician orders on the form specified by the agency
- All client communication on the form designated for that function by the agency
- Date documentation is completed

Sample Documentation (Inpatient Shift Report)
Date: 5/07/05
Time: 0530

Mr. Homes, Room 102, is a 75-year-old client of Dr. Smith admitted with diverticulitis; he has a history of hypertension and diabetes. He is slightly hard of hearing in his left ear. Priority nursing diagnosis: Altered comfort related to abdominal cramps. Mr. Homes complained of pain at 9 am and 2 pm, was medicated with 4 mg morphine sulfate IV each time, and experienced relief within 30 minutes. His potassium level was 3.7 this am, and the last fingerstick glucose level was 140. He is scheduled for a barium enema this pm at 5:00 and has received enemas till clear. Food and fluids are restricted (NPO). He has dextrose 5% in water (D_5W) infusing at 50 mL/hr, with 400 mL left to count. He is scheduled for a fingerstick glucose level test at 4 pm.

● **Nursing Procedure 2.4**

Following the Nursing Process (Preparing a Plan of Care)

Purpose

Provides a guiding foundation for individualized client care
(Display 2.6 describes the Nursing Process)
Facilitates continuity of nursing care

● Display 2.6 The Nursing Process

Assessment

Assessment includes gathering and analyzing client data and involves appraising areas in which the client might require nursing care or assistance to meet basic or higher-level needs. It provides direction for focus of individualized client care.

Diagnosis

Diagnosis involves using the data collected during assessment to identify actual and potential problems. Diagnosis guides the selection and implementation of care measures.

Planning (Outcome Identification)

Outcome identification includes prioritizing client needs and establishing key goals of care, with criteria for evaluating whether goals have been met. A goal is a statement of behavior that reflects measurable progress toward resolution of the problem. Outcome identification promotes involvement of the client and support person in the plan of care. Planning involves developing strategies to help the client meet goals and attain desired outcomes. Special consideration should be given to circumstances that might affect care strategies, such as age or transcultural or economic issues. Planning promotes the delivery of individualized, effective, outcome-focused nursing care and allows for tailoring of strategies to accommodate special circumstances.

Implementation

Implementation involves carrying out actions/nursing orders designed to help the client meet goals. Implementation helps achieve desired outcomes.

Evaluation

Evaluation is an ongoing step of reassessment and interpretation of new data to determine whether goals are being met fully, partially, or not at all. Evaluation ensures that the client is receiving proper care and his or her needs are being met.

Equipment

- Pencil or pen (if plan of care is permanent part of chart)
- Client Kardex or plan of care
- Appropriate reference books

Assessment

Assessment should focus on the following:
- Data gathered from client environment
- Client history

- Physical and mental status
- Social supports

Nursing Diagnoses

Will vary depending on client's circumstances (see individual procedures)

Outcome Identification and Planning

Desired Outcomes

Sample desired outcomes include the following:
- Individualized client care is planned and implemented.
- Client receives consistent, continuous care as designated in the plan of care.

Special Considerations in Planning and Implementation

General

Always consider the safety and privacy needs of the client. Involve client/family as much as possible in all stages of the nursing process.

End-of-Life Care

The plan of care for dying clients should focus on supporting the wishes of the client and family and providing palliative care (e.g., pain management) and correcting problems that are resolvable (e.g., fluid deficiencies, electrolyte imbalances). Ascertain the status of advance directives and ensure that the plan of care for the client is consistent; consult physician and agency policies as needed if clarifications are needed relative to potential conflicts with agency policies.

Home Health

In the home setting, a plan of care acts as the physician's orders for the client. The nurse must be able to complete the plan of care and turn it in to the agency for mailing to the physician in a timely manner. In the home setting, the plan of care reflects the client's condition, need for skilled care, schedule of visits, functional limitations, care needs, and general living situation. The plan includes all necessary information to meet agency policy, regulatory requirements, and payer source needs. Supplies needed should be noted on the plan of care to meet the requirement of some reimbursement agencies.

🏃 Transcultural

The client's cultural orientation should always be taken into consideration when planning care.

Cost-Cutting Tips

Care should be planned to avoid wasting time, resources, and expense while maximizing client care. A well-thought-out plan of care accurately designates client acuity levels and appropriate staffing types and numbers for various types of clients.

Implementation

Action	Rationale
Assessment	
1. Systematically gather data: assess the client's status from the admission history, physical examination, and diagnostic tests (may use body systems or basic needs areas).	*Organizes data*
2. Underline any abnormal data or note on separate pad.	*Designates areas of concern and probable causes*
3. Interview client regarding perceptions of condition and need priorities.	*Determines what needs client believes are of highest priority and how those needs might be met*
4. Organize and group areas of concern.	*Facilitates clear definition of needs or problems*
5. Determine client's ability to meet identified needs; match client strengths and supports to needs.	*Determines level of nursing care needed: teaching, guidance, or direct nursing intervention*
Diagnosis	
6. Determine nursing diagnoses centering on needs requiring nursing intervention or teaching. Write diagnoses with two parts and a connector:	
• Part 1: Actual or potential client problem (e.g., Noncompliance with diet therapy)	
• Part 2: Probable cause of problem (e.g., Knowledge deficit)	
• Connector: Connecting phrase such as "related to" or "associated with" (e.g., Impaired skin integrity related to immobility)	*Serves as guide for individualizing plan of care; clearly communicates problems*

Action	Rationale
Planning (and Outcome Identification)	
7. Prioritize diagnoses according to nature of problem and client's perceptions of need priority; life-threatening needs take first priority. Potential problems can often be addressed under a major actual concern (see goals).	*Determines priorities for plan of care*
8. Develop goals using these key elements: • Statement of what client is expected to accomplish (e.g., Demonstrates adequate tissue perfusion) • Goal criteria, in terms of measurable behaviors (e.g., As evidenced by capillary refill of 5–10 sec, 2+ or greater pulses, and warm skin) • Specific time/date at which expectation should be met (e.g., By discharge or by third postoperative day) • Conditions or special circumstances associated with meeting goal (e.g., With the assistance of vasodilator therapy)	*Expresses goals in concrete terms*
9. Use the guidelines in Display 2.7 when writing goals so that they are clear, concise, and realistic.	*Allows nurse to determine whether goals were met*
10. List actions needed to reach goals. Nursing actions may include supervising, teaching, assisting, monitoring, or direct intervention.	*Identifies actions needed to meet goals*
11. Determine who will perform actions to resolve problem. Consult client and support persons to determine their ability and willingness to perform actions.	*Designates locus of control of nursing interventions: client-centered (actions performed by client); shared (client and nurse jointly perform actions); nurse-centered (actions performed by nurse).*

● Display 2.7 Writing Goals

Use the following guidelines when writing goals so that they are clear, concise, and realistic:

- Goals should be client-centered (e.g., "The client will . . .").
- Goals should be written in active and measurable terms (e.g., "The client will walk . . ."). Avoid terms like understand or realize.
- Goals of health care and maintenance should be realistic.
- Time limits should be realistic and should include short- and long-term goals.
- One goal should be set at a time.
  Sample goal: By discharge, the client will demonstrate knowledge of diabetic self-care by giving own insulin and planning a 1,500-calorie ADA diet without assistance or coaching.

Action	Rationale
12. State actions clearly, including the following elements: • Who will perform the action (e.g., client, nurse, assistant) • How often or to what extent the action will be performed (e.g., three times daily; three out of four foods will be named) • Under what conditions action will be performed (e.g., with assistance, after instruction, with supervision)	*Clearly communicates planned interventions*
13. State actions one by one. Explain or clarify as needed.	
Implementation **14.** Perform action (nurse or designated health care team member).	
Evaluation **15.** Assess client in view of goals and criteria.	*Identifies progress toward goal*
16. Determine whether desired outcomes were achieved.	*Determines whether outcomes were achieved partially, fully, or not at all as a basis for plan revision*

Action	Rationale
17. Review behaviors and criteria.	
18. Revise plan as needed to maintain progress toward goal:	
• Continue effective actions.	
• Determine factors hindering the meeting of goal and remove or minimize them.	*Makes goal more reachable*
• Modify goal, if needed, by expanding time limits or lowering expectations.	*Makes goal more realistic for the client*
• Modify actions and eliminate those no longer indicated.	*Maintains current, relevant plan*
• Add new actions, if needed.	
• If indicated, shift locus of control.	
• Continuously assess client status using data-gathering process.	
Documentation	
19. Place documentation on appropriate temporary or permanent forms.	

Evaluation

Were desired outcomes achieved? Examples of evaluation include:
- Desired outcome met: Individualized client care was planned and implemented.
- Desired outcome met: Client received consistent, continuous care as designated in the plan of care.

Documentation

Components of documentation vary greatly based on diagnosis and procedures performed. See specific procedures for documentation guidelines.

Charting (Nurses' Progress Report)

Purpose

Facilitates comprehensive communication of relevant client data from one nursing caregiver to other nurses or members of health care team

Equipment

- Small pad and pencil (for client summary notes)
- Client Kardex or plan of care
- Pen (color per agency policy)
- Client-specific progress note or nurses' note sheets
- Computer (if using computerized charting system)

Assessment

Assessment should focus on the following:
- Previous notes from nurses, physicians, and other team members for an update on client status
- Current status, as indicated by:
  - Vital signs
  - Intake (infusion rates and amount remaining in tube feedings, IVs, and other infusions)
  - Output (drainage amounts); indicate locations of tubes and drains
  - Dressings (degree and type of soiling, frequency of changes, and status of underlying skin/wound)
  - Treatments (number of times performed, duration, and client response)

Outcome Identification and Planning

Desired Outcomes

A sample desired outcome is:
- Continuity of care is provided through dissemination of information in an accurate, comprehensive, and brief form.

Special Considerations in Planning and Implementation

General

Many facilities use computerized charting. It is important to use only the codes or passwords assigned to you individually to document on client records. NEVER allow someone else to document using your password. Ensure that the electronic charting is not being completed in a public location that would allow others to view the chart. Although the format is different for each system, the basic principles remain the same. Use computer checklists and client information data panels based on the instructions provided in the agency orientation to the system. Often you will need to document additional information that clarifies or amplifies the information provided in a computer; however, there may be a tendency to use only the basic checklists. When you need to provide more detailed information, always use the panels designated by the system for providing the information.

Charting must be complete regardless of the format. Assessment data should be obtained at the beginning of and throughout the shift and should be recorded in a small notebook until needed. Health care agencies may require that client data be recorded in a specialized format using the following categories: Subjective, Objective, Assessment, Planning, Implementation, and Evaluation. These categories may be used in whole (SOAPIE) or in part (SOAP, APIE). There are also other variations, such as DAR (Data/Action/Response); this form of charting includes subjective and objective data; implementation of actions; and evaluation of implementation to determine the degree to which the goals were met. You may organize data in your notebook by indicating the type with an initial (e.g., A for Assessment or Pl for Planning). If routine client care flow sheets or checklists are used, do not duplicate data. Use nurses' notes to record data not covered on flow sheets and to elaborate, if needed.

Home Health

Notations should be made for each care visit regarding the homebound status of the client. Content of notes should address how sick the client is. Report findings in objective and specific terminology. Notes should be directed toward justifying the reason for a home health visit.

Implementation

Action	Rationale
1. Designate body systems requiring detailed assessment and documentation.	*Provides framework for concise charting addressing only pertinent areas in great detail*
2. Assess client in an orderly manner (see Procedure 3.5), and record findings in a small notebook.	*Organizes notes and facilitates accuracy through minimum dependence on memory*
3. When time allows, record initial client assessments in a chart (Table 2.1 lists guidelines).	*Provides other health care team members with an update on pertinent client data*
4. As the day progresses, record in a small notebook	*Indicates possible changes in client's status requiring update*

● Table 2.1 Guidelines for Initial Assessment Notes

Assessment Area	Criteria
Neurological	Level of consciousness, orientation, verbal response, pupil size and reaction, incisions or head dressings, intracranial pressure monitor, sensory or mobility deficits (if applicable, expand musculoskeletal—mobility limitations, cast or traction, and extremity status). **Safety measures**—side rails, restraints (skin status and care).
Respiratory	Respiratory rate, depth, character, dyspnea, symmetry of chest movement, breath sounds, secretions, cough, incisions, dressings, oxygen therapy, and chest tubes
Circulatory	Skin color, temperature, capillary refill, heart sounds, pulse rate, rhythm, ECG pattern (if available), heart sounds, pulse assessment (absent to 4+), skin turgor, edema, neck vein distention, hemodynamic pressures (if available), intravenous therapy (with counts), incisions/dressings
Gastrointestinal	Bowel sounds, shape and feel of abdomen, tenderness, nausea, emesis, diet and intake, dysphagia, bowel movements, nasogastric tube/tube feeding, ostomy site, stoma, drainage and care, and incision/dressings
Genitourinary	Urinary output, continence, appearance of urine, Foley catheter status
Supportive therapy	Wound drains, irrigations, invasive lines, pain-control measures (transcutaneous electrical nerve stimulation unit, patient-controlled analgesia pump)

Action	Rationale
or bedside activity flow chart, if available, time of, precise details of, and client response to treatments or teaching. Also record occurrences pertinent to the client's physical or mental state. For computerized charting, access the appropriate documentation panel and record information as designated by the computer system.	*in documentation; provides prompt and accurate recording of client data*

Action	Rationale
5. Record pertinent observations in chart or on computer in an organized manner. USE ACTIVITY FLOW SHEETS, if available. Or use SOAPIE categories (in whole or in part) or other formats.	*Promotes problem-oriented charting and organized, thorough documentation; eliminates repetition and shortens notes*
6. Document any changes from initial assessment, or the absence of any changes, at least every 4 hours or according to client and agency policies.	*Indicates ongoing nursing assessment and care*
7. Use final note to highlight major shift events or progress toward goals.	*Emphasizes priority shift occurrences and facilitates rapid review of notes*
8. Document p.r.n. medication (medication given as necessary) in nurses' notes per agency policy.	*Demonstrates adherence to established policy*
9. Adhere to the following legal guidelines in documentation:	*Decreases indications of falsification or deception*
• Never erase or scratch out errors in charting (draw a line through the sentence and indicate the error with initials or according to agency policy).	*Erasures and scratching out are considered as illegal entries, unacceptable in a court of law. Agency procedure must be followed for the entry to be considered legal or permissible as an acceptable entry.*
• Check for and correct small errors (e.g., wrong time or date).	*Minimizes errors in charting that may decrease total credibility*
• When recording events not witnessed or performed by you, use following form: "[name] reported administering or witnessing . . ."	*Clarifies that recorder did not personally perform or view action*
• Draw a line through space at end of completed notes.	*Prevents someone else from adding information*
• Sign notes before chart leaves your possession.	*Avoids confusion of authorship should other people write on same form*
• Chart actions on completion, not before performing them.	*Avoids charting error due to delays in or cancellation of action*

Action	Rationale
• Use complete words or acceptable abbreviations only (see Appendix B).	*Eliminates miscommunication*
• For computerized charting, never give out your password for someone to chart for you or for any other reason.	*Prevents misuse; may be grounds for dismissal and has licensure implications; protects client privacy*

Evaluation

Were desired outcomes achieved? An example of evaluation is:
    Desired outcome met: Continuity of care was provided through dissemination of information in an accurate, comprehensive, and brief form.

Documentation

The following should be noted on the client's chart:
● Assessment data
● Planning
● Procedures performed and client's response
● Evaluation

Sample Documentation
Narrative Charting
Date: 1/23/05
Time: 1330

Alert, oriented X3. Family at bedside. Skin warm and dry, with capillary refill of less than 5 sec. Respirations even and nonlabored, with faint expiratory wheezes noted. Cough strong with scant, thin, yellow secretions produced. Pillow pressed to chest by client to splint incision site during cough. Abdomen soft with active bowel sounds. Voiding without difficulty. Chest tubes intact on right chest wall, with dressing clean and dry. Drainage serous and moderate—30 to 40 mL/hr. TENS unit intact at settings of 45 and 30. No complaints of severe pain.

Sample Documentation continued
Charting by Exception
Date: 1/23/05
Time: 1330

(Graphic sheet and assessment flow sheet or checklist are used to validate normal findings.) Faint expiratory wheezes noted bilaterally in lower lobes. Thin, yellow secretions produced with coughing. Moderate serous drainage—30 to 40 mL/hr noted from chest tubes. TENS unit in place at settings of 45 and 30.

SOAPIE Charting
Date: 1/23/05
Time: 1330

S "I don't have any pain."
O Skin warm and dry with capillary refill less than 5 sec; respirations even with expiratory wheezes; cough strong with scant, thin, yellow secretions produced; chest tubes intact with clean, dry dressing. Drainage is serous and moderate—30 to 40 mL/hr. TENS unit intact at settings of 45 and 30.
A Pain-free
P Continue supportive care with TENS unit. Encourage use of pillow to splint chest incision site when coughing.
I Pillow pressed to chest by client during deep-breathing and coughing exercises
E Verbalized lack of pain after coughing

DAR Charting
Date: 1/23/05
Time: 1330

Comfort:
D (S) "I'm having severe pain in my left knee, where I had the surgery."
   (O) Skin warm and dry with capillary refill less than 5 sec at (L) knee operative area; (L) and (R) leg pedal pulses 3+, no edema in left leg.
A Morphine 10 mg IM in right hip. Client repositioned.
R Verbalized complete pain relief in left leg area

Sample Documentation continued

Focus Charting

Date: 1/23/05
Time: 1330

Comfort:
Grimacing during and 15 min after deep-breathing and coughing exercises. Instructed to hold pillow to chest to splint incision when coughing; return demonstration from patient received. Verbalized decrease in discomfort when coughing.

● **Nursing Procedure 2.6**

Reporting Incidents (Variance or Unusual Occurrence Reporting)

Purpose

Documents for legal purposes any adverse event that occurs with a client, family, visitors, or health care personnel during clinical care activities

Provides documentation for improving quality of client care in a facility

Identifies need for changes in or reinforcement of procedures and guidelines for staff teaching through agency in-service education

Equipment

- Small pad and pencil (for event summary notes)
- Pen (color per agency policy)
- Appropriate form for incident reporting
- Client-specific progress note or nurses' note sheets

Assessment

Assessment should focus on the following findings related to the event:

- Persons involved in the event
- Condition of individual(s) involved

- Witnesses to the event
- Direct physical surroundings of the event
- Actions taken at time of event

Outcome Identification and Planning

Desired Outcomes

A sample desired outcome is:
- Information related to the event is documented and reported accurately and immediately.

Special Considerations in Planning and Implementation

General

Each agency has a specific policy and documentation form for reporting incidents. The policy should be followed. Before completing the report form, the nurse should take the necessary steps to assess the client and provide any care necessary to secure client safety, in addition to notifying the appropriate agency personnel and physician. If medical care is needed for a visitor or other personnel, follow the agency procedure for obtaining care for those individuals (which is generally directing them to their own physician or going through emergency services). Do not attempt to provide care outside of the agency policies. Information concerning the event should not be discussed with uninvolved persons, including other health care personnel, clients, and visitors; however, seek help as necessary and within policy guidelines to ascertain safety of client or other persons.

Home Health

Unless necessary for safety, do not discuss information concerning the event with uninvolved persons, including other health care personnel, clients, and visitors.

Implementation

Action	Rationale
1. Obtain correct agency-approved reporting form.	*Ascertains that correct form is used for legal purposes*
2. Jot in notebook pertinent observations related to each category of information.	*Organizes notes and facilitates accuracy*
3. Record pertinent observations and information on the event form. Provide only the information that is requested (e.g., immedi-	*Records the pertinent information without increasing liability by providing unnecessary information*

Action	Rationale
ate occurrences leading to the event, witnessed findings, follow-up nursing assessment).	
• When recording an event that you did not witness, such as a fall, state what the client or involved party states he or she was doing at the time of incident. DO NOT try to interpret what happened; just record the facts as requested.	*Clarifies that recorder did not personally view the event*
• Use complete words or acceptable abbreviations only.	*Eliminates miscommunication*
4. Provide signatures as requested.	*Provides a legal signature*
5. Submit form to appropriate agency personnel for follow-up and review.	*Promotes appropriate processing*
• Do not place the form in the client's chart and do not photocopy it.	*Maintains privacy; avoids exposure of client information to uninvolved individuals*
6. Record in the client's chart only the facts of your observations directly related to the client's condition or treatment and immediate steps taken to provide client safety. Do not emphasize, elaborate, or provide any explanatory information (see sample documentation note). DO NOT chart in the client's record that an incident report was completed.	*Minimizes legal ramifications*

Evaluation

Were desired outcomes achieved? Examples of evaluation include:
• Desired outcome partially met: Information related to the event was documented and reported accurately.

Documentation

The following should be noted on the client's chart:
- Facts directly related to the event (e.g., "client found on floor," NOT "client fell")
- Client assessment
- Actions taken to ensure safety or as follow-up to assessment findings
- Physician notification

Sample Documentation
Date: 2/19/05
Time : 1400

Client noted lying on floor. Assisted back to bed and side rails up ×4. Alert and oriented, PERLAC, strong equal hand grip; small 1-cm bruise noted on occipital area, no swelling noted. Safety precautions protocol instituted. Dr. Riggs notified for follow-up.

Essential Assessment Components

OVERVIEW

- In most situations, the trend of vital sign readings is more relevant than any individual reading.
- Pain assessment is considered to be the fifth vital sign. Early pain assessment allows the nurse to interpret other vital signs in the proper context (increased pulse and blood pressure may be secondary to pain).
- To obtain a true assessment of client status when using mechanical equipment, data must be correlated with clinical findings.
- Generally, the more acute the client and setting are, the more frequent and more in-depth the assessment must be.
- A thorough clinical assessment provides the foundation for competent and complete follow-up care.
- Assessment consists of objective and subjective data related to the client's present and past physical and mental health status.
- Performing assessment in a systematic manner helps to eliminate errors and oversights in data collection.
- Blood pressure and pulse may be obtained by a variety of methods to determine cardiac or vascular status. One method may be more appropriate in certain clinical situations than in others, but each method requires precision.
- Measuring the client's weight provides data about the client's current health state and provides cues for directing treatment.

Measuring Electronic Vital Signs

Purpose

Provides objective data for determining client's overall health status
Allows frequent monitoring of vital signs electronically through
  noninvasive means

Equipment

- Electronic vital sign machine with appropriate-sized blood
  pressure cuff for size and age
- Thermometer probe covers
- Noninvasive blood pressure printer (optional)
- Flow sheet for frequent readings (if printer is not used)
- Watch with second hand
- Nonsterile gloves

Assessment

Assessment should focus on the following:
- Ordered frequency of readings, if any
- Conditions that might indicate need for frequent readings
  (e.g., head injury, trauma, surgery)
- Skin integrity of arm (or extremity being used)
- Initial and previous vital sign readings
- Circulation in extremity in which readings are obtained (skin
  color and temperature, pulse volume, capillary refill)
- Presence of shunt, fistula, or graft in extremity
- History of mastectomy or lymph node removal from extremity
- Medication regimen including cardiac or blood pressure
  medications
- Appropriate site for temperature measurement: oral (unless
  contraindicated: oral surgery, combativeness, or inability to
  cooperate), axillary, or rectal (unless contraindicated: age,
  rectal surgery, or combativeness)
- Choice of extremity to use to obtain pulse and blood pressure (e.g., if arm cannot be used for brachial blood pressure,
  use leg for popliteal pressure)

Nursing Diagnoses

The nursing diagnoses may include the following:
- Decreased tissue perfusion related to hypovolemia
- Decreased cardiac output related to dehydration
- Risk for hyperthermia related to exposure to microorganisms
  during invasive procedures

Outcome Identification and Planning

Desired Outcomes

Sample desired outcomes include the following:
- Client demonstrates vital signs that are within client's baseline parameters.
- Client exhibits adequate cardiac output and tissue perfusion as evidenced by pink, warm, dry skin with a capillary refill < 3 seconds.

Special Considerations in Planning and Implementation

General

Wait at least 30 minutes after the client exercises, eats, or smokes before assessing vital signs so that readings reflect a resting state. Report readings reflecting a 20-mm Hg change in blood pressure or pulse below 60 or above 100 beats per minute. For clients at significant risk for fluid or blood loss, such as those at risk for gastrointestinal bleeding, a 10-mm Hg blood loss may be considered significant. Frequently assess clients who show any of these changes.

Perform vital sign assessments frequently for clients in the immediate postoperative period and after experiencing trauma, and for clients with acute neurologic deficits. If the client has had a mastectomy, do not take blood pressure in the affected extremity.

Avoid placing a blood pressure cuff on an extremity in which a hemodialysis shunt, fistula, graft, or IV infusion is being maintained. Ensure that the blood pressure cuff is the appropriate size and width (at least 40% of the circumference of the midpoint of the limb used). A cuff that is too small may result in elevation of blood pressure; a large cuff may excessively decrease blood pressure.

Pediatric

Perform less invasive assessments (respirations and pulse) first. Use games to encourage cooperation and decrease anxiety. Obtain apical pulse for newborns and infants, because this measurement is more accurate. Blood pressure is not routinely assessed for newborns and toddlers. If manual blood pressure is obtained in a small child, use of a Doppler may increase the accuracy of readings. A chemical dot thermometer may be preferred for children.

Geriatric

Be alert for orthostatic hypotension, a common finding in older adults. Older adults may have lower normal ranges for body temperature.

End-of-Life Care

Individualize the frequency of vital sign assessment for the dying client as much as possible within institutional policy. With the exception of pain assessment, vital signs are often assessed less frequently in this population. Consider client and family preferences and plan assessments to minimize disruption of family interactions and to facilitate client comfort.

Delegation

Unlicensed assistants or technicians may obtain vital signs. Significant changes or abnormal findings may warrant a follow-up or more detailed assessment by the RN or LPN. Trends should be addressed by the RN. When an automated vital sign machine is used, the nurse is responsible for monitoring the client's extremity regularly.

Implementation

Action	Rationale
1. Explain procedure to client.	*Reduces anxiety*
2. Perform hand hygiene and organize equipment.	*Reduces microorganism transfer; promotes efficiency*
Taking Electronic Blood Pressure and Pulse	
3. Check the cuff and tubing of automated vital signs machine for air leaks and kinks.	*Facilitates accurate readings*
4. Attach noninvasive blood pressure printer to blood pressure module (Fig. 3.1), if available, and turn both machines on.	*Allows continuous recording of vital signs; activates equipment*

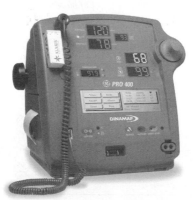

FIGURE 3.1

Action	Rationale
5. Place arm at level of heart in straight position (Fig. 3.2).	*Facilitates correct reading: if arm is below heart level, the blood pressure will be elevated; if above, the blood pressure will be decreased*
6. Palpate brachial pulse.	*Determines most accurate position for cuff placement*
7. Assess pulse and blood pressure manually, using the arm you will use for automated readings.	*Provides baseline vital signs for comparison to determine the accuracy of automated readings*
8. Remove manual cuff and place cuff of automated machine snugly around extremity (artery arrow) above brachial pulse.	*Places cuff pressure directly over artery*
9. Press MANUAL, STAT, or START button. Turning the machine on will often produce an initial reading.	*Obtains initial reading*
10. Obtain reading(s) from digital display panel: • Systolic pressure • Diastolic pressure • Mean arterial pressure • Pulse/heart rate	*Provides baseline data*
11. Compare manual blood pressure and pulse readings to those obtained from the automated vital signs machine.	*Assesses accuracy of monitor function*
12. Check cuff for full deflation.	*Prevents prolonged obstruction of blood flow in extremity*

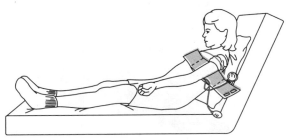

FIGURE 3.2

Action	Rationale
13. Set timer to recheck readings in 1 to 2 minutes, and check time interval with a reliable watch.	*Assesses accuracy of timing device*
14. Check new data readings and time elapsed since last reading.	*Assesses accuracy of machine functioning and verifies range of current blood pressure*
15. Set timer for frequency of readings as desired. (Method may vary, but time is usually set by increasing or decreasing minutes until desired time interval is obtained.)	*Regulates frequency of readings*
16. Set alarm limits with appropriate controls.	*Alerts nurse to readings that require immediate attention*
17. Reassess circulation status of extremity and cuff deflation with each reading.	*Prevents inadvertent compromise of circulation*

Taking an Electronic Temperature

Action	Rationale
18. Obtain disposable probe cover. Cover thermometer probe by sliding cover over probe until it snaps into place.	*Prevents contamination of thermometer probe*
19. Place covered probe into appropriate body orifice or at site (note additional preparation when indicated by route):	
Oral: Place probe in the posterior sublingual pocket and ask client to close lips around probe.	*Promotes contact with mucous membranes or skin for accurate reading*
Axillary: Place probe in axilla and hold arm down securely at client's side.	*Promotes continued contact with skin surface*
Rectal: Lubricate probe and gently insert past outer rectal sphincter.	*Prevents trauma to rectal tissues*
Tympanic: Push the "on" button (required with some units) and await the "ready" signal on the unit first. Pull the pinna of the ear up and back to promote visualization of the	*Detects the maximum tympanic membrane heat radiation*

Action	Rationale
tympanic membrane (for children <3 years of age, pull pinna down and back). Then insert the probe snugly in the external ear canal and aim it toward the tympanic membrane or as directed by the manufacturer.	
20. For oral, axillary, and rectal readings: Hold the probe in place until you hear a signal indicating that the reading is complete.	*Maintains contact until accurate reading is obtained*
For tympanic thermometer: Activate unit by pushing trigger button (located on top of some units), then remove the probe from the ear. The reading will be immediate.	*Initiates reading of heat radiated from the tympanic membrane*
21. Note the temperature reading, then discard the probe cover.	*Decreases spread of microorganisms*
22. Replace the thermometer in its charger/holder.	*Recharges thermometer for future use*

Evaluation

Were desired outcomes achieved? Examples of evaluation include:
- Desired outcome partially met: Blood pressure and pulse are within client's normal limits, but temperature is elevated at 100.4F.
- Desired outcome met: Skin is hot and dry, mucous membranes are flushed.

Documentation

The following should be noted on the client's chart:
- Vital sign readings (record in nurses' notes only if reading is significantly different from previous readings) and characteristics
- Summary of trends of readings
- Condition of extremity from which blood pressure was taken
- Need for increase or decrease in frequency of readings

Sample Documentation
Date: 2/24/05
Time: 1500

Oral temperature elevated at 100.4?, pulse 102 bpm and
thready. Left arm BP 120/80 mm Hg. Left hand pink
with brisk capillary refill.

Nursing Procedure 3.2

Palpating Blood Pressure

Purpose

Determines systolic pressure (the return of the pulse) when
blood pressure cannot be obtained by auscultation

Equipment

- Blood pressure cuff
- Sphygmomanometer
- Flow sheet for reading of frequent assessments

Assessment

Assessment should focus on the following:
- Ordered frequency of readings, if any, or conditions that
  might indicate need for frequent readings (e.g., cardiac
  failure, trauma, postoperative hemorrhage)
- Extremity being used to obtain blood pressure (e.g., if arm
  cannot be used for brachial blood pressure, use leg for
  popliteal pressure)
- Skin integrity of extremity being used
- Initial and previous blood pressure recordings
- Circulation in extremity in which readings are being
  obtained (skin color and temperature, color of mucous
  membranes, pulse volume, capillary refill)
- Medication regimen including cardiac drugs

Nursing Diagnoses

The nursing diagnoses may include the following:
- Ineffective peripheral tissue perfusion related to dehydration
- Decreased cardiac output related to excess blood loss

Outcome Identification and Planning

Desired Outcomes

Sample desired outcomes include the following:
- Client remains free of injury resulting from decreased cardiac output and significant changes in blood pressure.
- Client shows signs of adequate tissue perfusion evidenced by brisk capillary refill; normal heart rate; warm, pink, dry skin.

Special Considerations in Planning and Implementation

General

If the client's blood pressure could be auscultated previously but now can be obtained only via palpation, notify the physician and continue to monitor the client closely with blood pressure, pulse, and respirations every 5 to 10 minutes. Report any readings reflecting a 20-mm Hg change in blood pressure. Remember that systolic readings in the popliteal area are usually 10 to 40 mm Hg above brachial readings.

Keep in mind that although a diastolic pressure can be obtained by palpation, frequent errors occur in obtaining results. If unable to palpate blood pressure, try using a Doppler device (see Nursing Procedure 3.3, Doppler Pulse Assessment).

If the client has had a mastectomy or has a hemodialysis shunt or IV infusion, avoid taking blood pressure in the affected extremity.

Pediatric

In the young client, anticipate using the flush method to obtain blood pressures rather than the palpation method. Consult a nursing fundamentals text or agency policy manual for instructions.

Geriatric

Avoid leaving the blood pressure cuff on elderly clients because their skin may be thin and fragile. Be alert for orthostatic hypotension, a common finding in older adults.

Delegation

Blood pressure assessment by palpation should be performed by licensed personnel only since clients may have compromised circulation.

Implementation

Action	Rationale
1. Explain procedure to client and family.	*Decreases anxiety; promotes cooperation*

Action	Rationale
2. Perform hand hygiene and organize equipment.	*Reduces microorganism transfer; promotes efficiency*
3. Palpate for brachial or radial pulse.	*Finds pulse offering best palpable volume for procedure*
4. Place cuff on arm selected for blood pressure.	*Positions cuff for inflation*
5. Palpate again for pulse. Once pulse is obtained, continue to palpate.	*Once again locates pulse for procedure*
6. Inflate cuff until unable to palpate pulse.	*Occludes arterial blood flow*
7. Continue to inflate cuff until measurement gauge is 20 mm Hg past the point at which pulse was lost on palpation.	*Clearly identifies point of pulse return*
8. Slowly deflate cuff at rate of 2 to 3 mm Hg per second.	*Prevents missing first palpable beat*
9. Note reading on measurement gauge when pulse returns.	*Identifies systolic blood pressure reading*
10. Repeat steps 5 through 9.	*Confirms readings*
11. Deflate cuff completely and remove (or leave on if readings are being obtained at frequent intervals).	*Promotes comfort*
12. Restore equipment.	*Prepares for next use*
13. Perform hand hygiene.	*Reduces microorganisms*

Evaluation

Were desired outcomes achieved? Examples of evaluation include:

- Desired outcomes not met: Drop in blood pressure noted within 5 minutes, prior blood pressure 80 palpable, currently 70 palpable. Chest pain noted with activity.
- Desired outcome met: Client shows signs of adequate tissue perfusion with capillary refill < 3 seconds.

Documentation

The following should be noted on the client's chart:

- Systolic blood pressure measurement upon palpation
- Extremity from which blood pressure was obtained
- Circulatory indicators (capillary refill, color of skin and mucous membranes, skin temperature, quality of pulses)
- Level of consciousness

Sample Documentation
Date: 2/4/05
Time: 0830

Blood pressure by palpation, 80 mm Hg systolic from right arm. Client slightly lethargic at times. Skin cool to touch. Nailbeds and mucous membranes slightly pale. Capillary refill, 3 seconds.

● **Nursing Procedure 3.3**

Obtaining Doppler Pulse

Purpose

Determines presence of arterial blood flow when pulse is difficult to palpate or not palpable

Equipment

- Doppler
- Conductant gel
- Washcloth
- Small basin of warm water
- Soap
- Towel

Assessment

Assessment should focus on the following:
- Medical diagnosis
- History of medical problems related to cardiovascular deficits
- Medication regimen including cardiac drugs
- Quality of pulses in extremities
- Circulatory indicators of extremities (color, temperature, sensation, capillary refill)
- Pulse rate and blood pressure

Nursing Diagnoses

The nursing diagnoses may include the following:
- Ineffective tissue perfusion related to decreased blood flow to lower extremities
- Decreased cardiac output related to dehydration

Outcome Identification and Planning

Desired Outcomes

Sample desired outcomes include the following:
- Client remains free of injury from changes in pulse presence or quality due to early detection and prompt intervention.
- Client demonstrates adequate cardiac output and tissue perfusion as evidenced by warm skin and capillary refill < 3 seconds.

Special Considerations in Planning and Implementation

Delegation

The nurse should be the one who obtains a pulse using Doppler if the client's condition is unstable or circulatory problems are present. Doppler pulse may be delegated to a skilled technician certified by the facility, if protocol permits.

Implementation

Action	Rationale
1. Explain procedure to client and family.	*Decreases anxiety; promotes cooperation*
2. Perform hand hygiene and organize equipment.	*Reduces microorganism transfer; promotes efficiency*
3. Apply coupling gel over pulse area. Inform client that gel will be cold.	*Enhances transmission of vascular and pulse sounds*
4. If using portable manual Doppler, place eartips of Doppler scope in ears (similar to positioning stethoscope).	*Enables sound to be detected by nurse*
5. Place Doppler transducer over identified pulse area (Fig. 3.3).	*Places transducer over area that will transmit pulse sound*
6. Turn Doppler on until faint static sound is audible. Adjust volume with control knob.	*Activates system; sets volume to suit listener's hearing range*
7. Identify pulse by listening for a hollow, rushing, pulsatile sound (a "swooshing" sound).	*Confirms presence of pulse*
If pulse is not audible within 4 to 5 sec, slowly slide Doppler over a 1- to 2-inch radius within same pulse	*Locates pulse*

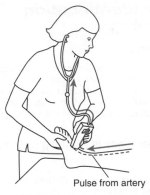

Pulse from artery

FIGURE 3.3

Action	Rationale
area. If pulse still is not audible, continue this step, increasing radius by 1 to 2 inches until pulse is audible or until you are convinced that pulse is not present.	
8. Wash gel from skin, rinse, and pat dry.	*Prevents skin irritation*
9. If pulse was difficult to obtain, draw a circle around pulse site or mark with an X.	*Outlines location of pulse for next assessment*
10. Restore equipment.	*Prepares for next use*
11. Perform hand hygiene.	*Promotes cleanliness*

Evaluation

Were desired outcomes achieved? Examples of evaluation include:

- Desired outcome met: Pulse diminished to detection by Doppler only during first hour after surgery, but restored to 1+ palpable after 1 liter of saline ordered by Dr. Peters.
- Desired outcome met: Skin warm and dry in right leg at 4-hour check after surgery.

Documentation

The following should be noted on the client's chart:
- Area in which pulse was obtained

- Circulatory indicators in all extremities (capillary refill, color and temperature of skin, quality of pulses)
- Pulse rate, blood pressure, respirations, temperature, pain level

---

Sample Documentation
Date: 1/3/05
Time: 0600

Right foot cool; nailbeds and sole of foot slightly bluish. Pedal pulse detectable only by Doppler. Left foot cool, with faint palpable pulse. Capillary refill, 6 sec in right foot and 3 sec in left foot.

● Nursing Procedure 3.4

Measuring Apical–Radial Pulse

Purpose

Detects presence of pulse deficit that is related to poor ventricular contractions or dysrhythmias

Equipment

- Stethoscope
- Watch with second hand

Assessment

Assessment should focus on the following:
- Ordered frequency of readings with follow-up orders
- History of dysrhythmias, cardiac conditions
- Pulse characteristics
- Previous pulse recordings
- Medication regimen including cardiac drugs

Nursing Diagnoses

The nursing diagnoses may include the following:
- Ineffective peripheral tissue perfusion related to hypovolemia
- Decreased cardiac output related to irregular heart rhythm

Outcome Identification and Planning

Desired Outcomes

Samples of desired outcomes include:
- Client exhibits regular, equal apical and radial pulse rates throughout treatment period.
- Client will experience no pulse deficit during immediate postoperative period.

Special Considerations in Planning and Implementation

General

Clients with ventricular (pump) pathologies and cardiac dysrhythmias are particularly prone to pulse deficits.

Pediatric

Remember that some infants and children experience occasional nonpathologic dysrhythmias, such as premature ventricular contractions (PVCs), which may cause an apical–radial pulse difference (pulse deficit). Obtain a baseline of pulse deficit occurrence, and note client response. Monitor for change in frequency of occurrence or response.

Geriatric

Assess apical–radial pulse every 24 hours in clients with such chronic conditions as diabetes and atherosclerosis because they are particularly prone to pulse deficits.

Home Health

Because the procedure requires two people, enlist and train a family member to assist. Encourage family members to perform the procedure between nurse visits.

Delegation

Apical–radial pulse measurement may be performed by a skilled technician with a nurse.

Implementation

Action	Rationale
1. Explain procedure to client.	*Decreases anxiety*
2. Perform hand hygiene and organize equipment.	*Reduces contamination; promotes efficiency*
3. Have one nurse position himself or herself to take radial pulse (at radial artery).	

Action	Rationale
4. Have second nurse place stethoscope under client's gown at apex (fifth intercostal space at midclavicular line) to obtain apical pulse. Maintain privacy.	*Locates apical pulse*
5. Place watch so both nurses can see second hand.	*Facilitates accuracy in beginning and ending*
6. State "begin" when ready to start (nurse counting apical pulse will state when to begin and end counting).	*Prevents error in count because nurse with stethoscope in ear cannot hear count call*
7. At the same time, both nurses count pulse for 1 full minute.	*Ensures accuracy of reading*
8. Call out "stop" when 1 minute has passed.	*Ends count*
9. Compare rates obtained.	*Determines whether pulse deficit exists*
If a difference is noted between apical and radial rates, subtract the radial rate from the apical rate.	*Calculates pulse deficit*
10. Repeat steps 6 through 9.	*Verifies results*
11. Readjust gown for comfort.	*Maintains privacy*
12. Perform hand hygiene.	*Reduces microorganisms*
13. Notify physician if pulse deficit was noted.	*Initiates prompt medical intervention*

Evaluation

Were desired outcomes achieved? Examples of evaluation include:

- Desired outcome met: Client remains free of pulse irregularities or pulse deficit throughout treatment period.
- Desired outcome met: Client remains free of pulse irregularities or pulse deficit during immediate postoperative period.

Documentation

The following should be noted on the client's chart:

- Apical–radial pulse rate
- Quality of pulse
- Irregularities of pulse rhythm (if present)
- Calculated pulse deficit, if present
- Response to deficit
- Current cardiac drugs

Sample Documentation
Date: 1/6/05
Time: 0830

Apical–radial pulse, 94 apical and 74 radial with pulse
deficit of 20. Pulse irregular. Client states no dizziness,
faintness, or chest discomfort. Physician notified.

● **Nursing Procedure 3.5**

Assessing Pain

Purpose

Determines the presence, location, quality, temporal pattern,
  and intensity (level) of client discomfort
Provides a basis for treatment and provision of comfort
  measures

Equipment

- Pain rating scale and pain description table
- Pain record form (optional)

Assessment

Assessment should focus on the following:
- Location of pain
- Intensity of pain: strength, power, or force of pain identified
  with numeric or verbal scale
- Quality of pain: characteristics of pain: searing, dull, throb-
  bing, sharp, burning, etc.
- Temporal pattern: acute/chronic, spasmodic, continuous,
  steady, intermittent, or transient, and changes noted
- Associated symptoms

Nursing Diagnoses

The nursing diagnoses may include the following:
- Pain (acute) related to stress on surgical incision when
  coughing
- Anxiety related to anticipation of discomfort

Outcome Identification and Planning

Desired Outcomes

Sample outcomes include the following:
- The client states pain has decreased from a level of 8 to a level of 2 or lower.
- The client verbalizes that anxiety level is lower related to pain.
- The client demonstrates nonverbal cues of comfort.

Special Considerations in Planning and Implementation

General

Remember that the client is the expert regarding pain. The nurse's direct observations should not be used to dispute the client's perception. Pain is present if the client says it is. Perform pain assessment with vital signs and additional times as indicated.

Pediatric

Use nonverbal cues to determine the presence of pain in newborns, infants, and toddlers. While children as young as 8 years can use a 0-to-10 scale, a graphic rating scale, such as a faces chart, can be quite effective.

Geriatric

Remember that elderly clients often have multiple sources of pain. Pain may be chronic, and the elderly client may demonstrate a stoic approach to pain. Observe for nonverbal cues of pain if cognitive impairment is present. Assess for altered pain sensation in some elderly clients, particularly if diabetes or neurovascular disease is present.

🎚 Transcultural

Consider the impact of the individual's culture when assessing pain level. Open expression of pain is encouraged in some cultures, while other cultures value stoic responses to pain as something to be ignored or endured in silence.

Delegation

Pain assessment should be performed by a nurse, particularly with ongoing pain management (i.e., PCA or epidural), and when interpretation of nonverbal cues is needed. In some facilities, unlicensed staff may be trained in basic pain assessment.

Implementation

Action	Rationale
1. Explain procedure to client, emphasizing the importance of the client's pain report.	*Decreases anxiety; reassures client that all pain reports will be believed*

Action	Rationale
2. Perform hand hygiene and organize equipment.	*Reduces contamination if physical exam is needed; promotes efficiency*
3. Ask client if pain or discomfort is or has been present. Ask client about pain at rest and with movement.	*Provides an indication of pain status and pain history; encourages client to report discomfort*
4. Determine location: use a form with a body outline (Fig. 3.4) and ask client to indicate where the pain is.	*Provides a way for client to show areas of discomfort*
5. Assess intensity: • Use a pain scale: Ask client what number best represents his or her level of pain (0 indicates no pain, the highest number indicates the strongest pain). OR • Use a graphic scale: Ask client to point to the picture (e.g., faces [Fig. 3.5]) or the number or stack of chips that indicate the level of pain experienced.	*Quantifies pain; provides a way to determine effectiveness of pain management therapies*

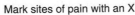

Mark sites of pain with an X

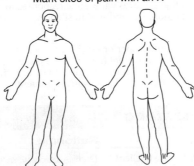

FIGURE 3.4

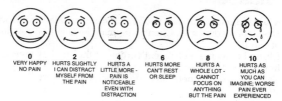

0	2	4	6	8	10
VERY HAPPY NO PAIN	HURTS SLIGHTLY I CAN DISTRACT MYSELF FROM THE PAIN	HURTS A LITTLE MORE - PAIN IS NOTICEABLE EVEN WITH DISTRACTION	HURTS MORE CAN'T REST OR SLEEP	HURTS A WHOLE LOT - CANNOT FOCUS ON ANYTHING BUT THE PAIN	HURTS AS MUCH AS YOU CAN IMAGINE; WORSE PAIN EVER EXPERIENCED

FIGURE 3.5

Action	Rationale
6. Ascertain quality: Ask client to choose from a list of descriptive terms (Appendix A). Read the list to client if client is blind or illiterate.	*Helps client describe pain with frequently used terms*
7. Assess temporal pattern. Ask the following questions: a. "When did/does the pain start?" b. "How long does the pain last?"	*Provides further information about pain; helps determine appropriate dosing schedule for pain medication*
c. "Does the pain recur before it's time for the next pain medication?"	*Indicates breakthrough pain*
8. Ask client if other symptoms accompany pain (Appendix A).	*Assists in determining causes of pain and additional treatments needed*
9. Inquire about alleviating or aggravating factors (movement, cough, repositioning).	*Indicates measures to be used in pain relief or pain prevention*
10. Initiate comfort measures: • Apply cool cloth to head for headache, and dim lights	*Reduces pain perception by decreasing noxious stimuli*
• Offer massage (see Appendix A for other measures).	*Decreases tension, which may aggravate pain*
• Administer analgesic as ordered.	*Relieves pain via various mechanisms*
11. Perform hand hygiene.	*Reduces microorganisms*
12. Reassess client; notify physician if pain is not relieved.	*Initiates prompt medical intervention*

Evaluation

Were desired outcomes achieved? Examples of evaluation include:
● Desired outcome met: Client states pain level is 1 on a scale of 1 to 10.
● Desired outcome met: Client verbalizes that anxiety level is lower related to pain.
● Desired outcome met: Client demonstrates nonverbal cues of comfort.

Documentation

The following should be noted on the client's chart:
● Pain severity or intensity (rating) and location
● Other pain assessment findings: quality of pain, temporal pattern, associated symptoms, alleviating and aggravating elements
● Vital signs
● Nonpharmacologic pain relief measures
● Pharmacologic pain relief measures
● Client's response to relief measures (current pain level)
● Vital signs after relief measures
● Notification of physician (if indicated)

Sample Documentation
Date: 1/6/05
Time: 0830

Client complained of pain at abdominal incision site, rating it as 8 on a 1-to-10-point scale. Blood pressure 138/82 mm Hg; pulse 90 bpm; resp 26 breaths/minute. Positioned on left side with slight relief. Morphine 4 mg given IV. States pain level is now 2. Resting quietly in bed with side rails up.

● **Nursing Procedure 3.6**

Obtaining Weight With a Sling Scale

Purpose

Measures body weight when client cannot stand or tolerate sitting position

Equipment

- Sling scale with sling (mat) (Fig. 3.6)
- Disposable cover for sling (or disinfectant and cleaning supplies)
- Washcloth
- Pen
- Graphic sheet or weight record

Assessment

Assessment should focus on the following:
- Doctor's orders regarding frequency and specified time of weighing
- Medical diagnosis
- Previous body weight
- Rationale for using bedscale (e.g., client's weakness or inability to stand; standing contraindicated)
- Type and amount of clothing being worn (client should always be weighed in same type and amount of clothing)
- Adequacy of bedscale function

Nursing Diagnoses

The nursing diagnoses may include the following:
- Imbalanced nutrition, more than body requirements related to poor dietary habits
- Risk for imbalanced fluid volume (excess) related to impaired renal function

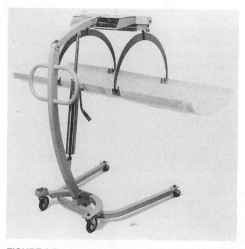

FIGURE 3.6

Outcome Identification and Planning

Desired Outcomes

Sample desired outcomes include:
- Client exhibits a 1-kg weight loss per sling scale weight after three series of dialysis exchanges.
- Client demonstrates a loss of 3 kg via sling scale in 1 week of beginning weight loss diet.

Special Considerations in Planning and Implementation

General

If the client cannot turn independently or has drainage tubes that could become dislodged, obtain assistance to move client. If client's weight may exceed capacity of sling scale, seek alternative means for weighing client.

Pediatric

Weigh infants and small toddlers on pediatric scale for accuracy.

Delegation

Weighing a client using a sling scale may be performed by an assistant, a skilled technician, or a nurse.

Implementation

Action	Rationale
1. Explain procedure to client.	*Decreases anxiety*
2. Perform hand hygiene and organize equipment.	*Reduces microorganism transfer; promotes efficiency*
3. Calibrate (zero balance) scales (with sling across stretcher frame) according to manufacturer's directions.	*Ensures accuracy of results*
4. Prepare the sling:	
• Remove sling from stretcher frame and cover with disposable cover.	*Reduces transfer of microorganisms between clients*
• Roll sling into tube and place in storage holder.	*Prepares the sling; secures it while moving the system into position*
• Leave scale close to bed.	*Allows for easy access to sling*
5. Raise height of bed to comfortable working level.	*Promotes use of good body mechanics*
6. Secure all tubes to avoid pulling during the procedure. Have an assistant hold tubes, if necessary.	*Prevents tube dislodgment and subsequent client injury*

Action	Rationale
7. Lower head of bed.	*Places client in position to roll onto sling*
8. Remove sling from storage holder.	
9. Lower bed rail on side of bed with clearest access or from which most tubing originates.	*Facilitates placement of base under bed without disrupting tubing or other equipment*
Be sure opposite side rail is in raised position.	*Prevents accidental falls*
10. To place client on sling: • Roll client to one side of bed.	*Positions client on sling with minimal disturbance*
• Place rolled sling on other side of bed and unroll partially.	
• Assist client to turn to opposite side of bed (over rolled portion of sling to flat portion)	
• Unroll entire sling until flat.	
• Turn client supine on sling.	
• Position top sheet over client.	*Maintains privacy*
• Be sure BED RAILS ARE UP on unattended side of bed!	*Prevents accidental falls*
11. Roll scale to bedside, lower bed rail, and roll caster base under bed.	*Facilitates connection of sling to scale*
12. Center stretcher frame over client.	*Ensures centering of body*
13. Widen stance of base with shifter handle of caster base.	*Provides support base for weight*
14. Slowly release control valve and lower stretcher frame. Tighten valve when frame reaches mattress level.	*Enables proper placement of hooks in holes*
15. Place rings (hooks) on end of stretcher frame into sling holes.	*Attaches sling to weighing portion of scale*
16. Have client fold arms across chest.	*Prevents injury to arms and provides balance of body weight*
17. Raise client up with hydraulic pump handle until body is clear of bed.	*Places weight of body and attached tubing on scale*

Action	Rationale
18. Hold all tubing, wires, and equipment above client's body.	*Removes weight from equipment*
19. Press button on readout console.	*Obtains weight (in pounds or kilograms)*
20. Lower client onto bed by slowly releasing control valve.	*Returns client to bed gently*
21. Remove client from sling, rolling from side to side.	*Decreases client discomfort while removing equipment*
22. Remove sling cover, roll sling, and place in storage holder (or place sling in holder for cleaning of sling cover at later time).	
23. Remove caster base from under bed.	*Permits movement of sling scale*
24. Lift side rails.	*Ensures safety*
25. Raise head of bed and lower height of bed. Place client in comfortable position.	*Restores bed to position of safety and comfort*
26. Replace covers.	*Ensures privacy*
27. Restore or discard all equipment appropriately.	*Reduces transfer of microorganisms between clients; prepares equipment for future use*
28. Perform hand hygiene.	*Reduces microorganisms*
29. Record weight immediately.	*Avoids loss of data and need for reweighing of client*

Evaluation

Were desired outcomes achieved? Examples of evaluation include:
- Desired outcome met: Client shows a 1-kg weight loss per sling scale weight after three series of dialysis exchanges.
- Desired outcome met: Client shows a 3-kg weight loss 1 week after beginning weight loss diet.

Documentation

The following should be noted on the client's chart:
- Weight obtained (in pounds or kilograms)
- Type (and number or location) of scale used for weighing (e.g., sling bedscale on unit)
- Client's tolerance of procedure

Sample Documentation
Date: 3/9/04
Time: 0600

Weight after third dialysis exchange: 82 kg on sling scale. Weight loss of 1 kg from predialysis weight. Client reported slight shortness of breath in flat position, although respirations were smooth and nonlabored during weighing process. Client resting quietly in semi-Fowler's position.

● **Nursing Procedure 3.7**

Performing Basic Health Assessment 🧤

Purpose

Determines strengths and weaknesses of physical and mental health status

Equipment

- Pen
- Appropriate assessment form
- Gown
- Drape or sheet
- Blood pressure cuff
- Stethoscope
- Penlight
- Sphygmomanometer
- Thermometer
- Scales
- Watch with second hand
- Measurement tape
- Cotton balls
- Nonsterile gloves

Assessment

Assessment should focus on the following:
- Medical diagnosis
- Source of information
- Information obtained on health history
- Need for partial versus in-depth assessment

Nursing Diagnoses

The nursing diagnoses may include the following:
- Acute confusion related to drug overdose

- Ineffective peripheral tissue perfusion related to low blood cell level

Outcome Identification and Planning

Desired Outcomes

Sample desired outcomes include:
- Client experiences no undetected signs and symptoms of underlying mental or physical alterations.
- Client maintains adequate tissue perfusion, as evidenced by alert and oriented mentation and warm skin with capillary refill < 3 seconds.

Special Considerations in Planning and Implementation

General

Clients with acute conditions may require a more in-depth (focused) assessment of specific systems. Assessment in acute situations should be prioritized to address life-threatening areas immediately, with assessment of other areas undertaken as soon as possible thereafter. After initial detailed assessment is obtained for baseline data, an abbreviated assessment of the problem areas noted from the initial assessment may be performed each shift. A detailed assessment may then be performed periodically (every 24 to 72 hours, depending on agency policy and client state of health).

Pediatric

Normal developmental stage and physiologic changes must be taken into consideration when assessing the client. Although most of the information in the history may be obtained from the parent(s), the child's perspective regarding illness and care will be valuable throughout treatment.

Geriatric

Normal developmental stage and physiologic changes must be taken into consideration when assessing the client. Information in the history should be obtained from the client when possible. If the client is incoherent, the family can provide baseline data regarding client abilities and valuable perspectives regarding illness and care throughout treatment.

Home Health

A complete assessment must be completed on the client initially, with abbreviated updates on each visit.

Transcultural

When interviewing clients for whom English is not their native language, securing the services of an interpreter helps to reduce the potential for mistaken interpretation of client responses. Biocultural norms should be determined before judging whether findings are pathologic (e.g., mongolian spots are a normal skin variation in children of African, Asian, or Latin cultural background but may be pathologic in Caucasian children). Color changes in persons of color may be best observed in areas of minimal pigmentation (sclera, conjunctiva, nailbeds, palms and soles, and mucosal areas). A bluish hue may be normal for persons of Mediterranean or African descent.

Delegation

An RN or an LPN (as specified by agency policy) should perform general assessment appropriate for the client and setting. Significant abnormal findings may warrant a follow-up or more detailed assessment by the RN when the initial assessment is performed by the LPN. Reports by unlicensed staff of indicators of acute changes such as client complaints of pain, abnormal vital signs, or other findings should be promptly addressed by a registered or licensed nurse.

Implementation

Action	Rationale
1. Perform hand hygiene, and organize equipment.	*Reduces microorganism transfer; promotes efficiency*
2. Explain procedure to client, emphasizing importance of accuracy of data.	*Decreases anxiety; increases compliance*
3. Provide for privacy.	*Decreases embarrassment*

Taking a Health History

4. Interview client using therapeutic communication techniques (see Nursing Procedure 2.1, Therapeutic Communication). Include the following areas:	*Provides baseline data for future reference when providing care*
• Biographic information (name, age, sex, race, marital status, informant)	*Identifies client*
• Chief complaint (as stated in client's own words)	*Explains why client sought health care and what problem means to client*
• History of present problem (date of onset; detailed description of problem nature, loca-*	*Defines details of problems; helps determine nursing diagnoses*

Action	Rationale
tion, severity, and duration, as well as associating, contributing, and precipitating factors)	
• Past medical and surgical history (date and description of problems, previous hospitalizations, doctor's name, allergies, as well as conditions or medications; current medications taken and time of last dose)	*Serves as baseline and guide for treatment decisions; identifies potential problems related to interactions*
• Family history of mental and physical conditions	*Identifies hereditary factors that may affect health status*
• Psychosocial history (occupation; educational level; abuse of alcohol and other substances; tobacco use; religious preference; cultural practices)	*Identifies psychosocial, spiritual, and educational factors that may contribute to state of health*
• Nutritional information (diet, food likes and dislikes, special requirements, compliance with diets)	*Identifies nutritional factors related to state of health*
• Review of body systems (client's self-report of conditions or problems)	*Detects subjective cues that may further define problem*

Performing Physical Assessment

Action	Rationale
5. Assess general appearance.	*Provides objective cues about overall health state*
6. Obtain vital signs, height, and weight.	*Provides objective data about health state*
7. Assess the following in relation to neuromuscular status:	*Detects cues to abnormalities of neurologic or muscular status*
• Level of consciousness: awake, alert, drowsy, lethargic, stuporous, or comatose	
• Orientation: oriented to person, time, and place or disoriented	

Action	Rationale
• Sensory function: able to distinguish various sensations on skin surface (e.g., hot/cold, sharp/dull, and awareness of when and where sensation occurred)	
• Motor function: muscle tone (as determined by strength of extremities against resistance), gait, coordination of hands and feet, and reflex responses	
• Range of motion	
• Structural abnormalities, such as burns, scarring, spinal curvatures, bone spurs, contractures	
8. While proceeding from head to toe, inspect skin of head, neck, and extremities.	*Detects skin abnormalities*
• Note color, lesions, tears, abrasions, ulcerations, scars, degree of moistness, edema, vascularity.	*Provides baseline data for comparison*
• Measure size of all abnormal lesions and scars with tape measure.	
9. Palpate skin, lymph nodes, pulses, capillary refill, and joints of head, neck, and extremities. Note temperature, turgor, raised skin lesions, or lumps. Assess:	*Detects skin abnormalities and lymph enlargement*
• Lymph node tenderness and enlargement (Fig. 3.7 identifies lymph node areas)	
• Pulse quality, rhythm, and strength (Fig. 3.8 identifies pulse sites)	*Determines quality and character of pulses*
• Crepitus, nodules, and mobility	
10. Complete assessment of head and neck, including eye, ear, nose, mouth, and throat:	*Detects cues to pathophysiologic abnormalities of eye, ear, nose, mouth, and throat*

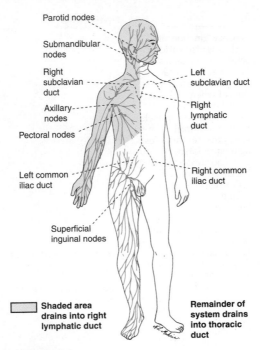

Parotid nodes

Submandibular nodes

Right subclavian duct

Axillary nodes

Pectoral nodes

Left common iliac duct

Superficial inguinal nodes

Left subclavian duct

Right lymphatic duct

Right common iliac duct

Shaded area drains into right lymphatic duct

Remainder of system drains into thoracic duct

FIGURE 3.7

Action	Rationale
Assess the eyes:	
• Note pupil status (size, shape, response to light and accommodation)	*Assesses cranial nerve status and pupil structure and function*
• Test visual acuity. Using adequate lighting, have client stand 20 feet from chart (glasses may be worn and should be noted in documentation). OR Have client read newspaper or other small print.	*Assesses visual acuity at a distance*
	Assesses acuity of vision within close proximity
• Assess condition of cornea and conjunctival sac.	*Detects injury or other complication*

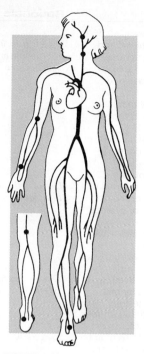

FIGURE 3.8

Action	Rationale
• Inspect for abrasions, discharge, and discoloration.	*Detects injury, inflammation, or infection*
Assess the ears:	
• Assess external ear structure (e.g., shape, presence of abnormalities on inspection and palpation).	*Detects injury or other complication*
• Test hearing acuity (ability of client to respond to normal sounds).	*Detects hearing impairment*
• Note presence of ear discharge and degree of wax buildup.	*Detects infection or excess wax*

Action	Rationale
Assess the nose: • Inspect external and internal structures. • Note presence of unusual or excessive discharge. • Test ability to inhale and exhale through each nostril. • Note ability to identify common odors correctly.	*Detects injury, infection, obstruction, or other complication*
Assess the mouth: • Inspect for internal or external lesions. • Note color of mucous membranes. • Inspect for abnormalities of teeth. • Note any unusual odor.	*Detects injury, inflammation, or infection*
Assess the throat: • Inspect for swelling, inflammation, or abnormal lesions. • Test ability to swallow without difficulty.	*Detects injury, inflammation, or infection*
11. Inspect skin status of anterior and posterior trunk and extremities, including feet.	*Detects skin abnormalities*
12. Palpate chest, breasts, axillary tail of Spence, and back. • Note raised lesions on any area and tenderness on palpation. • Inspect symmetry of breasts and nipples, skin status, lymph nodes, and presence of discharge, lumps, or nodules.	*Detects abnormal masses and lesions*
13. Assess cardiac status: • Note any unusual pulsations at precordium. • Note character of first (S_1) and second (S_2) heart sounds.	*Detects cues related to pathologic cardiac abnormalities*

Action	Rationale
• Auscultate for the presence or absence of third (S_3) or fourth (S_4) heart sounds. • Note presence of murmurs or rubs. • Auscultate heart sounds in the following areas (Fig. 3.9): *Aortic:* at second or third intercostal space just to right of sternum *Pulmonic:* at second or third intercostal space just to left of sternum *Tricuspid:* at fourth intercostal space just to left of sternum *Mitral:* in left midclavicular line at fifth intercostal space	
14. Assess respiratory status: • Note character of respirations and of anterior and posterior	*Determines if adventitious breath sounds (rales, rhonchi, or wheezes) are present, indicating abnormal pathophysiologic alterations*

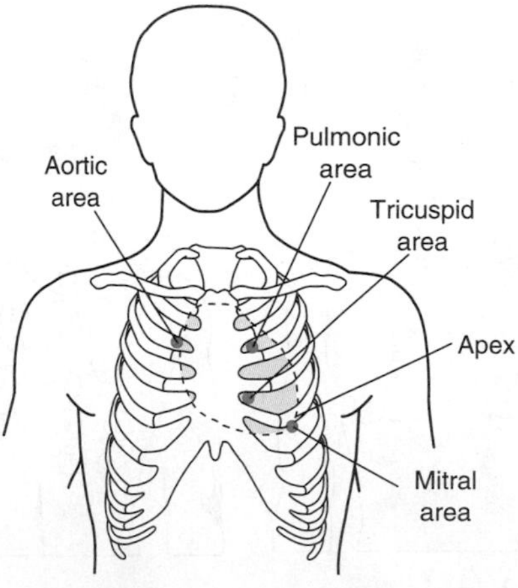

FIGURE 3.9

Action	Rationale
breath sounds in the following areas: *Bronchial:* over trachea *Bronchovesicular:* on each side of sternum between first and second intercostal spaces *Vesicular:* peripheral areas of the chest	
• When auscultating breath sounds, use side-to-side sequence to compare breath sounds on each side (Fig. 3.10). Avoid auscultating over bone or breast tissue.	*Increases possibility of detecting abnormalities*
15. Assess abdomen:	*Detects masses, abnormal fluid retention, or decrease or absence of peristalsis*
• Remember: Perform auscultation BEFORE palpation and percussion of abdomen.	*Palpation and percussion set underlying structures in motion, possibly interfering with character of bowel sounds*

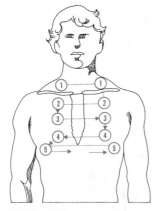 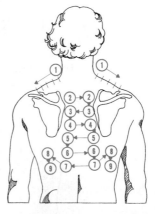

FIGURE 3.10

Action	Rationale
• Inspect size and contour. • Auscultate for bowel sounds in all quadrants. • Palpate tone of abdomen and check for underlying abnormalities (masses, pain, tenderness) and bladder distention.	
16. Assess genitalia and urethra: • Inspect for abnormalities in structure, discoloration, edema, abnormal discharge, or foul odor.	*Detects abnormalities of genitalia and urethral opening*
17. Restore or discard equipment properly.	*Removes microorganisms*
18. Perform hand hygiene.	*Prevents spread of microorganism*

Evaluation

Were desired outcomes achieved? Examples of evaluation include:
• Desired outcome met: Client exhibits no signs and symptoms of underlying mental or physical alterations.
• Desired outcome met: Client maintains adequate tissue perfusion, as evidenced by alert and oriented mentation and warm skin with capillary refill < 3 seconds.

Documentation

The following should be noted on the client's chart:
• Time of assessment
• Informant
• Chief complaint
• Information from client history
• Detailed description of assessment area related to chief complaint
• Detailed description of abnormalities
• Reports of abnormal subjective and objective data (pain, nausea, etc.)
• Priority areas of assessment
• Assessment procedures deferred to a later time
• Ability of client to assist with assessment

Sample Documentation
Date: 4/29/04
Time: 0830

A 44-year-old black man presented with nagging chest pain in center of chest that started 24 hours ago. He denies nausea, headache, or radiation of pain to arms or back. No abnormal heart sounds detected. Vital signs: blood pressure, 130/90; pulse, 82; temperature, 98.8 F; respirations, 22. Bedside oscilloscope displays normal sinus rhythm. No jugular vein distention. Pulses in upper and lower extremities weak (1+). Skin slightly moist but warm. No lower extremity edema noted.

Hygiene

OVERVIEW

- Hygiene is usually a private matter; consider the client's preference in terms of timing and personal items such as toiletries, as well as the amount of family assistance available or needed.
- Clients should be encouraged to perform as much hygiene care as possible within prescribed limitations.
- Maintaining good hygiene can promote the following:
  - Healthy skin, by preventing infections and skin breakdown
  - Improved circulation
  - Comfort and rest
  - Nutrition, by stimulating the appetite
  - Self-esteem, by improving the appearance
  - Sense of well-being
- Some major nursing diagnostic labels related to hygiene care are bathing/hygiene self-care deficit, dressing/grooming self-care deficit, risk of impaired skin integrity, and anxiety.
- Providing hygiene measures for clients receiving palliative end-of-life care promotes the major objective of comfort.
- Hygiene care should be provided at regular intervals while simultaneously balancing the need to conserve energy.
- When appropriate, family members can be taught hygiene care techniques and can be encouraged to assist with or perform this care; doing so provides an effective teaching experience and conserves staff time while the client is debilitated.

- All hygiene care procedures may be delegated to unlicensed assistive personnel. For clients with special needs such as special positioning or transfer during care, prevention of aspiration, or other concerns, additional instruction or supervision may be needed.

● **Nursing Procedure 4.1**

Providing Back Care 🖐

Purpose

Promotes comfort
Stimulates circulation
Relieves muscle tension
Facilitates therapeutic interaction

Equipment

- Lotion
- Soap
- Towel
- Washcloth
- Warm water
- Gloves, if the client's or nurse's skin is broken or if the client has an infectious skin disorder

Assessment

Assessment should focus on the following:
- Client's desire for back rub
- Client's knowledge of purpose of back rub
- Blood pressure and pulse rate and rhythm, if there is a history of cardiac or vascular problems
- Respiratory rate, if there is a history of respiratory problems
- Skin and bony prominences
- Client's ability to tolerate prone or lateral position
- Client's allergy to ingredients of lotion

Nursing Diagnoses

The nursing diagnoses may include the following:
- Chronic pain related to muscle tension, decreased mobility, or impaired circulation
- Risk of impaired skin integrity related to immobility or decreased circulation
- Anxiety related to fear of the unknown (tests, back rub)

Outcome Identification and Planning

Desired Outcomes

Sample desired outcomes include the following:
- Client expresses feelings of comfort with reduction in pain.
- Client exhibits calm, relaxed facial expression.
- Client verbalizes concerns during back rub.

Special Considerations in Planning and Implementation

General

Use the client's preferred substance for the back rub. Some clients may prefer baby oil or powder rather than lotion. Powder should be used sparingly, to avoid inhalation of powder. Use only light pressure for clients with back disorders; a doctor's order is required for a back rub for these clients.

Pediatric

Using total body massage with gentle conversation may be soothing and calming for a child and may help reduce the stress of hospitalization. Use gentler strokes with infants and young toddlers.

Geriatric

As their skin is drier, use baby oil or oil-based lotion for the skin of elderly clients. The skin of elderly clients is thinner, so avoid vigorous massage.

End-of-Life Care

Offer back rubs more often, when possible and desired. Comfort is a priority in end-of-life care. If opportunity exists, allow more time to do back rub and allow client time to verbalize concerns.

Home Health

Teach the procedure to a family member as a possible method of potentiating the effects of, or decreasing the need for, pain or sleeping medication.

Transcultural

Ascertain the client's desire for a back rub to avoid misunderstanding: some individuals may consider a back rub as gender-sensitive. Individuals from various cultures, especially males, may consider a back rub as an invasion of personal space. Use of various oils/substances on the body may have specific meaning in various cultures. Communicate with client to clarify desire before use.

Cost-Cutting Tip

Teach family members back care techniques and encourage them to perform care.

Delegation

Generally, back care may be delegated to unlicensed assistive personnel. However, the care of clients with back problems or those who need special positioning may require additional instruction or supervision. Instruct assistive personnel to report unusual findings. It is the nurse's responsibility to assess the skin and the effects of back care.

Implementation

Action	Rationale
1. Explain procedure to client.	*Promotes relaxation and compliance*
2. Maintain a quiet, relaxing atmosphere (temperature at a comfortable setting, lighting dim, room neat, noise eliminated, door closed).	*Promotes relaxation*
3. Wash hands and organize equipment.	*Reduces microorganism transfer; promotes efficiency*
4. Warm lotion by running bottle under warm water or placing bottle in a basin of warm water.	*Prevents discomfort and muscle spasms caused by cold lotion and hands*
5. Place client in prone or side-lying position.	*Provides easy access to back while maintaining a comfortable, relaxing position*
6. Drape with sheet or bath blanket.	*Provides warmth and privacy*
7. Wash back with soap and water; rinse and dry thoroughly. Use long, firm strokes.	*Removes dirt and perspiration; stimulates circulation*
8. Pour lotion into hands and rub hands together.	*Distributes lotion evenly*
9. Encourage client to take slow, deep breaths as you begin.	*Facilitates relaxation*
10. Place palms of hands on sacrococcygeal area. Once you have placed your hands on the client's back, don't remove them until you have completed the back rub.	*Facilitates circulation via upward massage* *Provides maximum soothing effect through continuous contact with skin. Effective back rubs have been associated with increased oxygen saturation, so maximum time for effect is important.*
11. Make long, firm strokes up the center of the back,	*Stimulates circulation and release of muscle tension*

Action	Rationale
moving toward shoulders, and back down toward buttocks, covering the lateral areas of the back. Repeat this step several times. It may be helpful to imagine a large heart on the client's back to accomplish this step.	
12. Move hands up the center of the back toward the neck and rub nape of neck with fingers; continue rubbing outward across shoulders.	*Releases tension in neck muscles and promotes relaxation*
13. Move hands down to scapulae and massage in a circular motion over both scapulae for several seconds.	*Stimulates circulation around pressure points*
14. Move hands down to buttocks and massage in a figure-eight motion over the buttocks; continue this step for several seconds (Fig. 4.1).	*Stimulates circulation around pressure points*
15. Lightly rub toward neck and shoulders, then back down toward buttocks for several	*Ends back rub with a calming, therapeutic effect*

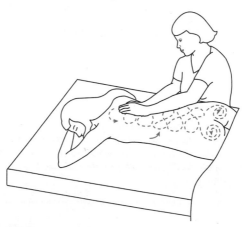

FIGURE 4.1

Action	Rationale
strokes (using lighter pressure and moving laterally with each stroke).	
16. Remove excessive lotion with towel.	*Reduces risk of skin breakdown and bacterial growth from excessive moisture*
17. Reposition client and replace covers.	*Promotes comfort and provides warmth*
18. Raise side rails and place call light within reach.	*Facilitates communication; promotes safety*

Evaluation

Were desired outcomes achieved? Examples of evaluation include:
- Desired outcome met: Client expressed feelings of comfort and reduction in pain.
- Desired outcome met: Client demonstrated a relaxed facial expression following back rub.
- Desired outcome met: Client verbalized concerns during back rub.

Documentation

The following should be noted on the client's chart:
- Client's response to back rub and ability to tolerate procedure
- Condition of skin and bony prominences
- Blood pressure, pulse, and respirations before and after procedure, if applicable
- Any abnormalities or problems encountered

Sample Documentation
Date: 12/3/05
Time: 2200

Back care, including back rub, given; activity tolerated without excessive fatigue, shortness of breath, or changes in vital signs. Client now in lateral recumbent position with call light within reach. Bilateral side rails up. Stated back rub was relaxing.

Preparing a Bed 🧤

Purpose

Promotes comfort
Promotes cleanliness

Equipment

- Bottom sheet (fitted, if available)
- Top sheet (regular sheet)
- Draw sheet (may use second regular sheet)
- Pillowcase for each pillow in the room
- Gloves to remove old linens
- Gown and gloves, if client has draining wound or is in isolation

Assessment

Assessment should focus on the following:
- Doctor's order for activity, impending surgery, or procedure
- Need, if any, for assistance in turning client
- Bladder and bowel continence
- Presence of surgical wound or drains
- Plans for client absence from room for a specified length of time or anticipation of new admission

Nursing Diagnoses

Nursing diagnoses may include the following:
- Disturbed sleep pattern related to excessive diaphoresis
- Sleep deprivation related to sustained environmental stimulation in ICU

Outcome Identification and Planning

Desired Outcomes

Sample desired outcomes include the following:
- Client rested quietly for 3 hours after linen change.
- Client is consistently sleeping 1 hour or more with implemented plan of more frequent linen changes.

Special Considerations in Planning and Implementation

General

Make the bed after the client's bath is completed. Anticipate the need for assistance when turning the client when making an occupied bed. If client has low activity tolerance and is fatigued, plan a rest period after the bath, then get assistance with the bed change to decrease client energy expenditure during the process. Plan more frequent linen changes for clients experiencing excessive perspiration.

Geriatric

Conserve client energy by planning adequate rest periods and obtaining assistance as needed. Ensure linens are secure to avoid wrinkling and subsequent skin indentations and tears because many elderly clients have decreased skin turgor.

End-of-Life Care

Conserve client energy as much as possible. Plan adequate rest periods and obtain assistance as needed. Ensure linens are secure to avoid wrinkling and subsequent skin indentations and tears, because decreased skin turgor is a problem for many clients at this stage.

 Cost-Cutting Tip

If client discharge is anticipated, do not apply fresh linen to bed.

Implementation

Action	Rationale
1. Assist client out of bed (e.g., to a chair).	*Provides easy access to bed for changing*
2. Don gloves, remove old linen, and place linen in pillowcase or linen bag. If bed is soiled or new client is due, spray or wash mattress with germicidal agent. If an egg crate mattress is used, place it on the bed. Remove gloves and wash hands.	*Reduces microorganism transfer*
3. Apply bottom sheet: • Place bottom sheet over mattress as evenly as possible, leaving 1 inch or less hanging over bottom edge.	*Ensures sheet can be tucked in on all sides*
• Tuck sheet at top and miter corners.	*Secures sheet to the bed*
• Move along the side of the bed, tucking the sheets securely and pulling tightly to remove wrinkles	*Ensures snug fit on mattress*

Action	Rationale
• If fitted sheets are supplied, pull each corner of the mattress up slightly and slip it into a corner of the fitted sheet. If necessary, pin the last two corners of the sheet to underside of mattress to keep sheets smooth.	*Secures sheet to bed*
4. Place a draw sheet or pull sheet on bed to assist in repositioning client:	
• Fold full-sized sheet into thirds.	
• Place sheet across bed 2 feet from the top, tucking it in or not, depending on activity level of client, agency policy, or preference (Fig. 4.2).	*Positions sheet under shoulders and hips of client*
5. Apply top sheet:	
• Place the top sheet over the bed with the top edge 2 inches over the top of the mattress.	*Ensures appropriate coverage*
• If blanket is used, place on top of sheet, tuck in and miter bottom corners of both.	*Secures sheet to bed*
• Make small fold or pleat at bottom edge of top linen.	*Provides room for feet*

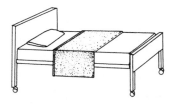

FIGURE 4.2

Action	Rationale
6. Place a clean pillowcase on each pillow in room.	*Completes bed preparation*
7. Assist client to bed and position for comfort or finish bed in appropriate manner for circumstances:	
• For a closed bed: Place pillow on bed with open end facing the wall or place pillow on the bedside table.	*Preserves bed when client is out of room for extended period or when new client is expected*
• For an open bed: Pull top of sheet (and blanket) to head of bed and fanfold both back neatly to bottom third of bed.	*Prepares bed for client when return is expected momentarily*
• For a post-operative bed: Make an open bed but do not tuck top sheet and blanket, leaving top sheet and blanket fanfolded to the side of bed opposite door (Fig. 4.3).	*Facilitates moving client from stretcher to bed without prolonged exposure or draft; prevents interference of client transfer to bed by bed linens and makes covering the client easy*
After client is transferred to bed, pull covers across bed and tuck and miter at bottom.	*Secures linen on bed*
8. Discard or restore linen appropriately and perform hand hygiene.	*Promotes clean environment*

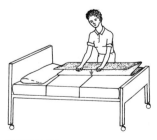

FIGURE 4.3

Evaluation

Were desired outcomes achieved? Examples of evaluation
include:
- Desired outcome met: Client verbalized comfort when linens
  were changed.
- Desired outcome met: Client experienced longer sleep period
  (3 hours) after linen change.

Documentation

The following should be noted on the client's chart:
- Bed linens changed
- Status of client (expected from surgery, discharged, or
  in bed)

Sample Documentation
A bed change is not usually documented in note form.
You may indicate with a brief note on the activity
checklist if the client's tolerance of the procedure is being
monitored.
Date: 12/3/05
Time: 1000

Client out of bed for 15 minutes while linens changed.
Client denied pain or dizziness. Assisted back to bed with
side rails up.

● **Nursing Procedure 4.3**

Providing Hair Care
Purpose

Improves client's appearance and self-esteem
Increases client's sense of well-being
Stimulates circulation to hair and scalp
Aids in relaxing client
Provides opportunity for therapeutic communication

Equipment

Equipment will vary with hairstyle desired:
- Comb (size of teeth varies with coarseness of hair)
- Setting gel and rollers with rolling papers (optional)
- Hair dryer with dome or heat cap (optional)
- Brush
- Hair net (optional)
- Moisturizers, oils (optional)
- Rubber bands, hair pins, clamps (optional)
- Nonsterile gloves

Assessment

Assessment should focus on the following:
- Contraindications to excessive movement and lowering or elevating head (e.g., skull fracture, neck injury)
- Knowledge of procedure for care
- Type of hair care needed or style desired
- Activity level and positions of comfort
- Allergy to ingredients of hair-care products
- Status of hair and scalp (presence of tangles, dandruff, lice, or need for shampoo)

Nursing Diagnoses

The nursing diagnoses may include the following:
- Impaired skin (scalp) integrity related to inadequate or excessive hair oils
- Risk for situational low self-esteem related to inability to perform grooming procedures
- Risk for infection related to scratching of scalp and head-lice infestation

Outcome Identification and Planning

Desired Outcomes

Sample desired outcomes include the following:
- Scalp is warm, with good capillary refill and no irritation.
- Client expresses satisfaction and suggests other self-care activities.
- Hair is clean, without tangles or infestation.

Special Considerations in Planning and Implementation

General

When the client is lying down, braids and knots from rubber bands and hair nets on the back of the head will press against the scalp, so they should be avoided. Check for pressure spots or irritation to the scalp and loosen or release braids in irritated areas.

Pediatric

Bind hair loosely and assess frequently for irritation or discomfort. Children cannot always express the discomfort caused by hair that is too tightly bound or braided.

Geriatric

Use a gentle technique when performing care; avoid tightly binding hair. An elderly client's skin is often thin, dry, and fragile, and the hair is brittle. Assess scalp for irritation frequently.

End-of-Life Care

Good grooming contributes to a sense of well-being and peace. It also portrays to family members a sense of caring.

 ### Transcultural

When in doubt about hair-care practices, ask the client or family members. Clients of different ethnic and cultural origins use different forms of basic hair care. For example, African American clients often add oils or moisturizers; Caucasian clients may shampoo daily or every other day to avoid buildup of hair oils.

 ### Cost-Cutting Tip

Encourage a family member to perform hair care when acceptable to client.

Implementation

Action	Rationale
1. Explain procedure to client.	*Increases cooperation and assistance*
2. Allow 15 to 30 minutes of uninterrupted time for hair care.	*Avoids rushing and possible injury to client*
3. Check and clean comb and brush before beginning (particularly if they are not the client's personal property).	*Prevents passing head lice or infection to client*
4. Perform hand hygiene and organize equipment.	*Reduces microorganism transfer; promotes efficiency*
5. Lower side rail.	*Depending on desired position (see below), allows easier access to client or facilitates moving the client into a chair*

Action	Rationale
6. Assist client into position (depends on the individual needs of the client):	
• Supine, with head of bed elevated and pillows under back	*Allows head to move freely and provides access to hair and towel under head*
• Sitting on a bedside chair, if able, with towel on shoulders	
• Side-lying position, with towel under head	
• Prone position	
7. Don gloves (if broken skin is present) and comb hair through with fingers.	*Prevents body fluid contact; assesses degree of tangling*
8. Massage scalp and observe status. Depress scalp and note for return of color in that area.	*Increases circulation; checks capillary refill*
9. Shampoo and dry hair, as needed and allowed (see Procedure 4.4, Shampooing a Bedridden Client).	*Improves appearance of hair; promotes scalp circulation*
10. Brush hair to remove as many tangles as possible:	
• Hold hair with one hand and brush with the other (Fig. 4.4).	*Decreases discomfort of hair care*
• If hair is coarse and kinky, processed for curls, or naturally curly, use a comb.	*Facilitates removal of tangles*
11. Divide hair into sections with comb and fingers.	*Provides for easier handling*
12. Comb one section through at a time:	
• Gently and slowly comb tangles loose from scalp.	*Removes tangles*
• Hold hair section stable (near the scalp) with one hand. Comb through hair with other hand (as when brushing).	*Prevents pulling during combing and decreases pain to client*

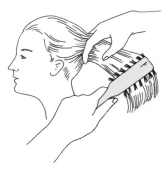

FIGURE 4.4

Action	Rationale
13. Keep hair loose at the scalp.	*Counteracts pulling from comb*
14. Style hair as client wishes.	*Enhances self-esteem*
15. Replace equipment and reposition client.	*Resets environment; allows for client comfort*
16. Remove gloves and perform hand hygiene.	*Reduces transfer of microorganisms*

Evaluation

Were desired outcomes achieved? Examples of evaluation include:
- Desired outcome met: Client requests mirror to observe appearance of hair and suggests other self-care activities.
- Desired outcome partially met: Scalp is cool, with sluggish capillary refill and no irritation.
- Desired outcome met: Hair is clean without tangles.

Documentation

The following should be noted on the client's chart:
- Response to hair care
- Condition of hair and scalp

Sample Documentation
Date: 11/3/04
Time: 1300

Hair combed with assistance of client. Client took active interest in grooming. Makeup applied by client. Scalp warm, without evidence of irritation or breakdown.

● **Nursing Procedure 4.4**

Shampooing a Bedridden Client 🖐

Purpose

Improves appearance and self-esteem
Promotes comfort and relaxation
Stimulates circulation to scalp
Aids in relaxing client

Equipment

- Shampoo
- Washcloth
- Shampoo board (or other assistive device)
- Two towels
- Nonsterile gloves
- Wash basin or plastic-lined trash can
- Water pitcher
- Linen saver or plastic trash bag
- Hair dryer (safety-approved and approved by agency)

Assessment

Assessment should focus on the following:
- Client need or desire for shampoo
- Client's knowledge of procedure of bed shampoo
- Blood pressure and pulse rate and rhythm if there is a history of cardiac or vascular problems
- Neurological status (e.g., increased intracranial pressure or other contraindications to manipulation of head)
- Client's ability to tolerate prone or side-lying position
- Client's allergy to ingredients of shampoo or need for medicated shampoo

Nursing Diagnoses

Nursing diagnoses may include the following:
● Risk for impaired skin integrity related to excessive buildup of hair debris and inadequate circulation at scalp area

Outcome Identification and Planning

Desired Outcomes

Sample desired outcomes include the following:
● Scalp is warm, with brisk capillary refill and no irritation.
● Client verbalizes comfort and expresses satisfaction after hair is washed.

Special Considerations in Planning and Implementation

General

Treat each case individually, because some clients require more frequent shampooing than others. Refer to basic hair-care techniques in Procedure 4.3 for considerations based on ethnic-cultural diversity. Avoid aerosol sprays or powders if client has a respiratory condition or tracheostomy.

Pediatric

Use a shampoo that is less harsh and less irritating to the eyes than regular shampoo. Obtain assistance as needed when shampooing the hair of infants and children to avoid excessive movement and wetting of covers.

Geriatric

Check scalp for irritation before shampooing. In the elderly client, skin is often thin and hair is brittle. Dry hair thoroughly to avoid chilling.

End-of-Life Care

Good grooming contributes to a sense of well-being and peace. It also portrays to family members a sense of caring. Avoid chilling; dry hair thoroughly.

Home Health

Teach proper hair-care techniques to family members for continued care. If client has lice, instruct family on need to treat all family members for lice, as well as need to clean home, linens, and personal items to prevent spread.

Transcultural

Clients of different ethnic and cultural origins require shampooing at different frequencies. For example, African American clients may shampoo every 1 to 2 weeks, while Caucasian clients may shampoo daily or every other day to avoid buildup of hair oils.

Cost-Cutting Tip

Encourage family members to perform hair-care techniques when acceptable to client.

Implementation

Action	Rationale
1. Prepare room environment (warm temperature, free of drafts).	*Avoids discomfort from chills*
2. Obtain doctor's orders for medicated shampoo, if needed.	*Provides scalp treatment*
3. Explain procedure to client and family members.	*Facilitates cooperation*
4. Wash hands and organize equipment.	*Reduces microorganism transfer; promotes efficiency*
5. Remove pillow from under client's head.	*Prevents soiling of pillow*
6. Place linen saver or plastic bag under shoulders and head of client.	*Avoids wetting of linens*
7. Place towel on top of linen saver.	*Absorbs water overflow*
8. Place shampoo board under client's neck and head.	*Facilitates drainage of water*
9. Position wash basin or trash can in direct line with spout of shampoo board.	*Provides reservoir for water*
10. Fill the pitcher with warm water (105°F to 110°F [40.5°C to 43.3°C]); check with thermometer or test for comfortable temperature with your inner wrist.	*Promotes scalp circulation; prevents chilling or skin injury from excess heat*
11. Ask client to hold washcloth over eyes during procedure.	*Prevents pain from shampoo in eyes*
12. Lower head of bed (infants may be held in your lap, with shampoo board under head); place supplies and sufficient water within easy reach.	*Facilitates downward flow of water; prevents delays in procedure*
13. Pour warm water over hair and moisten thoroughly (Fig. 4.5).	*Facilitates action of shampoo*

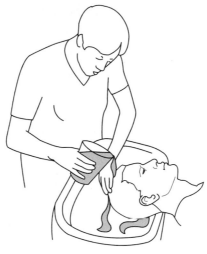

FIGURE 4.5

Action	Rationale
14. Don gloves and place small amount of shampoo in palms; massage shampoo into hair at front and back of head, working shampoo into a lather.	*Provides lather for removal of dirt and oils*
15. Massage lather over entire head in a slow, kneading motion.	*Cleans hair and scalp; promotes scalp circulation*
16. Rinse hair by pouring warm water over head several times.	*Removes shampoo and debris*
17. Repeat application of shampoo and massage hair and scalp vigorously with fingers for a longer period of time.	*Promotes thorough cleaning of hair and scalp*
18. Rinse thoroughly using several pitchers of water.	*Removes residue of shampoo*
19. If desired, apply a detangling conditioner to hair and leave on for 3 to 5 minutes per package instructions, then rinse thoroughly.	*Facilitates untangling*

Action	Rationale
20. Support client's head with your hand and remove shampoo board from bed.	*Prevents inadvertent injury; clears area for completion of procedure*
21. Position the client's head on the towel and cover head with it.	*Absorbs water from hair*
22. Briskly massage hair with towel.	*Removes water*
23. Replace wet towel with dry one and continue to rub hair.	*Promotes drying of hair*
24. Leave hair covered with towel until ready to use dryer.	*Provides for continued absorption of moisture; prevents chilling*
25. Thoroughly dry hands and/or replace gloves.	*Promotes safety in next steps*
26. Elevate head of bed to desired or prescribed angle.	*Promotes access to hair*
27. Turn on dryer to warm setting; feel heat to be sure it is not excessive.	*Prevents injury from dryer heat*
28. Blow hair until thoroughly dry; concentrate on one section of hair at a time, moving fingers or comb through hair while drying.	*Facilitates thorough drying of hair; removes tangles and ensures drying of all parts of hair*
29. Brush or comb hair.	*Removes tangles*
30. Oil or spray hair, as desired, and style.	*Facilitates styling*
31. Remove linen saver, linens, and other equipment from bedside.	*Provides clean environment*
32. Assist client to position of comfort, with side rails raised and call light within reach.	*Promotes safety; facilitates communication*
33. Remove gloves and perform hand hygiene.	*Reduces transmission of microorganisms*

Evaluation

Were desired outcomes achieved? Examples of evaluation include:

- Desired outcome met: Client verbalizes increased comfort after shampoo.
- Desired outcome met: Scalp is warm, with brisk capillary refill and no irritation.

Documentation

The following should be noted on the client's chart:
- When shampoo was done and if completed
- Client's response to activity
- Condition of hair and scalp
- Blood pressure, pulse, and neurological status before and after procedure, if applicable

Sample Documentation
Date: 1/3/05
Time: 0900

Shampoo performed in bed. Client tolerated supine position and procedure without distress. No scalp irritation noted. Client resting quietly, lying on left side with side rails up.

● **Nursing Procedure 4.5**

Providing Oral Care: Brushing and Flossing 🧤

Purpose

Decreases microorganisms in mouth and on teeth
Reduces the risk of cavities and mouth disease
Decreases buildup of food residue on teeth
Improves appetite and taste of food
Promotes comfort
Stimulates circulation to oral tissues, tongue, and gums
Improves appearance and self-esteem

Equipment

- Soft toothbrush
- Toothpaste
- Toothettes or swabs
- Emesis basin
- Nonsterile gloves
- Towel or linen saver and washcloth
- Cup of water
- Mouthwash (alcohol-free)
- Dental floss (optional)
- Suction and catheter (if client is unconscious)

Assessment

Assessment should focus on the following:
- Client's desire and need for oral care
- Client's usual routine for oral hygiene (method, frequency)
- Client's knowledge of purpose and procedure
- Client's ability to understand and follow instructions (e.g., to expectorate instead of swallowing mouthwash and toothpaste)
- Presence of dentures
- Status of palate, floor of mouth, throat, cheeks, tongue, gums, and teeth (e.g., presence of lesions, cavities)

Nursing Diagnoses

The nursing diagnoses may include the following:
- Impaired oral mucous membranes related to inadequate oral cleaning
- Impaired dentition related to lack of knowledge regarding dental health

Outcome Identification and Planning

Desired Outcomes

Sample desired outcomes include the following:
- Oral intake increased from 10% to 50%.
- Mucous membranes and lips are intact.
- Oral passage and teeth are clean.

Special Considerations in Planning and Implementation

General

Use a soft toothbrush or Toothette for client receiving anticoagulation therapy. Dilute mouthwash for clients with oral lesions or sensitive oral tissues.

Geriatric

Use extra care when performing oral care for elderly clients because they often have problems with loose teeth due to retracting gums. Good oral care may promote appetite.

End-of-Life Care

Pay special attention to the mouth and mucous membranes in clients who are mouth breathers to ensure that mucous membranes remain moist. Good grooming contributes to a sense of well-being and peace. It also portrays to family members a sense of caring.

 Cost-Cutting Tip

Encourage client to perform as much oral care as possible and encourage family members to assist, when necessary.

Implementation

Action	Rationale
1. Perform hand hygiene and organize equipment.	*Reduces microorganism transfer; promotes efficiency*
2. Explain procedure to client.	*Reduces anxiety; promotes compliance*
3. Lower side rail and position client in one of the following positions: supine at an angle greater than 45 degrees (if not contraindicated), side-lying position, or prone with head turned to side.	*Decreases risk of aspiration; promotes drainage of mouthwash from mouth*
4. Don gloves.	*Prevents exposure to body fluids*
5. Drape towel under client's neck and assist client to rinse mouth with water.	*Prevents secretions from wetting or soiling bedclothes; facilitates removal of secretions*

If Client Can Perform Self-Care

6. Assist the client in brushing teeth:	
• Provide a glass of water, toothbrush, and toothpaste.	*Gives client necessary equipment*
• Moisten the toothbrush with water and apply toothpaste to brush.	
• Allow client to brush teeth, and instruct on proper technique.	*Promotes self-care*
7. Assist the client in cleansing the oral cavity:	
• Provide mouthwash-soaked Toothette, or apply as appropriate.	*Freshens mouth*
• Encourage client to swab inner cheeks, lips, tongue, and gums, or perform these actions for client, if needed.	*Decreases microorganism growth in mouth*
• Instruct client to rinse with mouthwash and expectorate.	*Freshens mouth*
• Instruct client to rinse and expectorate any excess water.	*Removes residue*

Action	Rationale
If Client Cannot Perform Own Care	
6. Perform oral care on the client:	
• Prepare toothbrush as above.	
• Apply brush to back teeth and brush inside, top, and outside of teeth. Brush from back to front, using an up-and-down motion (Fig. 4.6). Repeat these steps, brushing teeth on opposite side of mouth.	*Permits cleaning back and sides of teeth*
• Allow client to expectorate or suction excess secretions.	*Removes toothpaste and oral secretions*
• Instruct client to clench teeth together, or grasp the mandible and brush outside of front lower teeth to upper teeth; brush the outside of the front and side teeth.	*Exposes front teeth for brushing*
• Open mouth and brush top and insides of teeth.	
• Rinse toothbrush and brush tongue.	*Decreases microorganisms living in the mouth*
• Rinse toothbrush and brush teeth again.	*Removes residual toothpaste*
• If use of dental floss is desired, provide care at this time.	*Cleans between teeth*
7. Cleanse the oral cavity:	
• Swab inner cheeks, lips, tongue, and gums.	*Decreases microorganism growth in mouth*

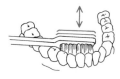 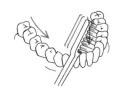

FIGURE 4.6

Action	Rationale
• Irrigate mouth with mouthwash and suction excess fluid.	*Freshens oral cavity*
• Rinse with water and suction excess.	*Removes residue*

If Client Is Unconscious
6. Provide oral care:

• Brush teeth with toothbrush and toothpaste as described above in step 6 in providing care for clients who can't provide their own care.	*Cleans teeth*
• Irrigate mouth with small amounts of water, suctioning constantly.	*Removes water and avoids pooling*

7. Cleanse the oral cavity:

• Swab mouth with Toothette moistened with mouthwash. Begin with inside of cheeks and lips; proceed to swab tongue and gums.	*Decreases microorganism growth in mouth*
• Rinse and suction excess toothpaste, mouthwash, water, and secretions.	
• Wipe lips with wet washcloth.	*Removes any residue*
• Apply petroleum jelly or mineral oil to lips.	*Moisturizes lips*
8. Discard soiled materials; restore supplies in proper place.	*Promotes clean environment*
9. Remove gloves and perform hand hygiene.	*Reduces transfer of microorganisms*
10. Position client for comfort with call button within reach.	*Promotes safety, comfort, and communication*

Evaluation

Were desired outcomes achieved? Examples of evaluation include:
- Desired outcome met: Oral intake increased from 10% to 50%.
- Desired outcome met: Mucous membranes and lips are intact.
- Desired outcome met: Oral passage and teeth are clean.

Documentation

The following should be noted on the client's chart:
- Amount of care done by client
- Client's response to activity
- Condition of oral cavity and lips

Sample Documentation
Date: 8/3/05
Time: 1000

Oral care performed with client assistance. Client fatigued after brushing back teeth but expressed interest in grooming activity. Makeup applied by client after rest period. Mucous membranes moist. Lips moist; skin intact.

● **Nursing Procedure 4.6**

Performing Denture Care

Purpose

Decreases microorganisms in mouth and on dentures
Decreases buildup of food residue on teeth or dentures
Improves appetite and taste of food
Promotes comfort
Stimulates circulation to oral tissues, tongue, and gums
Improves appearance and self-esteem

Equipment

- Denture brush
- Denture cream
- Denture cup
- Denture cleanser
- Emesis basin
- Nonsterile gloves
- Towel or linen saver and washcloth
- Cup of warm water

Assessment

Assessment should focus on the following:
- Client's desire and need for oral care

- Client's usual routine for oral hygiene and denture care (method, frequency)
- Client's knowledge of purpose and procedure
- Client's ability to understand and follow instructions
- Status of palate, floor of mouth, throat, cheeks, tongue, gums (e.g., presence of lesions)

Nursing Diagnoses

The nursing diagnoses may include the following:
- Impaired oral mucous membranes related to inadequate denture cleaning
- Hygiene self-care deficit related to lack of motivation

Outcome Identification and Planning

Desired Outcomes

Sample desired outcomes include the following:
- Mucous membranes and lips are intact.
- Oral passage and dentures are clean.
- Client expresses satisfaction with oral care and desire to maintain clean dentures.

Special Considerations in Planning and Implementation

Geriatric

Elderly clients often wear dentures. Assess their mouth for irritation from poorly fitting dentures.

 Cost-Cutting Tip

Encourage client to perform as much oral care as possible and encourage family members to assist, when necessary.

Implementation

Action	Rationale
1. Perform hand hygiene and organize supplies.	*Reduces microorganism transfer; promotes efficiency*
2. Explain procedure to client and encourage participation, if able.	*Promotes compliance*
3. Don gloves.	*Prevents contact with body secretions*
4. Assist client with denture removal: • Fill denture cup halfway with cool	*Prepares cleansing solution*

Action	Rationale
water and add denture cleanser to the water per manufacturer's instructions.	
• Give the client a glass of water. Instruct the client to take a sip. Ask the client to hold water in mouth and "float" dentures loose.	*Prevents dentures from breaking during removal*
• Allow client to remove dentures, or gently rock dentures back and forth until they are free from gums.	*Breaks seal created with dentures*
• To remove, lift bottom dentures up and pull top dentures down.	*Prevents undue pressure and injury to oral membranes*
• Place dentures in denture cup to soak. (If a denture cup is unavailable, use emesis basin or other receptacle and label clearly.)	*Facilitates removal of microorganisms*
5. Assist client with cleansing of oral cavity:	
• Provide a mouthwash-soaked Toothette.	*Freshens mouth*
• Encourage client to swab inner cheeks, lips, tongue, and gums.	*Decreases microorganism growth in mouth*
• Instruct client to swirl mouthwash in mouth and expectorate. Follow with water, as desired.	*Removes any residue*
6. Cleanse dentures:	
• Apply denture cleaner and brush using the technique described in Procedure 4.5.	*Facilitates removal of microorganisms*
• Thoroughly rinse paste from dentures with cool water.	*Removes cleaner and debris*
7. Reinsert dentures:	
• Apply denture cream to gum side of denture plate.	*Facilitates adherence*

Action	Rationale
• Insert upper plate and press firmly to gums. Repeat with lower plate.	*Adheres dentures to the gums*
8. Apply petroleum jelly or mineral oil to client's lips.	*Maintains skin integrity of lips*
9. Remove towel from client's chest. Discard soiled materials.	*Maintains clean environment*
10. Remove gloves and perform hand hygiene.	*Prevents transmission of microorganisms*
11. Position client for comfort, with side rails raised and call light within reach.	*Promotes comfort, safety, and communication*
12. Place personal hygiene items in client's drawer or on bedside table.	*Provides an orderly environment*

Evaluation

Were desired outcomes achieved? Examples of evaluation include:
- Desired outcome met: Mucous membranes and lips are intact.
- Desired outcome met: Oral passage and dentures are clean.
- Desired outcome met: Client demonstrates satisfaction and understanding of the need for good oral care.

Documentation

The following should be noted on the client's chart:
- Amount of care done by client
- Client's response to activity
- Condition of oral cavity and lips

Sample Documentation
Date: 9/30/04
Time: 1000

Denture care performed with client assistance. Client expressed interest in grooming activity. Mucous membranes moist. Lips moist; skin intact.

Caring for Contact Lenses and Artificial Eyes 🧤

Purpose

Contact lenses: prevents corneal damage
Artificial eyes: prevents damage to tissue

Equipment

- Container for lenses or prosthesis
- Saline solution
- Clean gloves

Assessment

Assessment should focus on the following:
- Client's or family's ability to understand and perform procedure
- For contact lenses: type of contact lenses and measures normally used by client for lens cleaning
- For artificial eye: care measures normally used by client for cleaning

Nursing Diagnoses

The nursing diagnoses may include the following:
- Impaired tissue integrity related to chemical irritants from medications
- Risk for injury related to excessive length of time wearing contact lenses
- Risk for infection related to knowledge deficit regarding proper care techniques for artificial eye

Outcome Identification and Planning

Desired Outcomes

Sample desired outcomes include the following:
- Client exhibits intact mucous membranes and tissues of eye and socket.
- Client/caregiver demonstrates ability to perform procedure and verbalizes importance of removing contact lenses on regular schedule.
- Client/caregiver demonstrates ability to perform procedure and verbalizes importance of artificial eye care.

Special Considerations in Planning and Implementation

General

If possible, have the client perform the procedure per his or her routine. If needed, offer suggestions on how to improve techniques.

End-of-Life Care

Contacts won't be worn by a client in the last stages of life; however, for general eye care, apply moisture with saline to conjunctiva and mucous membranes as needed to avoid drying out when needed as a palliative measure.

Home Health

If the client and/or family cannot remove a prosthesis or contact lens and the nurse has any doubt about his or her ability to perform the procedure, arrange a rapid referral to an ophthalmologist. Removing contact lenses or a prosthesis can be a difficult procedure for the nurse to perform in the home setting because of the lack of necessary resources.

Implementation

Action	Rationale
1. Assemble and organize supplies.	*Promotes efficiency*
2. Teach, perform, or observe good handwashing.	*Reduces microorganism transfer*
3. Discuss procedure with client and encourage participation, if able, and assist as client requires or desires.	*Promotes compliance*
4. If performing procedure, don gloves.	*Prevents contact with bodily fluids*
5. Position client in recumbent position; stand on right side to remove right contact lens or prosthesis. Stand on the left side to remove left contact lens or prosthesis.	*Improves access to eye*
6. Position left thumb on upper eyelid, right thumb on lower eyelid, and gently pull apart. (Reverse position of thumbs if removing a left lens or prosthesis.) NOTE: If lens is visible, proceed. If lens cannot be seen,	*Improves visualization* *Prevents probing and possible damage to the eye*

Action	Rationale
arrange for an ophthal-mologist to see the client.	
7. For hard lens or prosthesis:	
• Gently open the eye beyond the edges of the lens or prosthesis by pulling lids apart. Apply gentle pressure on the eyeball by press-ing down on the upper lid with the right thumb.	*Releases the suction holding the lens or prosthesis in place*
• Gently slide the lens or prosthesis out.	*Removes lens or prosthesis, facili-tating cleaning*
For soft lens:	
• Once lens is seen, gently pinch between thumb and forefinger and remove.	*Removes lens, facilitating cleaning*
8. Inspect the eye tissues for any damage.	*Identifies need for follow-up care*
9. Place lenses or prosthesis in appropriate container and perform cleaning.	*Reduces transmission of micro-organisms; maintains clean lenses or prosthesis*
10. If necessary, repeat steps for opposite eye.	
11. Replace prosthesis or lenses, if needed or desired.	
12. Dispose of soiled gloves appropriately; perform hand hygiene.	*Prevents spread of micro-organisms*

Evaluation

Were desired outcomes achieved? Examples of evaluation include:
- Desired outcome met: Client exhibited moist, intact mucous membranes and tissues of eye and socket.
- Desired outcome met: Client/caregiver demonstrated proce-dure and verbalized importance of removing lenses on a reg-ular schedule.
- Desired outcome partially met: Client failed to demonstrate proper artificial eye care, but he verbalized the importance of proper care.

Documentation

The following should be noted on the client's chart:
- Condition of eye and surrounding tissue
- Ability of client or caregiver to perform procedure properly
- Teaching performed regarding general care of artificial eye or contact lenses

Sample Documentation
Date: 9/6/04
Time: 1100

Left eye prosthesis removed. Eye socket cleaned per
physician's order and prosthesis replaced. Client
instructed on procedure, including handwashing before
and after procedure, cleaning of eye socket, storage and
cleaning of prosthesis. Verbalized understanding of
procedure.

● **Nursing Procedure 4.8**

Shaving a Client 🖐

Purpose

Improves client's appearance and self-esteem
Increases client's sense of well-being

Equipment

- Towel
- Shaving cream or soap
  as desired by client
- Disposable gloves
- 2 washcloths
- Small basin of warm water
- Appropriate razor with
  fresh, clean blade
- Aftershave lotion, if desired

Assessment

Assessment should focus on the following:
- Condition of skin (nicks, bruises, thin and fragile)
- Contraindications to shaving
- Type of razor or shaver to be used
- Use of anticoagulants
- Knowledge of procedure for care

Nursing Diagnoses

The nursing diagnoses may include the following:
- Grooming self-care deficit related to neuromuscular
  impairment
- Risk for injury, bleeding, related to use of anticoagulant

Outcome Identification and Planning

Desired Outcomes

Sample desired outcomes include the following:
● Client expresses satisfaction with grooming.
● Client demonstrates a face that is clean and shaved without any evidence of cuts or bruises.

Special Considerations in Planning and Implementation

General

If the client is taking an anticoagulant, check the agency's policy about the need to obtain a special doctor's order prior to shaving. When assessing drug profile, note drugs that contain aspirin or drugs that are not classified as anticoagulants but may cause bleeding. Obtain doctor's order or note agency's policy concerning shaving these clients.

Pediatric

If shaving is ordered before a procedure, maintain control of razor and child to avoid accidental cutting.

Geriatric

Be gentle when shaving. Shave only as often as necessary. The elderly client's skin is often thin, dry, and fragile, and the hair is brittle.

End-of-Life Care

Include shaving as part of a client's grooming as indicated. Doing so contributes to a sense of well-being and peace. It also portrays to family members a sense of caring.

Transcultural

When in doubt about a client's shaving practices, consult the client or a family member. For shaving not related to preparation for a procedure, clients of different ethnic and cultural origins may have objections to shaving of hair, as this may be the cultural norm.

🖘 Cost-Cutting Tip

Encourage a family member to perform shaving when acceptable to client.

Implementation

Action	Rationale
1. Explain procedure to client.	*Increases cooperation and assistance*

Action	Rationale
2. Allow 5 to 10 minutes of uninterrupted time for shaving.	*Avoids rushing and possible injury to client*
3. Perform hand hygiene and organize equipment.	*Reduces microorganism transfer; promotes efficiency*
4. Lower side rail.	*Allows easier access to client*
5. Assist client into position: supine position, with head of bed elevated or semi-Fowler's (for facial shave).	*Provides access to shaving area*
6. Don gloves.	*Prevents contact with body fluids*
7. Place towel across chest.	*Prevents client from getting wet*
8. Moisten face with warm, damp washcloth.	*Softens area to avoid cuts*
9. Apply generous amount of shaving cream or lathered soap.	*Softens area to avoid cuts and facilitates movement of razor*
10. Pull the skin taut.	*Eliminates excessive skin folding to avoid cutting client*
11. Shave in direction of hair growth, using short, smooth strokes.	*Follows natural hair direction to avoid nicks, cuts, or bruises; avoids irritation*
12. For manual disposable razors, dip razor into water periodically and shake off excess water.	*Removes hair debris and excessive cream or soap to facilitate smooth strokes*
13. Allow client to rinse face or use washcloth to clean area.	*Removes cream or soap and debris*
14. Pat area dry and apply aftershave lotion as desired.	*Provides comfort and reduces the risk of skin irritation from rubbing*
15. Reposition client and raise side rails.	*Provides for comfort and safety*
16. Discard equipment appropriately, remove gloves, and perform hand hygiene.	*Avoids spread of microorganisms*

Evaluation

Were desired outcomes achieved? Examples of evaluation include:
- Desired outcome met: Client demonstrates clean, shaved face without any cuts or bruises.
- Desired outcome met: Client expresses comfort after procedure.

Documentation

The following should be noted on the client's chart:
- Type of razor used
- Response to shave
- Condition of skin
- Nicks or bruises present
- Lotion or aftershave applied

Sample Documentation
Date: 12/31/04
Time: 1000

Face shaved using electric razor with doctor's order, as client is taking Coumadin. No bruising or cuts noted. Client verbalized comfort after procedure.

Medication Administration

OVERVIEW

- Medication administration is one of the most frequently performed nursing procedures.
- Precision is essential in administering medication to ensure the maximum therapeutic effectiveness of the medication. Under- or overdosage, inappropriate administration techniques, or inaccurate client identification can lead to numerous complications, including death.
- To administer drugs safely, the nurse must make decisions about altering technique based on the age, developmental stage, weight, physiologic status, mental status, educational level, and past physical history of the client.

- Legal liability remains a major concern in medication administration; however, using a few basic guidelines can significantly decrease the nurse's risk of involvement in a lawsuit:
  - Know the medication being administered.
  - Know the correct technique for administration.
  - Know client-related factors that might affect administration methodology (see above).
  - Know the agency policy on administering drugs by any technique.
  - Know the client's rights in relation to medication administration.
  - REMEMBER THE FIVE RIGHTS OF MEDICATION ADMINISTRATION EACH TIME DRUGS ARE ADMINISTERED: THE RIGHT CLIENT, DRUG, ROUTE, TIME, AND AMOUNT.
  - Document administration immediately after giving medication.
  - Always ask if you are unsure about any aspect of drug therapy or administration.
- Medications given by the oral route usually are the least expensive, but the oral route is the least dependable route of administration.
- Generally, medications given by parenteral routes act faster and have more reliable results than drugs given by other routes. Because errors in parenteral medication can quickly become debilitating or lethal, USE EXTREME CAUTION!
- Although exposure to blood is often minimal during parenteral medication injection, the use of gloves is recommended.
- Administration of parenteral medications may require manipulation of needles, placing the nurse at risk for a needlestick injury. When available, the nurse should use a needleless methodology and equipment for medication administration.
- Before administering ordered medication, check for use of complementary and alternative therapies such as herbal remedies and over-the-counter medications to decrease the risk of possible drug interactions.
- The nursing diagnostic labels applicable to medication administration vary greatly with type of drug and route. However, some of the more common diagnoses include acute pain, chronic pain, knowledge deficit, and anxiety.
- If nausea or pain medication has been ordered in multiple forms (oral, parenteral, or rectal), determine the client's preference before preparing the medication.
- As a basic standard of care, medication preparation, teaching, and administration are done by a licensed registered or vocational nurse. Some drugs may be given by registered nurses only. Policies vary by agency and state. BE SURE TO NOTE SPECIFIC AGENCY POLICIES FOR A GIVEN ROUTE AND DRUG BEFORE DELEGATING ADMINISTRATION!

Using Principles of Medication Administration

Purpose

Avoids client injury due to drug errors
Ensures adherence to basic safety factors of drug administration
  in preparing and administering medications

Equipment

- Physician's order
- Medication administration record, medication scanner, or
  computerized medication record
- Pen
- Disposable gloves
- Medication to be administered
- Drug reference book
- Medicine tray or medication cart

Optional Equipment (depending on route of administration)

- Syringes with
  appropriate-size needles
- Alcohol swabs
- Medication cups
- Cup of water
- Drinking straw
- Medication labels
- Calculator
- Lubricant
- Medicine dropper
- Needleless system
  equipment (e.g., access
  pins, caps)

Assessment

Assessment should focus on the following:
- Clarity and legibility of physician's order
- Age and weight of client
- Lighting in medication preparation area

Nursing Diagnoses

Nursing diagnoses may include the following:
- Acute pain related to back injury
- Risk for injury related to adverse effects of drug therapy
- Deficient knowledge related to lack of exposure to information
  about prescribed medication therapy
- Deficient knowledge related to lack of exposure to informa-
  tion about prescribed medication therapy
- Deficient knowledge related to lack of exposure to informa-
  tion about prescribed medication therapy

Outcome Identification and Planning

Desired Outcomes

Sample desired outcomes include the following:
- Client remains free of injury associated with medication therapy, receiving the correct drug and dosage at the correct time.
- Client verbalizes correct information about medication therapy and dosing procedure.

Special Considerations in Planning and Implementation

General

Consult a drug reference manual or pharmacist for information on drugs with which you are unfamiliar. Instruct client and family to monitor for side effects and possible reactions to medications.

Pediatric

Infants and children often require very small doses of medications. Using a syringe instead of a medication cup provides the most accurate measurement of liquid medications.

Home Health

See Display 5.1 for home health considerations.

Delegation

As a general standard, *only* licensed nurses may administer medications. In most agencies, drugs administered by intravenous (IV) route may be administered only by registered nurses. POLICIES VARY BY AGENCY AND STATE, HOWEVER. BE SURE TO CONSULT SPECIFIC AGENCY POLICIES FOR DELEGATION OF DRUG ADMINISTRATION FOR A GIVEN ROUTE OR DRUG. Registered nurses generally administer IV push medications and medications given through central line catheters and PICC lines. IV sedation drugs are given by registered nurses. In many facilities, selected IV piggyback medications and peripheral IV saline flush solutions may be given by licensed vocational nurses. BE SURE TO CHECK AGENCY POLICY BEFORE DELEGATING *ANY* DRUG ADMINISTRATION TO OTHER PERSONNEL!

Implementation

Action	Rationale
1. Perform hand hygiene.	*Reduces microorganism transfer*
2. Gather equipment and unlock medication cart or cabinet.	*Promotes efficiency*

> ● **Display 5.1** Principles of Management, Storage, and Disposal of Medications in the Home Setting

- Administer medications only to the client admitted to the home-health service (i.e., not to a spouse or relative).
- Administer only those drugs prescribed by the attending physician.
- Prepare a written schedule of medications that is developed based on client's schedule of activities and sleeping patterns.
- Post a schedule on the refrigerator to help remind the client of medication administration times.
- For clients at home who have problems with memory, use devices that remind them when drugs must be taken (e.g., calendars, daily pill dispensers).
- Try taping single pills to a piece of cardboard (out of reach of children) to help increase client recognition and understanding of each medication and its appropriate administration.
- Use a color code or notation on each pill bottle to help with recognition. A 7-day pill administration box may be helpful.
- If working with a client to use a medication box that is set up once a week, ensure that a family member or caregiver is available who can continue to set up the medication box after the client has been discharged from nursing services (this may be necessary to meet requirements of some insurance companies for coverage).
- Review the schedule of administration on each visit and with each change in medication.
- Instruct clients to store medications in original labeled containers, with containers for current medications grouped close together.
- Highlight the number of refills on a prescription bottle with a marker to assist the client in timely reordering of medications.
- If refrigeration is needed, store medications away from food items in an area of limited access.
- Teach how to determine expiration dates.
- Instruct to flush old pills down toilet and discard bottle.

Action	Rationale
3. Compare medication administration record to physician's order, adhering to the five rights of drug administration; use these	*Promotes safety; avoids client injury related to wrong dose, drug, route, time, or client*

Action	Rationale
principles throughout preparation and administration. Check for the right: • *Client*—includes checking name, identification number, room number, prescribing physician's name on the order, medication administration record, and client identification band • *Drug*—includes ascertaining that generic names are compatible with brand names (if both are used) and that client has no allergies to ingredients of ordered medications; includes checking drug labels with medication administration record or electronic medication record • *Dosage*—includes determining that dosage ordered is within usual dosage range for route of administration, weight, and age of client; checking dosages on drug labels for compatibility with dosages written on medication administration record or electronic medication record; and performing accurate dose calculations • *Time*—includes checking that medication administration frequency (e.g., "every 12 hours" [q12h] or "three times a day" [tid]) is compatible with times (e.g., 6 AM and 6 PM or 10 AM, 2 PM, and 6 PM) listed on medication administration record or electronic medication record	

Action	Rationale
• *Route*—includes checking drug label to ascertain if medication can be administered by ordered route and checking that route recorded on medication administration record or electronic medication record corresponds to the physician's order	
4. Notify physician if client has allergy to any ordered medication.	*Prevents client injury resulting from allergic reactions*
5. Focusing on one medication at a time, begin label checks by comparing the actual drug labels to the order, as transcribed on the medication administration record; if using a medication administration record, begin at the top and systematically move down the page; if using computer or scanner, scan or focus on one drug at a time.	*Promotes systematic preparation; prevents error in preparation by adhering to the five rights of medication administration*
6. Compare drug labels with the orders on the medication administration record or computer and determine if dosage calculations are necessary.	*Verifies correct medication; ensures preparation of correct dose*
7. Perform calculations using one of the following formulas in Display 5.2. IF YOU ARE UNCERTAIN OF THE ACCURACY OF YOUR CALCULATIONS, CHECK WITH ANOTHER NURSE.	*Provides safety check*
8. Check label on each medication: • Before removing drug from drawer or storage area • Before pouring or drawing up medication	*Prevents administration of wrong drug to client or administration of drug to wrong client*

● **Display 5.2** Methods of Dosage Calculation

Desired dosage (D) is the dosage ordered

Available dosage (H) equals the dosage on hand (e.g., the number of milligrams or the number of milliequivalents) or *available volume* (H) is the amount of solution or number of tablets containing the drug (e.g., mL, minims, tablets) on hand

Vehicle (V) is the drug form (number of tablets or amount of solution containing the available dosage)

Amount (A) is the volume/amount of the drug to be administered (e.g., number of mL, minims, tablets)

Method 1: Basic Equation

$$\frac{D}{H} \times V = A$$

Example
The physician's order (D) is 400 mg. The available dosage (H) is 200 mg available in the vehicle (V) of one tablet.

$$\frac{400}{200} \times 1 \text{ tablet} = A$$

2×1 tablet = A

A = 2 tablets

Method 2: Ratio and Proportion

H:V :: D:A

Example
The physician's order (D) is 400 mg. The available dosage (H) is 200 mg available in the vehicle (V) of one tablet.

200:1 :: 400:A

$$\frac{200}{1} = \frac{400}{A}$$

Cross multiply to find A:

$200 \text{ A} = 400 \times 1$

$$A = \frac{400}{200}$$

A = 2 tablets

Action	Rationale
(or once medication is in hand, if unit dose) • Before replacing multiple-dose containers on shelf (or before removing your hands from the drug once it is on the medicine tray, if unit dose)	
9. Recheck medication administration record for appropriate client identification or scan client's arm band as scanner system requires.	*Ensures that nurse is focusing on right client record*
10. Using aseptic technique, pour or draw up each medication after second label check (Fig. 5.1); use guidelines in Table 5.1 when preparing drugs for various routes of administration.	*Reduces risk of contamination; ensures accurate measurement of drug*
11. Place each drug on medication tray after checking label a third time and before proceeding to prepare the next drug. If using scanner system to give medications at bedside, administer medication after scanning drug and client.	*Provides third label check*
12. Recheck medication record or computer with each drug on tray.	*Provides safety check*
13. Place all administration equipment on tray.	*Ensures organization of proper equipment for administration*
14. Lock medication cart or cabinet.	*Adheres to institution accreditation guidelines*

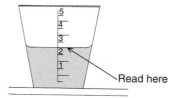

Read here

FIGURE 5.1

● **Table 5.1** Guidelines for Preparing Various Forms of Medication

Guideline	Rationale
1. Most agencies require that certain medications (such as heparin, insulin, IV digoxin) be checked by a second nurse during preparation. Check agency policy and procedure manuals for the full listing of these drugs.	Prevents error in preparation of drugs with potentially lethal effects
2. Do not open unit-dose packages in advance if dosages are exact (i.e., pills, oral liquids, and suppositories). Open just before administering.	Provides identifying drug information Prevents waste
3. When preparing topical, nasal, ophthalmic, and other boxed medications, remove medication from box and check labels of actual containers.	Prevents administration of wrong drug
4. If pouring pills from multiple-dose containers, pour pill into cap and then into medicine cup. Pour liquids with label facing palm of hand. Read amount of medication poured in medicine cups at bottom of meniscus (see Fig. 5.1).	Maintains asepsis Prevents destruction of label Measures liquid drug correctly
5. Separate drugs requiring preassessment data, such as vital signs.	Prevents administration before vital sign assessment
6. When preparing any drug, check for expiration date.	Eliminates administering drugs that no longer have full therapeutic effect

Evaluation

Were desired outcomes achieved? Examples of evaluation include:
● Desired outcome met: Client remains free of injury associated with medication therapy, receiving the correct drug and dosage at the correct time.
● Desired outcome met: Client accurately stated purpose of medication and dosing regimen for self-administration.

Documentation

The following should be noted on the client's chart:
● Medication ordered
● The right client and the right drug, route, time, and amount of medication

- Any reaction to medication
- Client's tolerance to medication
- Any complaints of pain or discomfort

Sample Documentation
Date: 2/17/05
Time: 2100

Doctor's order noted for initiation of new antibiotic. Client received 1 Bactrim DS via intravenous infusion over 30 minutes at 8 a.m. as ordered. Client demonstrated no reaction on initiation or during infusion, or after completion of infusion. No complaint of pain or discomfort verbalized.

Nursing Procedure 5.2

Administering Eye (Ophthalmic) Drops

Purpose

Instills medications in mucous membranes of eye for various therapeutic effects, such as decreasing inflammatory and infectious processes and preventing drying of cornea, conjunctiva, and other delicate eye structures

Equipment

- Two to six cotton balls, one to three per eye (some agencies recommend use of sterile cotton balls)
- Disposable gloves
- Medication record or electronic medication record
- Pen
- Medication to be administered

Assessment

Assessment should focus on the following:
- Evidence of lesions, redness, or drainage in structures of eye (sclera, cornea, conjunctival sacs, eyelids)

- Status of vision before drug administration
- Complaints of pain or eye discomfort
- Client's ability to administer eye medications
- Client's knowledge about eye medication and reason for use

Nursing Diagnoses

Nursing diagnoses may include the following:
- Acute pain related to swelling and irritation in left eye
- Ineffective therapeutic regimen management related to lack of recall of proper technique for self-instillation

Outcome Identification and Planning

Desired Outcomes

Sample desired outcomes include the following:
- Client shows no redness, edema, or drainage from eye.
- Client demonstrates correct procedure for self-instillation of medication.

Special Considerations in Planning and Implementation

Geriatric

For older clients who have difficulty remembering, use a calendar to remind them when to administer eye medication.

Transcultural

Instilling eye medications involves touching the client's head, and in some cultures (e.g., Vietnamese), touching the head may be viewed as taking away the spirit. The nurse should consult the client, or parents if a child is involved, regarding what is culturally appropriate. Ask a family member to assist in positioning the client's head if necessary or desired.

Delegation

As a basic standard, medication preparation, teaching, and administration are done by a licensed registered or vocational nurse. Some drugs may be given by registered nurses only. Policies vary by agency and state. BE SURE TO NOTE SPECIFIC AGENCY POLICIES FOR A GIVEN ROUTE AND DRUG BEFORE DELEGATING ADMINISTRATION!

Implementation

Action	Rationale
1. Perform hand hygiene.	*Decreases microorganism transfer*
2. Prepare drug to be administered according to	*Promotes safe drug administration*

Action	Rationale
the five rights of drug administration (see Procedure 5.1).	
3. Identify client by checking identification bracelet and by addressing client by name.	*Verifies identity of client*
4. Explain procedure and purpose of medication to client.	*Reduces anxiety; promotes cooperation*
5. Don gloves.	*Prevents exposure to secretions from eye*
6. Position client in supine or sitting position, with forehead tilted back slightly.	*Facilitates proper placement of medication*
7. If drainage or excess tearing is noted around lower lashes and eyelids, wipe eye with cotton ball from the inner to outer aspect (if both eyes need to be wiped, use a separate cotton ball for each eye).	*Removes excess secretions and debris to facilitate absorption of medication through mucous membranes; prevents cross-contamination*
8. If using bottle with a dropper, squeeze top of medication dropper to aspirate solution into dropper tube. If using ointment, remove cap from container tube.	*Prepares medication for administration*
9. Holding dropper or ointment to be administered in dominant hand, place heel of dominant hand on client's forehead (Fig. 5.2).	*Stabilizes hand for administering eye medication; helps to prevent accidental injury to client's eye*

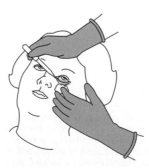

FIGURE 5.2

Action	Rationale
10. Using cotton ball, gently pull lower eyelid down.	*Exposes lower conjunctival sac for placement of medication*
11. Instruct client to look up toward forehead.	*Eliminates corneal-reflex stimulation*
12. Administer ordered number of drops (or quantity of ointment) into conjunctival sac of appropriate eye without letting dropper touch client (see Fig. 5.2); apply a thin line of ointment from inner to outer canthus without letting ointment tube tip touch the client, ending administration smoothly with a twisting motion.	*Places medication in conjunctival sac for absorption without contaminating dropper or ointment tip*
13. Remove hands and instruct client to close and roll eyes around, unless prohibited or unless client cannot do so.	*Spreads medication evenly over eye*
14. Remove excess medication and secretions from around eye with cotton balls.	*Prevents local irritation and discomfort*
15. Discard gloves and perform hand hygiene.	*Reduces microorganism transfer*
16. If ointments or drops temporarily affect vision, instruct client not to move about until vision is clearer.	*Prevents accidental injury*
17. Lift side rails.	*Reduces risk of falls*
18. Place call light within reach.	*Promotes ready access to communication and reduces risk of injury from falling when trying to get out of bed*
19. Discard or restore equipment properly.	*Facilitates clean and orderly environment*
20. Document administration on medication record.	*Provides legal record of medication administration; prevents accidental remedication*

Evaluation

Were desired outcomes achieved? Examples of evaluation include:
* Desired outcome met: Client shows no redness, edema, or drainage from eye after instillation process.
* Desired outcome met: Client administered medication correctly without assistance and verbalized procedure accurately.

Documentation

The following should be noted on the client's chart:
- Condition of eye structures (appearance of skin, presence of drainage, redness, lesions)
- Status of vision before and after medication administration
- Reports of eye pain or tenderness
- Eye in which drug was instilled
- Name of drug, amount, and date and time administered
- Adverse reactions to medication
- Effects of drug
- Teaching regarding drug and self-administration of medications

---

Sample Documentation
Date: 2/17/05
Time: 2100

One drop of gentamicin solution (3 mg/mL) administered in each eye as initial dose of medication. Client states left eye is slightly painful but reports no blurred vision. Slight redness in right eye and small amount of creamy, mucous-colored secretions from right eye. Client expressed some discomfort during the administration of the ophthalmic solution.

● **Nursing Procedure 5.3**

Administering Ear (Otic) Drops

Purpose

Instills liquid medication into external auditory canal for such therapeutic effects as decreasing inflammation and infection and softening ear wax for easy removal

Equipment

- Two or three cotton balls or tissues
- Disposable gloves
- Small basin of warm water
- Soap
- Washcloth

- Small dry towel
- Medication record or electronic medication record
- Pen
- Medication to be administered

Assessment

Assessment should focus on the following:
- Condition of external ear (excess wax production, cleanliness, drainage, and odor)
- Hearing ability of client
- Client's balance and coordination
- Ability of client to follow instructions
- Client's ability to self-administer ear medication
- Client's knowledge about ear medication and reason for use

Nursing Diagnoses

Nursing diagnoses may include the following:
- Acute pain related to inner ear inflammation
- Impaired verbal communication related to decreased hearing and excessive wax buildup

Outcome Identification and Planning

Desired Outcomes

Sample desired outcomes include the following:
- Client states that pain is relieved following administration of ear medication.
- Client exhibits absence of redness, edema, or discharge from the affected ear.
- Ear canal is clear, with no excess wax buildup.
- Client reports that hearing has returned to pre-illness level.

Special Considerations in Planning and Implementation

General

Clients should be cautioned not to insert cotton swabs or any other object into the ear canal to avoid injuring the eardrum.

Pediatric

If necessary, have a parent assist by holding the child in the proper position to minimize the risk of ear damage when administering ear medications.

Geriatric

For older clients who have difficulty remembering, use a calendar to remind them when to administer ear medication.

♦♦♦ Transcultural

Instilling ear medications involves touching the client's head, and in some cultures (e.g., Vietnamese), touching the head may be viewed as taking away the spirit. The nurse should consult the client, or parents if a child is involved, regarding what is culturally appropriate. Ask a family member to assist in positioning the client's head if necessary or desired.

Delegation

As a basic standard, medication preparation, teaching, and administration are done by a licensed registered or vocational nurse. Some drugs may be given by registered nurses only. Policies vary by agency and state. BE SURE TO NOTE SPECIFIC AGENCY POLICIES FOR A GIVEN ROUTE AND DRUG BEFORE DELEGATING ADMINISTRATION!

Implementation

Action	Rationale
1. Perform hand hygiene.	*Reduces spread of microorganisms*
2. Prepare medication, adhering to the five rights of drug administration (see Nursing Procedure 5.1).	*Decreases chance of drug error*
3. Identify client by reading identification bracelet and by addressing client by name.	*Confirms identity of client*
4. Explain procedure and purpose of drug.	*Decreases anxiety*
5. Verify whether client has allergies.	*Prevents allergic reactions and injury*
6. Don gloves.	*Decreases nurse's exposure to ear secretions*
7. Wash ear if excess wax is noted.	*Helps clear path for channeling of drug into ear canal*
8. Assist client into side-lying, sitting, or semi-Fowler's position. Position the ear to receive medication either facing directly upward (in side-lying position) or position forehead tilted upward and turned toward opposite side (in sitting or semi-Fowler's position).	*Positions client for channeling of drug into ear canal*
9. Using nondominant hand, gently pull auricle of the ear up and back (for adults	*Straightens ear canal for channeling of drug into ear*

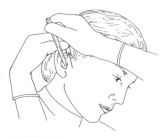

FIGURE 5.3

Action	Rationale
and children older than 3 years) or down and back (for children younger than 3 years).	
10. While resting heel of dominant hand on side of client's face near temporal area, drop ordered number of ear drops into ear canal without touching ear with medicine dropper (Fig. 5.3).	*Prevents accidental injury to tympanic membrane; delivers medication; avoids contaminating solution remaining in bottle*
11. Release ear and remove excess medication from around outside of ear with cotton ball or tissue.	*Reduces skin irritation; promotes comfort*
12. Replace cap on medicine container.	*Maintains medication sterility*
13. Instruct client to remain in position for 3 to 5 minutes.	*Allows time for medication to be absorbed*
14. Remove gloves and discard with soiled materials.	*Reduces transfer of microorganisms*
15. Raise side rails and place call light within reach.	*Prevents falls; promotes ready access for communication*
16. Perform hand hygiene.	*Reduces spread of microorganisms*
17. Document administration on medication record.	*Provides legal record of medication administration; prevents accidental remedication*

Evaluation

Were desired outcomes achieved? Examples of evaluation include:

- Desired outcome met: Client states that pain is relieved following treatment.

- Desired outcome met: Client exhibits absence of redness, edema, or discharge from affected ear.
- Desired outcome met: Ear canal is clear, with no excess wax buildup.
- Desired outcome met: Client reports that hearing has returned to pre-illness level.

Documentation

The following should be noted on the client's chart:
- Condition of ear (appearance of skin, presence of drainage, redness, edema, excess wax buildup)
- Status of hearing
- Reports of pain or tenderness
- Ear in which drug was instilled
- Name and amount of drug
- Adverse reactions to medication
- Effects of drug
- Teaching regarding drug information and techniques for self-administration of medications

Sample Documentation
Date: 2/17/05
Time: 2100

Client received first dose of neomycin (0.01%) ear drops. Given 2 drops in right ear, without report of pain. Slight redness noted in ear canal and a small amount of yellowish discharge from ear noted on cotton ball. No excess wax buildup noted. Client able to repeat statements without visual cues, indicating unimpaired hearing.

● **Nursing Procedure 5.4**

Administering Nasal Medication 🖑
Purpose

Delivers medication for local or systemic absorption through nasal membranes for such therapeutic effects as resolving infections, treating inflammation, and relieving congestion

Equipment

- Nasal drops to be given
- Medication record or electronic medication record
- Pen
- Disposable gloves
- Tissue
- Pillow roll (or large towel made into pillow roll)
- Wet washcloth

Assessment

Assessment should focus on the following:
- Condition of nasal mucosa
- Patency of nasal airway
- Evidence of bleeding or discharge
- Respiratory character
- Contraindications, if any, to client blowing nose
- Client's ability to administer nasal medication
- Client's knowledge about nasal medication and reason for use

Nursing Diagnoses

Nursing diagnoses may include the following:
- Ineffective breathing pattern related to bronchial congestion and nasal inflammation

Outcome Identification and Planning

Desired Outcomes

Sample desired outcomes include the following:
- Client's respirations are even and smooth, at rate of 16 breaths per minute.
- Client demonstrates clear nasal passage with pink septum.

Special Considerations in Planning and Implementation

Pediatric

If necessary, obtain the assistance of a parent to hold the child in position.

Geriatric

For older clients who have difficulty remembering, use a calendar to remind them when to use nose drops.

Home Health

Instruct client on how to administer nasal medications and provide information about the drugs involved. Caution client against overuse of nasal medications.

iii Transcultural

Instilling nasal medications involves touching the client's head, and in some cultures (e.g., Vietnamese), touching the head may be viewed as taking away the spirit. Consult the client, or parent if a child is involved, regarding what is culturally appropriate. Ask a family member to assist in positioning the client's head if necessary or desired.

Delegation

As a basic standard, medication preparation, teaching, and administration are done by a licensed registered or vocational nurse. Some drugs may be given by registered nurses only. Policies vary by agency and state. BE SURE TO NOTE SPECIFIC AGENCY POLICIES FOR A GIVEN ROUTE AND DRUG BEFORE DELEGATING ADMINISTRATION!

Implementation

Action	Rationale
1. Perform hand hygiene.	*Reduces microorganism transfer*
2. Prepare medication, adhering to the five rights of drug administration (see Nursing Procedure 5.1).	*Decreases chance of drug error*
3. Identify client by reading identification bracelet and by addressing client by name.	*Confirms identity of client*
4. Explain procedure and purpose of drug.	*Decreases anxiety*
5. Verify client's allergies listed on medication record or electronic medication record.	*Prevents allergic reactions and injury*
6. Don gloves.	*Decreases nurse's exposure to nasal secretions*
7. If excess mucus is noted in nares, instruct client to blow nose gently (unless contraindicated).	*Clears nares for proper medication absorption*
8. Wipe excess secretions with tissue.	*Removes secretions and cleans skin*
9. Place client in sitting position with head tilted slightly backward, or supine with head tilted back in a slightly hyperextended position (it may be necessary to place a	*Facilitates channeling of drug through nasal passage for optimal absorption*

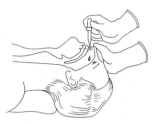

FIGURE 5.4

Action	Rationale
pillow roll or rolled towel under client's neck).	
10. Squeeze top of medication dropper with dominant hand.	*Suctions solution into dropper*
11. Stabilize client's forehead with palm of nondominant hand while gently lifting nose open.	*Prevents accidental damage to nasal mucosa if client suddenly tries to move head when dropper is in place*
12. Without touching client's nose or skin with dropper, hold dropper about ¼ to ½ inch above naris and tilt tip of dropper toward nasal septum (center of nose) (Fig. 5.4).	*Maintains asepsis of remaining drug; directs dropper to center of nose for proper placement of drug*
13. Squeeze top of dropper and deliver the appropriate number of drops.	*Delivers correct dose of medication*
14. Instruct client to take one short, deep breath and to remain in position for 3 to 5 minutes.	*Facilitates full absorption of drug*
15. Replace dropper in bottle.	*Maintains medication sterility*
16. Remove nasal secretions or solution from client's skin (use warm, wet washcloth, if necessary).	*Prevents local skin irritation and discomfort*
17. Lift side rails and place call light within reach.	*Promotes ready access for communication and client safety*
18. Discard gloves and restore other equipment properly.	*Promotes cleanliness; facilitates organization for future medication administration*
19. Perform hand hygiene.	*Prevents spread of infection*
20. Document administration on medication administration record.	*Serves as legal record of medication administration; prevents accidental remedication*

Evaluation

Were desired outcomes achieved? Examples of evaluation include:
- Desired outcome met: Client exhibits respirations that are even and smooth, at rate of 16 breaths per minute.
- Desired outcome met: Nasal passage is clear; septum is pink.

Documentation

The following should be noted on the client's chart:
- Name, dosage, and route of medication
- Assessment data relevant to purpose of medication
- Effects of medication
- Teaching of information about drug used and techniques of self-administration of medication

> *Sample Documentation*
> Date: 2/17/05
> Time: 2100
>
> Client received final dose of Neo-Synephrine nasally, 2 drops in right naris. Client states pain in nose relieved. No redness or swelling of nasal mucosa noted. No drainage from nares visible. Respirations smooth and even.

● Nursing Procedure 5.5

Administering Nebulizer Medication 🖐

Purpose

Delivers an inhaled dose of medication into the mucosa and bloodstream to ease respiratory distress

Equipment

Hand-Held Nebulizer

- Nebulizer set (cup, tubing, cap, T-shaped tube, mouthpiece or mask)
- Medication(s)

- Saline
- Air compressor, wall air or wall oxygen

Metered-Dose Inhaler

- Metered-dose inhaler
- Spacer device such as Aerochamber (if indicated)

Assessment

Assessment should focus on the following:
- Client's respiratory status, including underlying condition necessitating use of nebulized medication
- Medication allergies or sensitivity to latex (if latex gloves used)
- Client's ability to use nebulizer or metered-dose inhaler
- Client's knowledge about medication and the use of the nebulizer or metered-dose inhaler

Nursing Diagnoses

Nursing diagnoses may include the following:
- Impaired gas exchange related to airway blockage
- Ineffective breathing pattern related to airway spasms
- Ineffective airway clearance related to excessive mucus production

Outcome Identification and Planning

Desired Outcomes

Sample desired outcomes include:
- The client will experience improved gas exchange with pulse oximetry value within normal range.
- The client's breathing pattern will improve after treatment, with respiratory rate of 18 to 24.
- The client demonstrates correct use of nebulizer or metered-dose inhaler.

Special Considerations in Planning and Implementation

General

Encourage clients to perform good oral hygiene after using a nebulizer. Observe for signs of fungal infection (e.g., white patches). Instruct client to rise mouth thoroughly with water or ordered solution after using a nebulizer.

Pediatric

Children may cry when they see the mist from the nebulizer, but crying is actually beneficial because it can increase the chance of the medication getting into the airways and lungs. Use a mask instead of mouthpiece for infants and very small children to facilitate inhalation. To provide additional inhalation time, use a spacer for young children who don't have the manual dexterity and ability to coordinate depressing the canister and inhaling at the same time.

Geriatric

Use a mask instead of a mouthpiece for older clients with a disabling condition such as arthritis who find it difficult to use the nebulizer. To provide additional inhalation time, use a spacer for older clients who don't have the manual dexterity and ability to coordinate depressing the canister and inhaling at the same time.

Home Care

Suggest the use of a multi-dose nebulizer for a client at home. Encourage clients receiving nebulizer therapy in the home to clean and disinfect the nebulizer after each use and change the nebulizer set every 6 months.

Delegation

As a basic standard, medication preparation, teaching, and administration are done by a licensed registered or vocational nurse. Some drugs may be given by registered nurses or respiratory therapists only. A registered nurse should observe the client for untoward reactions if there are potential medication side effects. Policies vary by agency and state. BE SURE TO NOTE SPECIFIC AGENCY POLICIES FOR A GIVEN ROUTE AND DRUG BEFORE DELEGATING ADMINISTRATION!

Implementation

Action	Rationale
Using a Hand-Held Nebulizer	
1. Explain to the client the process of using the nebulizer.	*Promotes compliance*
2. Check physician orders.	*Ensures that the right dose is administered to the right client*
3. Perform hand hygiene.	*Decreases spread of microorganisms*
4. Pour the entire dose of the drug into the nebulizer cup.	*Ensures accurate dosing of drug*
5. Cover the cup with cap and fasten the T-piece to the cap. Attach the large tubing to one end of the T-piece and fasten the mouthpiece to the other end of the T-piece. Do not touch the interior parts of the mask or mouthpiece.	*Provides dead space to prevent room air from entering system and medicated aerosol from escaping; prevents introduction of organisms*

Action	Rationale
6. Attach oxygen tubing to the bottom of the nebulizer cup and attach the other end to the compressed air source.	*Provides conduit for compressed air*
7. Adjust wall oxygen to 6 L/min or less as ordered (Fig. 5.5) and turn air on until medication begins to mist. Leave the air on for about 6 or 7 minutes, until all of the medication is inhaled.	*Delivers a low dose of oxygen with treatment; air flow drives medication into aerosolized form*
8. Instruct client to breathe with lips tightly sealed around the mouthpiece; if a mask is used, ensure that the mask is properly applied to the client's face and encourage the client to take slow, deep breaths in through the mouth and out through the nose (Fig. 5.6).	*Promotes efficacy of medication; increases delivery of medication into lungs*
9. When medication is complete, perform hand hygiene and don gloves.	*Reduces transmission of microorganisms*

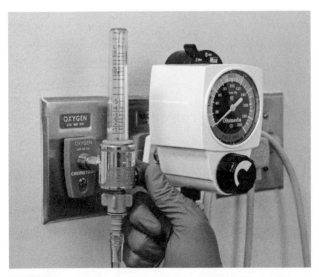

FIGURE 5.5

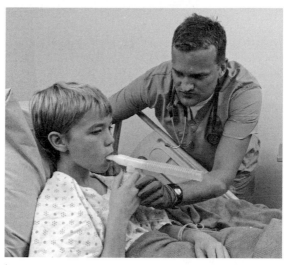

FIGURE 5.6

Action	Rationale
10. Detach tubing from compressed air source and nebulizer cup. If nebulizer is disposable, dispose of nebulizer in appropriate container. If nebulizer is to be reused, carefully wash with soapy water, rinse, and dry nebulizer components.	*Reduces transmission of microorganisms*
11. Observe client for several minutes to assess response to medication.	*Notes possible adverse reactions*
12. Remove gloves and perform hand hygiene.	*Reduces microorganism transfer*
13. Document procedure appropriately.	*Serves as legal record of medication administration*

Administering Metered-Dose Inhalation

Action	Rationale
1. Remove cap and hold inhaler upright.	*Allows proper administration of drug*
2. Shake inhaler and attach spacer/Aerochamber (optional).	*Mixes medication well*
3. Instruct client to tilt head back slightly and breathe out.	*Allows proper medication administration*

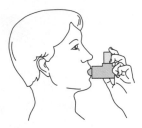

FIGURE 5.7

Action	Rationale
4. Position inhaler in client's mouth with lips sealed around mouthpiece (Fig. 5.7).	*Allows proper medication administration*
5. Press down on the inhaler to release medication as client starts to breathe in. Instruct client to breathe in slowly.	*Delivers medication to lungs*
6. Instruct client to breathe in slowly over 3 to 5 seconds; a longer deeper breath may be taken with spacer. If a second puff is ordered, repeat administration after client fully exhales with the first administration. If the medication is a dry powder capsule, have the client close the mouth tightly around the mouthpiece and inhale rapidly.	*Promotes medication distribution to lungs; administers full treatment; prevents loss of medication*
7. Recap medication and store appropriately.	*Allows for future use*
8. Observe client for several minutes to assess response to medication.	*Notes possible adverse reactions*
9. Remove gloves and perform hand hygiene.	*Reduces microorganism transfer*
10. Document procedure appropriately.	*Serves as legal record of medication administration*

Evaluation

Were desired outcomes achieved? Examples of evaluation include:
● Desired outcome met: Client states that breathing has improved.

- Desired outcome met: Client exhibits no signs and symptoms of respiratory distress.
- Desired outcome met: Client demonstrates correct use of nebulizer or metered-dose inhaler.

Documentation

The following should be noted on the client's chart:
- Name, amount, and route of drug given
- Purpose of administration if drug is given on a when-needed (p.r.n.) basis
- Assessment data relevant to purpose of medication
- Effects of medication on client
- Teaching of information about drug used or about self-administration technique

---

Sample Documentation

Date: 2/17/05
Time: 2100

Client complaining of shortness of breath; respirations 38 per minute, shallow and labored; wheezing noted on auscultation. Albuterol 1 puff administered as ordered PRN. Client voices understanding about use of self-administered technique. Client asleep; respiratory rate 22 breaths per minute, even and nonlabored.

● Nursing Procedure 5.6

Administering Oral Medication 🧤

Purpose

Delivers medication for absorption through alimentary tract

Equipment

- Medication record or electronic medication record
- Pen
- Disposable gloves, if possibility of exposure to oral secretions
- Medication to be administered
- Medication cup
- Water, juice, or beverage
- Drinking straw (optional)

Assessment

Assessment should focus on the following:
- Complete medication order
- Condition of client's mouth (presence of lesions, tears, bleeding, tenderness)
- Ability of client to swallow without difficulty
- Client's allergies
- Client's complaints of nausea or inability to retain oral medications
- Client's knowledge about medication and reason for use

Nursing Diagnoses

Nursing diagnoses may include the following:
- Acute pain related to surgical incision
- Disturbed sleep pattern related to unfamiliarity with hospital environment

Outcome Identification and Planning

Desired Outcomes

Sample desired outcomes include:
- Client states that pain is relieved within an hour of administration of analgesic.
- Client falls asleep within 1 hour of administration of sleep enhancer.

Special Considerations in Planning and Implementation

General

To ensure adequate drug absorption and proper action:
- Do not crush or allow client to chew certain solid forms of medication, such as capsules, enteric-coated tablets, or extended-release medications.
- Give medications that may cause gastric irritation with milk.
- Consult with physician to obtain a liquid or alternative form of a medication if client has difficulty swallowing pills and they cannot be crushed.
- Be alert for an increase or decrease in effect(s) when several oral medications are given at the same time.
- When a client receives a medication for the first time, monitor the client closely for an adverse reaction or sensitivity.
- If a new drug is being given, give it at a different time from other medications to obtain a clear picture of the client's response to the new drug.

Pediatric

Try holding and cuddling an infant to elicit a cooperative, non-combative response when administering oral medications. If necessary and appropriate, mix the medication with food or liquid, using as small an amount as possible to ensure that the child takes all of the drug. For very small or young children, administer oral liquid medications using a dropper or nipple device. Encourage toddlers' cooperation by giving them a choice of method of drug delivery—spoon, dropper, syringe—and allow them to help with administration by holding the pills and taking them without assistance.

Geriatric

For older clients who have difficulty remembering, use reminder devices such as daily pill dispensers and calendars.

Home Health

Be alert for self-prescribed medications, usually obtained from previous doctors, friends, or family members. These medications may interact with current medications, leading to potentially serious or even fatal adverse reactions. Ask to see all drugs taken within the past 24 to 72 hours, including any herbal remedies, which the client may not consider as drugs or medications.

Transcultural

To prevent drug interactions, ask whether the client has taken any complementary or alternative medications, such as herbal drugs, before administering ordered medications. Consult pharmacy and the physician as indicated.

Delegation

As a basic standard, medication preparation, teaching, and administration are done by a licensed registered or vocational nurse. Some drugs may be given by registered nurses only. Policies vary by agency and state. BE SURE TO NOTE SPECIFIC AGENCY POLICIES FOR A GIVEN ROUTE AND DRUG BEFORE DELEGATING ADMINISTRATION!

Implementation

Action	Rationale
1. Perform hand hygiene.	*Reduces microorganism transfer*
2. Prepare medication, adhering to the five rights of drug administration (see Procedure 5.1).	*Prepares drug; decreases chance of drug error*
3. Identify client by reading identification bracelet and by addressing client by name.	*Confirms identity of client*
4. Explain procedure and purpose of drug.	*Decreases anxiety; promotes cooperation*

Action	Rationale
5. Verify any allergies listed on medication record or electronic medication record.	*Alerts nurse to potential allergic reaction*
6. Obtain preassessment data.	*Determines if medication should be held or given*
7. Separate drugs that might be withheld based on preassessment data.	*Prevents inadvertent administration of drugs that may lead to client injury if administered*
8. Assist client into semi-Fowler's or sitting position.	*Prevents aspiration*
9. Don gloves if there is a possibility of exposure to oral secretions.	*Avoids exposure to client secretions*
10. Open unit-dose packages and place one drug in client's hand or pour in medication cup and give to client; provide assistance if needed.	*Maintains asepsis while administering medication*
11. Instruct client to place tablets or capsules into mouth and to follow with enough liquid to ensure that drug is swallowed.	*Ensures that liquid carries drug into the GI tract, preventing tablets from lodging in throat or esophagus*
12. Administer liquid medications after pills, instructing client to drink all of the solution; provide assistance if needed.	*Facilitates proper absorption of liquids that are not to be followed by a beverage*
13. Remain with client until all medications are taken; check client's mouth if there is any question of whether drug has been swallowed.	*Ensures that drug is taken and client is not "cheeking" the medication*
14. Reposition client and place call light within reach.	*Facilitates comfort; provides ready access for communication*
15. Lift side rails.	*Prevents accidental falls*
16. Discard or restore equipment properly:	*Promotes clean environment with necessary equipment ready for future use*
• If client refuses drug or drug has not been given for any reason, DO NOT leave drug at the bedside.	*Eliminates question of what happened to drug at later time*
• Remove drug from room and restore in medication drawer or cabinet only if in unopened unit-dose package.	*Allows nurse to administer drug at later date*

Action	Rationale
• If unit-dose package has been opened, discard in sink or flush down toilet, with witness present if necessary.	*Ensures that drug is destroyed; promotes compliance with federal regulations if medication is a controlled substance*
17. Remove gloves and perform hand hygiene.	*Prevents spread of infection*
18. Document administration on medication record.	*Serves as legal record of medication administration; prevents accidental remedication*
19. Assess client 30 to 60 minutes after administration and document client response to medication.	*Evaluates client's response to medication, helping to identify therapeutic or possible toxic effects*

Evaluation

Were the desired outcomes achieved? Examples of evaluation include:
- Desired outcome met: Client states that pain is relieved within an hour of administration of analgesic.
- Desired outcome met: Client falls asleep within 1 hour of administration of sleep enhancer.

Documentation

The following should be noted on the client's chart:
- Name, amount, and route of drug given
- Purpose of administration if drug is given on a when-needed (p.r.n.) basis
- Assessment data relevant to purpose of medication
- Effects of medication on client
- Teaching of information about drug used or about self-administration technique

---

Sample Documentation

Date: 2/17/05
Time: 2200

Client complaining of inability to sleep at 2100. Dalmane 15 mg PO given. Client asleep, with even, nonlabored respirations; rate 16. Client voices understanding about purpose of medication and correct dosing schedule for medication.

Administering Buccal and Sublingual Medication

Purpose

Delivers medication for absorption through oral mucous
  membranes

Equipment

- Medication record or electronic medication record
- Pen
- Disposable gloves
- Medication to be administered

Assessment

Assessment should focus on the following:
- Complete medication order
- Condition of mouth (presence of lesions, tears, bleeding,
  tenderness)
- Client's allergies
- Client's knowledge about the medication and reason for
  medication

Nursing Diagnoses

Nursing diagnoses may include the following:
- Acute pain related to myocardial ischemia
- Anxiety related to uncertainty of prognosis and results of
  diagnostic tests

Outcome Identification and Planning

Desired Outcomes

Sample desired outcomes include the following:
- Client states pain is relieved within 5 minutes of administration of one sublingual nitroglycerin tablet.
- Client demonstrates signs of decreased anxiety (relaxed facial
  expression and respiratory rate of 20 breaths per minute).

Special Considerations in Planning and Implementation

Geriatric

For older clients who have difficulty remembering, use devices
that remind the client when to take medications, such as calendars and daily pill dispensers.

Delegation

As a basic standard, medication preparation, teaching, and administration are done by a licensed registered or vocational nurse. Some drugs may be given by registered nurses only. Policies vary by agency and state. BE SURE TO NOTE SPECIFIC AGENCY POLICIES FOR A GIVEN ROUTE AND DRUG BEFORE DELEGATING ADMINISTRATION!

Implementation

Action	Rationale
1. Perform hand hygiene.	*Reduces microorganism transfer*
2. Prepare medication, adhering to the five rights of drug administration (see Procedure 5.1).	*Allows safe drug preparation, decreasing chance of drug error*
3. Identify client by reading identification bracelet and addressing client by name.	*Confirms identity of client*
4. Explain procedure and purpose of drug.	*Decreases anxiety; promotes cooperation*
5. Verify allergies listed on medication record or electronic medication record.	*Prevents administration of drug that might result in an allergic reaction*
6. Don gloves.	*Decreases nurse's exposure to client's body secretions*
7. Place tablet:	
• Under tongue for sublingual medication.	*Facilitates dissolving and absorption through oral mucous membranes*
• Between cheek and gum on either side of mouth for buccal administration (avoid broken or irritated buccal or sublingual areas).	*Reduces additional irritation*
If mucous membranes are dry, offer a sip of water before giving medication.	*Prevents medication from sticking to mouth; facilitates absorption of medication*
8. Instruct client not to swallow drug but to let drug dissolve.	*Facilitates absorption by proper route*
9. Discard gloves and perform hand hygiene.	*Reduces transfer of microorganisms*
10. Document administration on medication record.	*Serves as legal record of medication administration; prevents accidental remedication*

Evaluation

Were desired outcomes achieved? Examples of evaluation include:
- Desired outcome met: Client states pain is relieved within 5 minutes of administration of one sublingual nitroglycerin tablet.
- Desired outcome met: Client demonstrates signs of decreased anxiety (relaxed facial expression and respiratory rate of 20 breaths per minute).

Documentation

The following should be noted on the client's chart:
- Name, amount, and route of drug given
- Purpose of administration if drug is given on a when-needed (p.r.n.) basis
- Assessment data relevant to purpose of medication
- Effects of medication on client
- Teaching of information about drug used or about self-administration of medication

---

Sample Documentation
Date: 2/17/05
Time: 2100

Nitroglycerin gr. 1/150 SL for c/o sharp, nonradiating, midsternal chest pain, with relief in 2 minutes. No dysrhythmias noted. Blood pressure 110/70 after 1 tablet.

● **Nursing Procedure 5.8**

Preparing Medication From a Vial

Purpose

Obtains medication from a vial, using aseptic technique, for administration by a parenteral route

Equipment

- Medication administration record or electronic medication record

- Vial with prescribed medication
- Appropriate-size syringe and needle for type of injection and viscosity of solution
- Extra needle
- Alcohol swabs
- Medication label or small piece of tape
- Medication tray
- Access pin and sterile cap (for needleless system and multi-dose vials)

Assessment

Assessment should focus on the following:
- Appearance of solution (clarity, absence of sediment, color indicated on instruction label)
- Vial label for expiration date of drug

Outcome Identification and Planning

Desired Outcomes

Sample desired outcomes include:
- Client received correct amount, type and dose of drug.
- Client relates procedure for medication preparation with multiuse vials without contaminating remaining medication.

Special Considerations in Planning and Implementation

General

If medication requires reconstitution, follow guidelines on vial. Maintain sterility of syringe, needle, and medication while preparing the drug. Figure 5.8 identifies the parts of a syringe and needle assembly that must be kept sterile. When using a needleless system, replace the needle with an access pin with a sterile cap to allow frequent withdrawal of medication. Although exposure to a contaminated needle by the nurse is unlikely at this point in the medication administration procedure, use of a needleless system minimizes the nurse's risk of a needlestick injury.

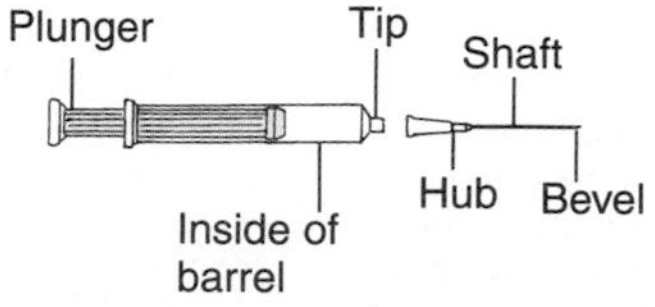

FIGURE 5.8

Geriatric

For older clients who have difficulty remembering, use devices that remind them when to take medications, such as calendars and daily medication dispensers. For clients with visual deficits, note whether client is able to withdraw an accurate amount of solution from the vial. Determine support person who can prepare medication for client as needed.

Home Health

Assess area in which client or family member will be preparing drug for adequacy of lighting. Instruct client to discard used needles, syringes, and empty vials by dropping into large coffee can with hole cut in lid. Urge client to store can in a safe place (away from children) until it becomes full, then transfer to garbage. Instruct client to secure clean needles and syringes in a locked container or cabinet to prevent unauthorized use.

Delegation

As a basic standard, medication preparation, teaching, and administration are done by a licensed registered or vocational nurse. Some drugs may be given by registered nurses only. Policies vary by agency and state. BE SURE TO NOTE SPECIFIC AGENCY POLICIES FOR A GIVEN ROUTE AND DRUG BEFORE DELEGATING ADMINISTRATION!

Implementation

Action	Rationale
1. Perform hand hygiene.	*Reduces microorganism transfer*
2. Organize equipment.	*Promotes efficiency*
3. Check label of medication vial with medication record or electronic medication record, using the five rights of drug administration (see Procedure 5.1).	*Avoids client injury from wrong drug or dosage*
4. Perform dosage calculations if vial contains more medication than client requires.	*Determines correct amount of solution to be given*
5. Remove thin seal cap from top of vial without touching rubber stopper.	*Exposes rubber top for insertion of needle while maintaining asepsis*
6. Firmly wipe rubber stopper on top of vial with alcohol swab. If needleless system is used, insert the spike of the access pin into the vial until the "wing" of	*Ensures asepsis; permits access to the fluid in the vial using a syringe only*

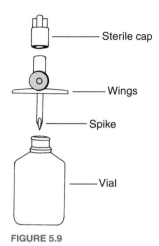

FIGURE 5.9

Action	Rationale
the pin touches the vial's rubber stopper (Fig. 5.9). Remove sterile cap without touching top of access pin.	
7. Pull end of plunger back to fill syringe with a volume of air equal to the amount of solution to be drawn up (Fig. 5.10); do not touch inside of plunger.	*Draws air into syringe to create positive pressure in vial; maintains plunger sterility*

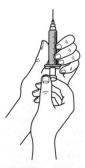

FIGURE 5.10

Action	Rationale
8. Remove needle cap. (For needleless systems, use syringe only. Remove cap and needle [if attached], if necessary. Connect syringe onto access pin and skip steps 9 and 10.)	*Prepares for insertion*
9. Using a slightly slanted angle, firmly insert needle into center of rubber top of vial, with the sharpest point of the needle (tip of bevel) entering first.	*Prevents solution from becoming contamination with sediment from rubber top*
10. Continue insertion until needle is securely in vial yet above the level of fluid.	*Prevents needle from slipping out of vial*
11. Press end of plunger down to instill air into vial.	*Infuses air to create positive pressure in vial*
12. Hold vial with nondominant hand and turn it up, keeping needle/spike inserted; control syringe with dominant hand and keep plunger down with thumb.	*Moves solution to area of vial closest to rubber stopper for easy removal*
13. Pull needle/spike back to point at which bevel is beneath fluid level; keep needle/spike beneath fluid level as long as fluid is being withdrawn.	*Places needle in position in which fluid can be obtained (below level of fluid)*
14. Slowly pull end of plunger back until appropriate amount of solution is aspirated into syringe.	*Ensures delivery of prescribed amount of medication*
15. If air bubbles enter syringe, gently flick syringe barrel with fingers of dominant hand; keep a finger on end of plunger; continue holding vial with nondominant hand.	*Congregates bubbles in one area for removal; prevents plunger from popping out of barrel*
16. Push plunger in until air is out of syringe.	*Displaces bubble of air into vial*
17. Withdraw additional solution, if needed.	*Replaces solution lost when clearing bubbles*
18. Pull needle out of bottle while keeping a finger on end of plunger. (For needleless systems, detach syringe	*Prevents plunger from popping out of barrel*

Action	Rationale
from access pin; cover pin with sterile cap. Apply sterile needle to syringe if IM/SQ or intradermal injection will be given.)	
19. If bubbles remain in syringe: <ul><li>Hold syringe vertically (with needle pointing up, if attached).</li><li>Pull back slightly on plunger and flick syringe with fingers.</li><li>Slowly push plunger up to release air, but not to the point of expelling the solution.</li></ul>	*Removes remaining air bubbles from syringe using principle that air rises*
20. Recheck amount of solution in syringe, comparing with drug volume required.	*Ensures that correct amount of drug has been prepared*
21. Compare drug label with medication record or electronic record.	*Provides additional identification check*
22. Change needle, if used to withdraw the solution from the vial and drug is known to be irritating to tissue; replace cap (cap replacement is unnecessary if the needleless system is used).	*Prevents tissue irritation due to drug clinging to outer surfaces of needle when solution is injected into skin*
23. Label syringe with drug name and amount of drug.	*Provides identification information at client's bedside*
24. Place syringe, medication record, and additional alcohol swabs on medication tray.	*Organizes equipment for administration of drug*
25. Discard or restore all equipment appropriately.	*Promotes clean and organized environment*
26. Perform hand hygiene.	*Prevents spread of microorganisms*

Evaluation

Were desired outcomes achieved? Examples of evaluation include:
- Desired outcome met: Client received correct amount, type, and dose of drug.
- Desired outcome met: Client accurately related the procedure for aseptically preparing dose of medication from a multidose vial without contaminating remaining medication.

Documentation

The following should be noted on the client's chart:
- Name of medication
- Date and time medication was prepared
- Dosage prepared
- In addition, if the medication is a controlled substance, follow agency policy and procedure for recording medication in Controlled Substance Record Book. Note any amount of the controlled substance that was wasted, the name of the nurse preparing the controlled substance, and the name of the nurse witnessing use and, if appropriate, witnessing the discarding of the wasted amount.

Sample Documentation
Date: 2/17/05
Time: 2100

Client instructed on method for insulin preparation from multiuse vial. Client prepared correct dose of medication from vial using sterile technique.

● **Nursing Procedure 5.9**

Preparing Medication From an Ampule

Purpose

Obtains medication from ampule, using aseptic technique, for administration by a parenteral route

Equipment

- Medication administration record or electronic medication record
- Ampule with prescribed medication
- Appropriate-size syringe and needle for type of injection and viscosity of solution (use filtered needle, if available)

- Medication label or small piece of tape
- Extra needle
- Medication tray
- Alcohol swabs
- Paper towel

Assessment

Assessment should focus on the following:
- Appearance of solution (clarity, absence of sediment, color indicated on instruction label)
- Ampule label for expiration date of drug

Nursing Diagnoses

Nursing diagnoses may include the following:
- Acute pain related to muscle strain
- Deficient knowledge related to procedure for preparing medication dose from an ampule

Outcome Identification and Planning

Desired Outcomes

Sample desired outcomes include:
- Client verbalizes pain level reduced to 0 within 30 minutes after medication is administered.
- Client prepares correct amount and type of drug from a vial using aseptic technique.

Special Considerations in Planning and Implementation

General

Maintain the sterility of syringe, needle, and medication while preparing the drug using principles of asepsis.

Home Health

Instruct client to discard ampules by wrapping in paper towel and dropping into large coffee can with hole cut in lid. Instruct client also to discard used syringes and needles in the can. Urge client to store can in safe place (away from children) until it becomes full, then transfer to garbage.

Delegation

As a basic standard, medication preparation, teaching, and administration are done by a licensed registered or vocational nurse. Some drugs may be given by registered nurses only. Policies vary by agency and state. BE SURE TO NOTE SPECIFIC AGENCY POLICIES FOR A GIVEN ROUTE AND DRUG BEFORE DELEGATING ADMINISTRATION!

Implementation

Action	Rationale
1. Perform hand hygiene.	*Reduces microorganism transfer*
2. Organize equipment.	*Promotes efficiency*
3. Check label of medication vial with medication record or electronic medication record, using the five rights of drug administration (see Procedure 5.1).	*Avoids client injury from wrong drug or dosage*
4. Perform dosage calculation if dosage in ampule differs from amount required.	*Determines correct amount of solution to be withdrawn*
5. Holding ampule, gently tap neck (top of ampule) with fingers (Fig. 5.11) or make a complete circle with the ampule by rotating wrist.	*Displaces solution from top of ampule to bottom; prevents drug waste and ensures that all of the drug is in the base of the ampule for withdrawal*
6. Place alcohol swab or gauze pad around neck of ampule with fingers of dominant hand; firmly place fingers of nondominant hand around lower part of ampule with thumb placed against junction.	*Promotes easy opening of ampule; helps to stabilize vial, providing protection against finger cuts*
7. With a quick snapping motion of the wrist, break top of ampule away from you and others who may be near you (Fig. 5.12).	*Opens ampule; prevents injury from glass pieces*
8. Place top of ampule on paper towel or immediately discard.	*Prevents injury from broken glass*
9. Remove needle cap.	

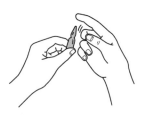

FIGURE 5.11

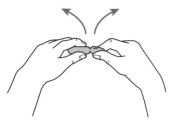

FIGURE 5.12

Action	Rationale
10. Press plunger of syringe all the way down; do not aspirate air into syringe.	*Prevents accidental displacement and waste of solution*
11. Place needle into ampule without letting needle or hub touch cut edges of the ampule.	*Maintains needle sterility*
12. Withdraw appropriate amount of solution into syringe (Fig. 5.13) and remove needle from ampule.	*Provides proper dosage of medication in syringe*
13. Place ampule on paper towel until ready to discard, or discard immediately.	*Prevents injury from jagged glass*

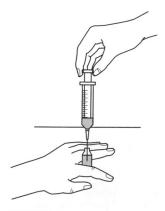

FIGURE 5.13

Action	Rationale
14. If bubbles are in syringe: • Hold syringe vertically, with needle pointing up. • Pull back slightly on plunger and flick syringe with fingers. • Slowly push plunger up to release air, but not to the point of expelling the solution.	*Removes remaining air bubbles from syringe using principle that air rises*
15. Recheck amount of solution in syringe, comparing with drug volume required.	*Ensures that correct amount of drug has been prepared*
16. Compare drug label with medication record or electronic medication record.	*Provides additional identification check*
17. Change needle if drug is known to cause tissue irritation; replace cap.	*Prevents tissue irritation from drug clinging to outer surfaces injected into skin*
18. Label syringe with drug name and dose amount.	*Provides identification information once at client bedside*
19. Place syringe, medication record, and additional alcohol swabs on medication tray.	*Organizes equipment for administration of drug*
20. Discard or restore all equipment appropriately.	*Promotes clean and organized environment*
21. Perform hand hygiene.	*Prevents spread of microorganisms*

Evaluation

Were desired outcomes achieved? Examples of evaluation include:
• Desired outcome met: Client verbalizes pain level reduced to 0 within 30 minutes after medication is administered.
• Desired outcome met: Client prepares correct amount and type of drug from a vial using aseptic technique.

Documentation

The following should be noted on the client's chart:
• Name of medication
• Date and time medication was drawn
• Dosage drawn
• In addition, if the medication is a controlled substance, follow agency policy and procedure for recording medication

in Controlled Substance Record Book. Include any amount of the controlled substance that was wasted, the name of the nurse preparing the controlled substance, and the name of the nurse witnessing use and, if appropriate, witnessing the discarding of the wasted amount.

Sample Documentation
Date: 2/17/05
Time: 2100

Daily injections of Demerol ordered. Client instructed on procedure for administration. Client correctly demonstrated procedure and prepared correct dose of medication from an ampule.

● **Nursing Procedure 5.10**

Preparing Medication With the Needleless System

Purpose

Delivers medication with minimal risk of needlestick injury for the nurse

Equipment

- Medication administration record or electronic medication record
- Prescribed medication
- Appropriate-size needleless syringe system
- Alcohol swabs
- Medication for administration
- Saline solution (if indicated)
- Medication tray

Assessment

Assessment should focus on the following:
- Medication and client assessment (see Procedure 5.1)
- Appearance of solution (clarity, absence of sediment, color indicated on instruction label)

- Medication compatibility with primary solution or flush solution
- Medication label for expiration date

Nursing Diagnoses

Nursing diagnoses may include the following:
- Risk of infection related to invasive procedure
- Deficient knowledge related to use of needleless equipment in medication administration

Outcome Identification and Planning

Desired Outcomes

Sample desired outcomes include the following:
- Client demonstrates no signs of infection of IV site or systemic sepsis.
- Client demonstrates correct procedure for medication preparation using needleless equipment.

Special Considerations in Planning and Implementation

Delegation

In most cases, IV medications may be given by registered nurses only. Policies vary by agency and state. BE SURE TO NOTE SPECIFIC AGENCY POLICIES FOR A GIVEN ROUTE AND DRUG BEFORE DELEGATING ADMINISTRATION!

Implementation

Action	Rationale
1. Perform hand hygiene.	*Reduces microorganism transfer*
2. Organize equipment.	*Promotes efficiency*
3. Check label of medications to be administered against medication record, using the five rights of drug administration (see Procedure 5.1).	*Avoids client injury from wrong drug or dosage*
4. Verify allergies listed on medication record or electronic medication record.	*Alerts nurse to possibility of allergic reaction*
5. Perform dosage calculations, if needed.	*Determines correct amount of solution to be prepared*

Action	Rationale
6. Assess IV site for redness and puffiness and palpate for tenderness.	*Reveals signs of infiltration or infection*
7. Administer medication: For secondary/piggyback medication:	
• Connect secondary set tubing to secondary medication bag, then hang secondary medication bag on IV pole. Add needleless locking cannula, if not built into tubing.	*Provides easy access for preparation*
• Prime tubing (see Nursing Procedure 7.8).	
• Affix a needleless locking cannula at the end of the secondary infusion tubing to the medication port on the primary tubing.	*Decreases risk of IV needle exposure*
• Close primary fluid regulator or clamp (particularly if infusion pump will be used), or lower the primary bag/bottle. Open secondary tubing clamp and adjust drip rate to desired infusion rate.	*Directs fluid flow from secondary bag; permits solution to infuse at prescribed rate*
For IV push medication:	
• Prepare medication in syringe, along with two syringes of normal saline or flush (see Nursing Procedures 5.7 and 5.8). Verify infusion rate and drug compatibility with primary fluid (refer to medication reference book).	*Prevents rapid infusion of drug or drug interaction with fluid*
• Clean connector site (saline lock) with alcohol swab. Use the medication port closest to the catheter insertion.	*Decreases risk of transmission of microorganisms; infuses medication at closest entry point into the bloodstream*

Action	Rationale
If injecting fluid into IV line, kink tubing.	
• Connect needleless syringe with saline; check for blood return; then flush line with 1 mL saline.	*Verifies patency of IV catheter*
• Remove needleless syringe used for saline flush.	*Prepares for medication administration*
• Clean connector site with alcohol swab.	*Decreases risk for transmission of microorganisms*
• Connect medication syringe; inject medication at prescribed rate; remove medication syringe.	*Promotes safe medication infusion; overly rapid infusion may be fatal*
• Connect syringe with normal saline and flush the line slowly with 1 to 3 cc.	*Delivers remaining medication; clears the line, preventing medication from mixing with other IV fluids; maintains line patency*
8. Observe client for adverse reactions.	*Provides opportunity for immediate intervention*
9. Perform hand hygiene.	*Decreases transfer of microorganisms*
10. Document administration on medication record.	*Serves as legal record of administration; prevents accidental remediation*

Evaluation

Were desired outcomes achieved? Examples of evaluation include:
- Desired outcome met: Client demonstrates no signs of infection at IV site or systemic sepsis.
- Desired outcome met: Client demonstrates correct procedure for medication preparation using needleless equipment.

Documentation

The following should be noted on the client's chart:
- Name of medication, dosage, route, rate of administration
- Assessment and laboratory data relevant to purpose of medication
- Effects of medication
- Teaching of information about drug or injection technique

Sample Documentation
Date: 2/17/05
Time: 2100

Client received initial dose of vancomycin 500 mg IV piggyback infusion. No redness or swelling seen at IV site. Client tolerated medication without any evidence of adverse reactions.

● **Nursing Procedure 5.11**

Mixing Medications

Purpose

Allows medications from multiple containers to be combined in one syringe for parenteral administration

Equipment

- Medication administration record or electronic medication record
- Prescribed medication
- Appropriate-size syringe and three needles for type of injection and viscosity of solutions
- Medication label or small piece of tape
- Alcohol swabs
- Medication tray

Assessment

Assessment should focus on the following:
- Appearance of solutions (clarity, absence of sediment, color indicated on instruction labels)
- Drug labels for expiration dates
- Parenteral drug compatibility charts
- Client allergies
- Drug compatibility with medications and primary infusion
- Appropriate infusion rate (refer to medication reference book)

Nursing Diagnoses

Nursing diagnoses may include the following:
- Deficient knowledge related to procedure for mixing medications

Outcome Identification and Planning

Desired Outcomes

Sample desired outcomes include the following:
- Client demonstrates proper procedure for mixing medications.

Special Considerations in Planning and Implementation

General

If a medication requires reconstitution, follow the guidelines on the vial. If you are uncomfortable with the mixing process described in this procedure, draw up medications using two separate syringes, remove cap from one syringe, and aspirate medication into the other syringe. When adding air to vial, make sure needle is not below fluid level.

Delegation

As a basic standard, medication preparation, teaching, and administration are done by a licensed registered or vocational nurse. Some drugs may be given by registered nurses only. Policies vary by agency and state. BE SURE TO NOTE SPECIFIC AGENCY POLICIES FOR A GIVEN ROUTE AND DRUG BEFORE DELEGATING ADMINISTRATION!

Implementation

Action	Rationale
1. Perform hand hygiene.	*Reduces microorganism transfer*
2. Organize equipment.	*Promotes efficiency*
3. Check labels of medications to be mixed with medication record or electronic medication record, using the five rights of drug administration (see Procedure 5.1).	*Avoids client injury from wrong drug or dosage*
4. Perform dosage calculations, if needed.	*Determines correct amount of solution to be prepared*
5. Remove thin seal caps from tops of both vials without touching rubber stoppers.	*Exposes rubber tops; maintains asepsis*

Action	Rationale
6. Firmly wipe top of each rubber stopper with alcohol swabs.	*Maintains asepsis*
7. Pull end of plunger of syringe back to fill syringe with an amount of air equal to amount of solution to be drawn from first vial.	*Draws air into syringe, which is needed for creating positive pressure in vial*
• If one solution is colored and the other is clear, the colored solution should be vial B and the clear solution should be vial A (Fig. 5.14A). Insulin is often the exception (check agency policy);	*Allows nurse to determine if clear solution has been contaminated with other solution; prevents contamination of short-acting Regular insulin, which is often used in acute situations, with NPH insulin.*

A Two multiple-dose vials

B A: Single-dose vial
B: Multiple-dose vial

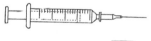

C

D

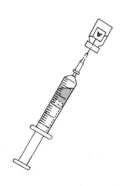

FIGURE 5.14

Action	Rationale
when mixing NPH and Regular insulin, Regular insulin should be vial B and NPH insulin should be vial A.	
• If one vial is multiple dose and one is single dose, the single-dose vial will be vial A and the multiple-dose vial will be vial B (see Fig. 5.14B).	*Prevents contamination of solution in multiple-dose container with other solution*
8. Insert air into vial A equal to the volume of solution to be withdrawn.	*Creates positive pressure in vial; prevents excess pressure on plunger that could cause plunger to pop out of barrel when withdrawing solution*
9. Remove needle from vial A and complete additional steps using same syringe.	
10. Pull end of plunger back to fill syringe with air equal to amount of solution to be drawn up from vial B.	*Draws air into syringe sufficient to create positive pressure in vial*
11. Insert air into vial B in same manner as first vial; do not, however, remove needle from vial B when air insertion is completed.	*Creates positive pressure in vial*
12. Invert vial, keeping needle in solution, and withdraw exact amount of solution needed from vial B (see Fig. 5.14C).	*Aspirates solution into syringe*
13. Attach new needle to syringe and remove cap.	*Prevents dull needle from pushing pieces of rubber top into vial and contaminating solution*
14. Insert needle into vial A, gently holding finger on plunger.	*Stabilizes plunger so drug in syringe is not pulled into vial*
15. Invert vial, keeping needle in solution, and withdraw exact amount of solution needed from vial A (see Fig. 5.14D).	*Withdraws solution from vial A*
16. Attach new capped needle to same syringe.	*Prevents tissue irritation from dull needle and medication on needle*

Action	Rationale
17. Recheck amount of solution in syringe.	*Ensures that correct amount of drug has been prepared*
18. Compare drug labels with medication record or electronic medication record.	*Provides additional identification check of drug*
19. Label syringe with drug name, date prepared, and dose.	*Provides identification information*
20. Place syringe, medication record, and additional alcohol swabs on medication tray.	*Organizes equipment for administration of drug*
21. Discard or restore all equipment appropriately.	*Promotes clean and organized environment*
22. Perform hand hygiene.	*Prevents spread of micro-organisms*

Evaluation

Were desired outcomes achieved? Examples of evaluation include:
- Desired outcome partially met: Client demonstrates the procedure for mixing of medications but required reteaching of process for withdrawing medication from second vial without contamination.

Documentation

The following should be noted on the client's chart:
- Names and dosages of medications mixed
- Site of intended injection and abnormal findings in local skin area
- Teaching provided to client about mixing medications

Sample Documentation
Date: 2/17/05
Time: 2100

10 units Regular insulin and 20 units Humulin NPH provided in one injection. Medications mixed well and administered without reaction around injection site.

Administering Intradermal Medications 👆

Purpose

Permits administration of small amounts of toxins or medication deposited under the skin for absorption

Serves as method of diagnostic testing for allergens or for exposure to specific diseases

Equipment

- Medication record or electronic medication record
- Pen
- Two alcohol swabs
- Disposable gloves
- Medication to be administered
- 1-mL syringe with 26- to 28-gauge needle
- Medication tray

Assessment

Assessment should focus on the following:
- Complete medication order
- Agency protocol regarding specific sites of skin tests
- Condition of client's skin (e.g., presence of redness, hematomas, scarring, swelling, tears, abrasions, lesions, excoriation, excessive hair)
- Client allergies

Nursing Diagnoses

Nursing diagnoses may include the following:
- Risk for injury related to allergen sensitivity

Outcome Identification and Planning

Desired Outcomes

A sample desired outcome is:
- Client shows no signs of local or systemic reaction to dermal injection.

Special Considerations in Planning and Implementation

General

Be certain that appropriate antidotes (usually epinephrine hydrochloride, a bronchodilator, and an antihistamine) are available on the unit before beginning. Allergens used in testing could cause a sensitivity or anaphylactic reaction that could be fatal.

Geriatric

Apply gentle pressure to the injection site; older clients often have fragile skin.

Delegation

As a basic standard, medication preparation, teaching, and administration are done by a licensed registered or vocational nurse. Some drugs may be given by registered nurses only. Policies vary by agency and state. BE SURE TO NOTE SPECIFIC AGENCY POLICIES FOR A GIVEN ROUTE AND DRUG BEFORE DELEGATING ADMINISTRATION!

Implementation

Action	Rationale
1. Perform hand hygiene.	*Decreases microorganism transfer*
2. Prepare drug to be administered according to the five rights of drug administration (see Nursing Procedure 5.1).	*Promotes safe drug administration*
3. Identify client by checking identification bracelet and by addressing client by name.	*Verifies identity of client*
4. Explain procedure and purpose of medication to client.	*Reduces anxiety; promotes cooperation*
5. Verify allergies listed on medication record or electronic medication record.	*Alerts nurse to possibility of allergic reaction*
6. Don gloves.	*Prevents direct contact with body contaminants*
7. Select injection site on forearm if no other site is required by agency policy or doctor's orders; use alternative sites (Fig. 5.15) if forearm cannot be used.	*Forearm is standard beginning point for intradermal injections and the area in which subcutaneous fat is least likely to interfere with administration and absorption.*
8. Position client with forearm facing up.	*Accesses injection area*
9. Cleanse site with alcohol, using a circular motion starting from the center and working outward. Allow alcohol to dry.	*Decreases microorganisms*
10. Remove needle cap.	

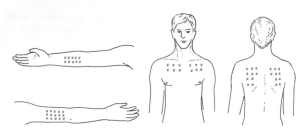

FIGURE 5.15

Action	Rationale
11. Place nondominant thumb about 1 inch below insertion site and pull skin down (toward hand).	*Pulls skin taut for injection*
12. Talk to client and warn of impending needlestick.	*Provides distraction; prevents jerking response*
13. With bevel up and using dominant hand, insert needle just below the skin at a 10- to 15-degree angle (Fig. 5.16).	*Places needle just below epidermis*
14. Once entry into skin surface is made, advance needle another ⅛ inch.	*Prevents leakage of medication*
15. Inject drug slowly and smoothly while observing for bleb (a raised welt) to form (the bleb should be present).	*Delivers medication slowly and allows nurse to stop administration if systemic reaction begins; provides visual feedback of proper drug administration*
16. Remove needle at same angle that it was inserted.	*Prevents tearing of skin*

Intradermal

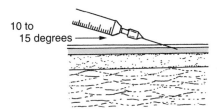

10 to
15 degrees →

FIGURE 5.16

Action	Rationale
17. Gently remove blood, if any, by dabbing with second alcohol swab.	*Cleans area while avoiding pushing medication out*
18. Observe skin for redness or swelling; if this is an allergy test, observe for systemic reaction (e.g., respiratory difficulty, sweating, faintness, decreased blood pressure, nausea, vomiting, cyanosis).	*Provides visual assessment of local or systemic reaction*
19. Reassess client and injection site after 5 minutes, after 15 minutes, then periodically while client remains in clinic.	*Detects subsequent reaction*
20. Place uncapped needle on tray.	*Prevents needlesticks*
21. Mark a 1-inch circle around bleb and instruct client not to rub the area.	*Serves as guide in locating and reassessing area later; prevents disruption of medication absorption*
22. Reposition client.	*Promotes comfort*
23. Discard equipment appropriately.	*Promotes clean and organized environment*
24. Perform hand hygiene.	*Decreases transfer of microorganisms*
25. Document administration on medication record.	*Serves as legal record of administration; prevents accidental remedication*

Evaluation

Were desired outcomes achieved? Examples of evaluation include:
- Desired outcome met: Client shows no signs of local or systemic reaction.

Documentation

The following should be noted on the client's chart:
- Name of allergen or toxin, dosage, injection site, and route of administration
- Indicators of local or systemic reaction, if any
- Abnormal findings in local skin area
- Results of test 24 to 48 h after administration
- Teaching of information about drug or injection technique

Sample Documentation
Date: 2/17/05
Time: 2100

Tuberculin skin test (0.1 mL) given intradermally in right lower forearm and circled. Noted a 0.5-cm reddened area surrounding injection site after injection, but no other reactions noted. Client tolerated procedure well; denies any complaints.

● **Nursing Procedure 5.13**

Administering Subcutaneous Medications 🖐

Purpose

Delivers medication into subcutaneous tissues for absorption

Equipment

- Medication record or electronic medication record
- Two alcohol swabs
- Nonsterile gloves
- Adhesive bandage
- Medication to be administered
- 2- to 3-mL syringe with ½- to ⅞-inch needle (25, 26, or 27 gauge) or insulin syringe
- Medication tray

Assessment

Assessment should focus on the following:
- Complete medication order
- Agency protocol regarding specific sites of subcutaneous injection
- Condition of client's skin (e.g., presence of redness, hematomas, scarring, swelling, tears, abrasions, lesions, excoriation, excessive hair)
- Client allergies

Nursing Diagnoses

Nursing diagnoses may include the following:

- Deficient knowledge regarding procedure for administration of insulin
- Risk for noncompliance related to complexity and chronicity of prescribed regimen

Outcome Identification and Planning

Desired Outcomes

Sample desired outcomes include the following:
- Client performs insulin self-injection with 100% accuracy within 1 week of receiving instructions.
- Client demonstrates adherence to medication regimen at checkup 6 weeks after discharge.

Special Considerations in Planning and Implementation

General

Check agency procedure manual before heparin or insulin administration. Some agencies recommend that aspiration after needle insertion should NOT be performed with heparin administration. Many agencies require that heparin and insulin be double-checked by another nurse during preparation.

Pediatric

For clients less than 1 year old, the vastus lateralis muscle is the preferred site. Limit the volume of injection to 0.5 mL for small children. Have an assistant hold the child and keep him or her from moving suddenly during the procedure to avoid tissue damage from needle.

Geriatric

The technique may need to be adapted in older clients, who often have less subcutaneous fat tissue. Choose needle length carefully to avoid pain and trauma to the underlying bone.

Home Health

Arrange supplies (e.g., insulin, alcohol, needles) in a line on a table to help client and family learn the sequence of steps in the procedure. Help client establish a pattern for ordering medication and supplies to avoid running out of needed materials. Instruct client to store supplies in a secure location and discard used supplies in a can until proper disposal.

Delegation

As a basic standard, medication preparation, teaching, and administration are done by a licensed registered or vocational nurse. Some drugs may be given by registered nurses only. Policies vary by agency and state. BE SURE TO NOTE SPECIFIC AGENCY POLICIES FOR A GIVEN ROUTE AND DRUG BEFORE DELEGATING ADMINISTRATION!

Implementation

Action	Rationale
1. Perform hand hygiene.	*Reduces spread of micro-organisms*
2. Prepare medication, adhering to the five rights of drug administration (see Nursing Procedure 5.1).	*Decreases chance of drug error*
3. Identify client by reading identification bracelet and by addressing client by name.	*Confirms identity of client*
4. Explain procedure and purpose of drug.	*Decreases anxiety*
5. Verify allergies listed on medication record or electronic medication record.	*Alerts nurse to possible allergic reaction*
6. Provide privacy.	*Decreases embarrassment*
7. Don gloves.	*Prevents direct contact with body fluids*
8. Perform or instruct client to perform the remaining steps.	*Helps client learn procedures*
9. Select injection site on upper arm or abdomen, away from the site of a previous injection. If administering heparin, select a site on the abdomen. Use alternative sites (e.g., thigh, upper chest, or scapular area) if arm or abdomen is not available because of tissue irritation, scarring, tubes, or dressings. Rotate sites. Figure 5.17 depicts various sites.	*Prevents repeated and permanent tissue damage; ensures that medication is administered at site with optimal absorption*
10. Position client for site selected.	*Allows nurse to access injection area; promotes comfort*
11. Cleanse site with alcohol and allow alcohol to dry.	*Reduces microorganism transfer; prevents irritation at injection site from alcohol*
12. Remove needle cap.	
13. Grasp about 1 inch of skin and fatty tissue between thumb and fingers. If administering heparin, hold skin gently; do not pinch.	*Prevents trauma to tissue*

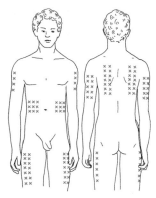

FIGURE 5.17

Action	Rationale
14. Talk to client and warn of impending needlestick.	*Provides distraction; prevents jerking response*
15. With dominant hand, insert needle at a 45-degree angle quickly and smoothly; for a client with more fatty tissue, insert at a 90-degree angle (Fig. 5.18).	*Facilitates injection into subcutaneous tissue (a heavier person has a thicker layer of subcutaneous tissue)*
16. Quickly release skin fold with nondominant hand.	*Allows spread of medication*
17. Aspirate with plunger and observe barrel of syringe for blood return. If administering heparin, do not aspirate.	*Determines if needle is in a blood vessel; with heparin, avoids traumatizing tissue and hemorrhage due to anticoagulant*

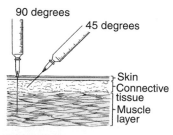

FIGURE 5.18

Action	Rationale
18. If blood does not return, inject drug slowly and smoothly.	*Delivers the medication*
19. If blood returns: • Withdraw needle from skin. • Apply pressure to site for about 2 minutes. • Observe for hematoma or bruising. • Apply adhesive bandage, if needed. • Prepare new medication, beginning with step 1, and select new site.	*Prevents injection into blood vessels*
20. After medication is injected, remove needle at same angle at which it was inserted.	*Prevents tissue damage*
21. Cleanse injection site with second alcohol swab and lightly massage. DO NOT massage after heparin injection.	*Promotes comfort; with heparin, prevents bruising and tissue damage*
22. Apply adhesive bandage, if needed.	*Contains residual bleeding*
23. Place uncapped needle on tray.	*Prevents needlestick*
24. Reassess client and injection site after 5 minutes, after 15 minutes, then periodically while client remains in clinic.	*Detects subsequent reaction*
25. Discard all equipment appropriately.	*Promotes cleanliness*
26. Remove gloves and perform hand hygiene.	*Decreases microorganism transfer*
27. Document administration on medication record.	*Serves as legal record of administration; prevents accidental remediation*

Evaluation

Were desired outcomes achieved? Examples of evaluation include:
• Desired outcome met: Client performs insulin self-injection with 100% accuracy 1 week after receiving instructions.
• Desired outcome met: Client demonstrates adherence to medication regimen at checkup 6 weeks after discharge.

Documentation

The following should be noted on the client's chart:
- Name, dosage, and route of medication; site of injection
- Assessment and laboratory data relevant to purpose of medication
- Effects of medication
- Teaching of information about drug or injection technique

Sample Documentation
Date: 2/17/05
Time: 2100

Client received first dose of regular insulin, 15 units subcutaneously in right upper arm. No scars, abrasions, or lumps noted on skin. Tolerated medication with no untoward response noted during 15-minute, 30-minute, and hourly follow-up assessments.

● Nursing Procedure 5.14

Using a Continuous Subcutaneous Insulin Pump

Purpose

Provides consistent delivery of insulin to control blood glucose levels more effectively
Allows freedom from rigid multi-injection schedule

Equipment

- Medication administration record or electronic medication record
- Prefilled insulin pump reservoir or syringe and a micro-computer that lets you adjust how much insulin is to be delivered (connected to infusion set)
- Infusion set (line with a plastic cannula; needle/cannula form may vary)
- Alcohol pads
- Tape

Assessment

Assessment should focus on the following:
- Sterility of needle on medication reservoir or syringe
- Adequacy of infusion line and insertion site
- Type of insulin (use only buffered short-acting or rapid-acting insulin)
- Expiration date of medication
- Sterility of infusion set
- Client's knowledge of and ability to manage insulin pump therapy

Nursing Diagnoses

Nursing diagnoses may include the following:
- Risk for injury related to altered mental status secondary to excessive insulin and hypoglycemia
- Ineffective management of therapeutic regimen related to deficient knowledge

Outcome Identification and Planning

Desired Outcomes

Sample desired outcomes include the following:
- Client will maintain blood glucose level within normal range during 6-week period after discharge.
- Client will demonstrate accurate procedure for maintenance of insulin pump and cannula insertion site before discharge.

Special Considerations in Planning and Implementation

General

Do not use infusion line if there is any question of the sterility of the components or if there is inflammation at the cannula insertion site (usually taped low on abdomen). Inform the physician if the site is inflamed or painful. Discard insulin if there is any indication of previous opening, inappropriate color, or sediment or if expiration date has passed. Change infusion pump set tubing every 2 to 4 days.

Home Health

Instruct client and caregiver in management of insulin pump before discharge from hospital; observe return demonstration by client and caregiver. Stress the importance of aseptic technique and monitoring site for infection, as well as need to change infusion after 3 or 4 days to avoid complications. Help client to determine where and how to obtain required medication and supplies.

Delegation

As a basic standard, medication preparation, teaching, and administration are done by a licensed registered or vocational nurse. Some drugs may be given by registered nurses only. Policies vary by agency and state. BE SURE TO NOTE SPECIFIC AGENCY POLICIES FOR A GIVEN ROUTE AND DRUG BEFORE DELEGATING ADMINISTRATION!

Implementation

Action	Rationale
1. Perform hand hygiene.	*Reduces microorganism transfer*
2. Organize equipment.	*Promotes efficiency*
3. Check label of prefilled medication container with medication record or electronic medication record, using the five rights of drug administration (see Nursing Procedure 5.1).	*Avoids client injury from wrong drug or dosage*
4. Program the insulin pump attached to infusion set tubing (or verify that insulin pump has been programmed) for basal rate insulin dose.	*Prepares for delivery of accurate basal insulin dose each hour*
5. Locate an area (usually on abdomen, buttocks, or hip) for insertion of infusion set (needle or soft cannula at end of long soft tubing).	*Delivers insulin into subcutaneous tissue for absorption; promotes comfort for prolonged infusion*
6. Cleanse skin area. Use the infusion needle to insert the flexible plastic tubing just under the skin. Remove the needle (if set permits) and tape the infusion set in place. Prime the tubing.	*Decreases microorganisms on skin; secures infusion tubing in subcutaneous tissue for medication absorption; removes air from tubing*
7. Secure beeper-sized insulin pump using a clip or by placing case in client's pocket.	*Prevents dislodgment of insulin cannula*
8. Monitor insulin level in pump and replace or refill as needed.	*Prevents disruption of insulin delivery*
9. Instruct client to administer bolus insulin dosages based on carbohydrate in-	*Provides insulin needed for proper blood sugar regulation with meals*

Action	Rationale
gestion (varies, but commonly 1 unit per 15 grams carbohydrate), if ordered.	
10. Monitor blood glucose levels every 4 hours or as ordered (fingerstick or venipuncture).	*Allows adjustment of treatment as needed to maintain adequate blood glucose level*
11. Observe the client for side effects or adverse reactions.	*Identifies complications and determines if medication adjustments are needed*
12. Instruct client and caregiver in medication purpose and effects, and observe return demonstration of injection set management.	*Ensures client is aware of what to expect with pump therapy and can manage care*

Evaluation

Were desired outcomes achieved? Examples of evaluation include:
- Desired outcome met: Client maintains blood glucose level within normal range over 6-week period after discharge.
- Desired outcome met: Client and caregiver demonstrated accurate procedure for maintenance of the insulin pump and cannula insertion site before discharge.

Documentation

The following should be noted on the client's chart:
- Name of medication
- Date and time medication was drawn
- Dosage drawn

Sample Documentation
Date: 2/17/05
Time: 2100

Client started on Regular insulin via insulin pump.
Fingerstick blood glucose before therapy: 260 mg/dl.
Client without signs and symptoms of hypoglycemia.
Follow-up fingerstick blood glucose level 110 mg/dl
1 hour after initiation of therapy.

Administering Intramuscular Medications 🖐

Purpose

Delivers ordered medication into muscle tissue

Equipment

- Medication record or electronic medication record
- Pen
- Two alcohol swabs
- Disposable gloves
- Medication tray
- Medication to be administered
- 3-mL syringe with 1-, 1.5-, or 2-inch needle (21, 22, or 23 gauge)

Assessment

Assessment should focus on the following:
- Medication order
- Site of last injection
- Allergies
- Client's response to previous injections, as noted in chart
- Intended injection site and condition (e.g., presence of bruises, tenderness, skin breaks, nodules, or edema)
- Factors affecting size and gauge of needle (client's size and age, site of injection, viscosity and residual effects of medication)

Nursing Diagnoses

Nursing diagnoses may include the following:
- Acute pain related to abdominal incision
- Anxiety related to fear of pain from invasive procedure

Outcome Identification and Planning

Desired Outcomes

Sample desired outcomes include the following:
- Client exhibits no signs of redness, edema, or pain at injection site.
- Client correctly states purpose of injection and understanding that pain will be minimal.
- Client states that pain decreased from level 8 to level 2 30 minutes after injection.

Special Considerations in Planning and Implementation

General

If nausea or pain medication has been ordered in multiple forms (oral, parenteral, or rectal), determine client's preference before preparing the medication.

Pediatric

If client is uncooperative or combative, obtain assistance to stabilize the injection site and avoid tissue damage from the needle.

Geriatric

If client is confused or combative, obtain assistance to stabilize the injection site and avoid tissue damage from the needle.

Delegation

As a basic standard, medication preparation, teaching, and administration are done by a licensed registered or vocational nurse. Some drugs may be given by registered nurses only. Policies vary by agency and state. BE SURE TO NOTE SPECIFIC AGENCY POLICIES FOR A GIVEN ROUTE AND DRUG BEFORE DELEGATING ADMINISTRATION!

Implementation

Action	Rationale
1. Perform hand hygiene.	*Reduces microorganism transfer*
2. Prepare medication, adhering to the five rights of drug administration (see Nursing Procedure 5.1).	*Decreases chance of drug error*
3. Identify client by reading identification bracelet and by addressing client by name.	*Confirms identity of client*
4. Explain procedure and purpose of drug to client.	*Decreases anxiety*
5. Verify allergies listed on medication record or electronic medication record.	*Alerts nurse to possibility of allergic reaction*
6. Don gloves.	*Decreases nurse's exposure to secretions*
7. Select injection site appropriate for client's size and age. Figure 5.19 depicts sites with anatomical landmarks.	*Provides sufficient muscle mass for medication absorption*
8. Assist client into position for comfort and easy visibility of injection site.	*Facilitates administration of injection*

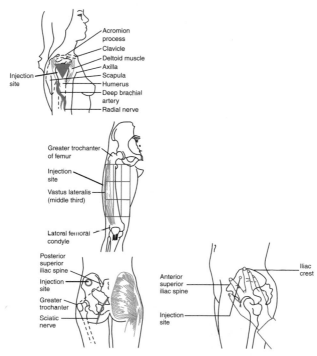

FIGURE 5.19

Action	Rationale
9. Clean site with alcohol.	*Maintains asepsis*
10. Remove needle cap.	
11. Pull skin taut at insertion area by using the following sequence:	*Facilitates smooth and complete insertion of needle into muscle*
• Place thumb and index finger of nondominant hand over injection site (taking care not to touch cleaned area) to form a V.	
• Pull thumb and index finger in opposing directions, spreading fingers about 3 inches apart.	

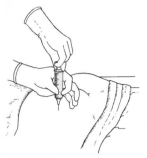

FIGURE 5.20

Action	Rationale
12. Talk to client and warn of impending needlestick.	*Provides distraction; prevents jerking response*
13. Quickly insert needle at a 90-degree angle with dominant hand (as if throwing a dart).	*Minimizes pain from needle insertion*
14. Move thumb and first finger of nondominant hand from skin to support barrel of syringe; place fingers on barrel (Fig. 5.20).	*Maintains steady position of needle and prevents tearing of tissue; allows observation of barrel when aspirating*
15. Pull back on plunger and aspirate for blood return in syringe (Fig. 5.21).	*Determines if needle is in a blood vessel rather than in muscle*
16. If blood does return when aspirating, pull the needle	*Prevents IV injection*

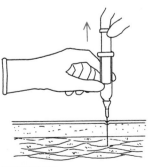

FIGURE 5.21

Action	Rationale
out, apply pressure to the insertion site, and repeat injection steps.	
17. If no blood returns, push plunger down slowly and smoothly; encourage client to talk or take deep breaths.	*Delivers medication; decreases client anxiety*
18. Remove needle at same angle as it was inserted.	*Prevents tearing of tissue*
19. Massage and clean insertion area with second alcohol wipe (if contraindicated for drug, apply firm pressure instead).	*Prevents drug from escaping into subcutaneous tissue*
20. Place needle on tray; do not recap.	*Prevents needlestick*
21. Remove gloves.	
22. Reposition client; raise side rails and place bed in lowest position with call light within reach.	*Maintains safety and comfort; allows communication*
23. Dispose of equipment properly.	*Prevents injury and spread of infection*
24. Perform hand hygiene.	*Reduces microorganism transfer*
25. Document administration on medication record.	*Serves as legal record of administration; prevents accidental remedication*

Evaluation

Were desired outcomes achieved? Examples of evaluation include:
- Desired outcome met: Client exhibits no redness, edema, or pain at injection site.
- Desired outcome met: Client correctly verbalizes purpose of injection.
- Desired outcome met: Client states that minimal pain was experienced during injection.

Documentation

The following should be noted on the client's chart:
- Name, dosage, and route of medication
- Assessment data relevant to purpose of medication
- Assessment of site before and after injection
- Effects of medication and client's response to medication
- Teaching of information about drug and techniques of administration by self or caregiver, if indicated

Sample Documentation
Date: 2/17/05
Time: 2100

Demerol 50 mg given intramuscularly in right deltoid for
c/o nagging pain in left hip. No local redness or swelling
after injection. Client tolerated injection well. Client
reports pain decreased from level 9 to level 2 within
30 minutes after administration of medication. Side
rails up and bed in low position.

● **Nursing Procedure 5.16**

Administering a Z-Track Injection 🖐

Purpose

Delivers irritating or caustic medications deep into muscle tissue
to prevent seepage

Equipment

- Medication record or
  electronic medication
  record
- Pen
- Two alcohol swabs
- Disposable gloves

- Medication tray
- Medication to be
  administered
- 3-mL syringe with 1- to
  1.5-inch needle
  (20 to 22 gauge)

Assessment

Assessment should focus on the following
- Complete medication order
- Intended injection site and condition of site (e.g., bruising,
  tenderness, skin breaks, nodules, or edema)
- Site of last injection
- Allergies
- Client's response to previous injections
- Factors affecting size and gauge of needle (e.g., client's size
  and age, site of injection, viscosity and residual effects of
  medication)
- Client's knowledge about medication and reason for use

Nursing Diagnoses

Nursing diagnoses may include the following:
- Imbalanced nutrition, less than body requirements, related to inability to absorb nutrients
- Risk for injury related to irritating effects of medication

Outcome Identification and Planning

Desired Outcomes

Sample desired outcomes include the following:
- Client makes no complaint of extreme pain after medication is administered by Z-track method.
- Client exhibits intact skin without bruising or hematoma formation.

Special Considerations in Planning and Implementation

General

Administer iron using the Z-track technique to avoid skin staining. Use a large muscle mass (i.e., ventral or dorsal gluteal muscle) for this technique. Drugs are given by this method because they are generally so irritating to the skin and subcutaneous tissue that sloughing may occur.

Delegation

As a basic standard, medication preparation, teaching, and administration are done by a licensed registered or vocational nurse. Some drugs may be given by registered nurses only. Policies vary by agency and state. BE SURE TO NOTE SPECIFIC AGENCY POLICIES FOR A GIVEN ROUTE AND DRUG BEFORE DELEGATING ADMINISTRATION!

Implementation

Action	Rationale
1. Perform hand hygiene.	Reduces microorganism transfer
2. Prepare syringe with medication, adhering to the five rights of drug administration (see Nursing Procedures 5.1, 5.8, 5.9, 5.10, and 5.11).	Prepares drug properly; decreases chance of drug error
3. Change needle after drug has been fully drawn up.	Prevents staining and irritation of skin and subcutaneous tissue when needle is inserted into skin

Action	Rationale
4. Pull plunger back another 0.1 mL.	*Makes air lock in syringe*
5. Identify client by reading identification bracelet and addressing client by name.	*Confirms identity of client*
6. Explain procedure and purpose of drug.	*Decreases anxiety; promotes cooperation*
7. Verify allergies listed on medication record or electronic medication record.	*Alerts nurse to possibility of allergic reaction*
8. Provide privacy.	*Decreases embarrassment*
9. Don gloves.	*Prevents direct contact with body secretions*
10. Assist client into prone position with toes pointed inward.	*Promotes comfort by relaxing gluteal muscles*
11. Outline dorsogluteal site by identifying appropriate landmarks; alternatively, use ventrogluteal or vastus lateralis area (see Nursing Procedure 5.15 and Fig. 5.21).	*Prevents sciatic nerve damage*
12. Clean site with alcohol and allow site to dry.	*Maintains asepsis*
13. Remove needle cap.	
14. Hold syringe with needle pointed down and observe for air bubble to rise to top (away from needle).	*Ensures that air clears needle after drug is administered so that drug can be "sealed" into muscle tissue*
15. Using fingers of nondominant hand, pull skin laterally (away from midline) about 1 inch and down (Fig. 5.22).	*Retracts skin and subcutaneous tissue from muscle*

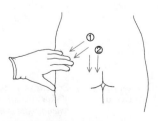

FIGURE 5.22

Action	Rationale
16. While maintaining skin re-traction, rest heel of non-dominant hand on skin below fingers (Fig. 5.23).	*Allows nurse to maintain retrac-tion and stability of needle while aspirating or if client suddenly moves*
17. Talk to client and warn of impending needlestick.	*Provides distraction; prevents jerking response*
18. With dominant hand, quickly insert needle at a 90-degree angle (as if throwing a dart) while maintaining traction on site with heel of non-dominant hand.	*Minimizes pain from insertion; ensures that needle enters muscle mass*
19. Pull plunger back and aspirate for blood return.	*Determines if accidental insertion into blood vessel has occurred*
20. If blood returns, remove needle, clean site with anti-septic swab, assess site, apply adhesive bandage, and begin injection pro-cedure again.	
21. If no blood returns, inject drug slowly, holding needle in place for 10 seconds.	*Prevents leakage into subcuta-neous tissue; allows adequate absorption time*
22. Remove needle at same angle as angle of insertion while releasing skin at the same time.	*Prevents tearing of tissue; avoids direct track between muscle and surface of skin*
23. Place alcohol swab over in-sertion area but do not massage.	*Avoids displacing drug into tis-sues, which would cause irrita-tion and pain*

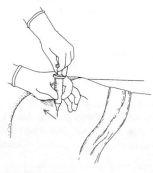

FIGURE 5.23

Action	Rationale
24. Place needle on tray; do not recap.	*Prevents needlestick*
25. Reposition client, raise side rails, and lower bed to lowest position; place call light within reach.	*Maintains safety and comfort; allows communication*
26. Dispose of equipment properly.	*Prevents injury and spread of infection*
27. Remove gloves and perform hand hygiene.	*Reduces microorganism transfer*
28. Document administration on medication record.	*Serves as legal record of administration; prevents accidental remedication.*
29. Check site 15 to 30 minutes later for pain, bleeding, fluid drainage, or bruising.	*Verifies that no seepage of medication has occurred*

Evaluation

Were desired outcomes achieved? Examples of evaluation include:
- Desired outcome met: Client states no pain present 5 minutes after injection.
- Desired outcome met: Client exhibits intact skin without bruising or hematoma formation at dorsogluteal injection site.

Documentation

The following should be noted on the client's chart:
- Name of medication, dosage, route, and site of injection
- Assessment and laboratory data relevant to purpose of medication
- Effects of medication and client's response to medication
- Condition of site before and after injection
- Teaching of information about drug or injection technique

Sample Documentation

Date: 2/17/05
Time: 2100

Client received first dose of Imferon 150 mg by Z-track injection in left dorsogluteal area. No local redness, swelling, or skin stain noted. Client tolerated procedure well. No complaints of pain, nausea, or headache.

Administering Intermittent Intravenous Medications 🧤

Purpose

Intermittently delivers medication through IV route for various therapeutic effects, most frequently treatment of infections

Equipment

- Medication record or electronic medication record
- Pen
- Disposable gloves
- Four or five alcohol swabs
- Medication to be administered mixed in 50 to 100 mL appropriate IV fluid (usually 0.9% saline or 5% dextrose) and attached to 22- or 23-gauge needle, or syringe with medication diluted in 10 to 30 mL appropriate solute
- Primary infusion setup/infusion lock (verify infusion and IV site are intact, or initiate if needed)
- Syringe with 10 mL saline for flush
- Small roll of ½- to 1-inch-wide tape

Assessment

Assessment should focus on the following:
- Complete medication order
- Condition of IV site, including patency and any discoloration, edema, or pain
- Appearance of primary IV fluid (e.g., presence of added medication, discoloration, sediment)
- Expiration dates on medication that has been mixed
- Condition of tubing already hanging, if any

Nursing Diagnoses

Nursing diagnoses may include the following:
- Risk for infection related to loss of skin integrity
- Pain related to tissue trauma secondary to burns

Outcome Identification and Planning

Desired Outcomes

Sample desired outcomes include the following:
- Client demonstrates decreased signs of infection after administration of IV medications.

- Client exhibits a patent IV site without evidence of redness, inflammation, or pain throughout therapy.
- Client reports a decrease in pain rating 30 minutes after administration of IV medication.
- Client states that upper abdominal pain has decreased within 2 days of beginning cimetidine infusions.

Special Considerations in Planning and Implementation

General

Verify the compatibility of the medication with primary infusion, flush, or admixtures in infusion.

Home Health

Instruct client and caregiver, when applicable, in medication management before discharge; observe return demonstration of administration procedure by client and caregiver.

Pediatric

When infusing intermittent medications in children, always use an infusion pump or controller and a volume-controlled chamber (such as a Buretrol or Volutrol) to prevent infusion errors related to increased rates or volumes. Check agency procedure manuals. Use the smallest amount of solution necessary to administer the medication safely and comfortably to avoid fluid overload while minimizing irritation to the blood vessels.

Geriatric

Use the smallest amount of solution necessary to administer the medication to avoid fluid overload, while using a sufficient volume to administer the medication with minimal irritation to the blood vessels (consult procedure manual, drug chart/book, or pharmacist).

Delegation

In most agencies, drugs given by the IV route may be administered by registered nurses only. POLICIES VARY BY AGENCY AND STATE, HOWEVER. CONSULT AGENCY POLICIES FOR DELEGATION OF DRUG ADMINISTRATION FOR A GIVEN ROUTE OR DRUG. Registered nurses generally administer IV push medications and medications given through central line catheters and PICC lines. IV sedation drugs are given by registered nurses. In some facilities, selected IV piggyback medications and peripheral IV saline flush solutions may be given by licensed vocational nurses with agency certification. BE SURE TO CHECK AGENCY POLICY BEFORE DELEGATING ANY DRUG ADMINISTRATION!

Implementation

Action	Rationale
1. Perform hand hygiene.	*Reduces microorganism transfer*
2. Prepare medication, adhering to the five rights of drug administration (see Nursing Procedure 5.1).	*Ensures drug is prepared safely; decreases chance of drug error*
3. Calculate infusion flow rate.	*Determines accurate infusion rate*
4. Identify client by reading identification bracelet and addressing client by name.	*Confirms identity of client*
5. Explain procedure and purpose of drug.	*Decreases anxiety; promotes cooperation*
6. Verify allergies listed on medication record or electronic medication record.	*Alerts nurse to possibility of allergic reaction*
7. Hang medication with attached tubing and needle on IV pole. If IV bolus, place syringe with prepared medication at bedside for easy access.	
8. Don gloves at any point during procedure when there is a risk of exposure to blood or body secretions (such as when untaping site for in-depth assessment).	*Decreases risk of exposure to body secretions*
9. Assess patency of IV catheter or infusion lock. Proceed to Step 10 for either IV lock or IV infusion line currently running.	*Confirms that established IV line is open*

For an IV Lock

Action	Rationale
10. Cleanse rubber port of IV lock with alcohol.	*Reduces microorganisms*
11. Stabilize lock with thumb and first finger of nondominant hand.	*Prevents pulling out of catheter*
12. Insert needle of sterile saline syringe into lock (use needleless syringe if available).	

Action	Rationale
13. Pull back on end of plunger and observe for blood return.	*Aspirates blood; ensures catheter is functional and patent*
14. If no blood returns, reposition extremity in which catheter is placed and reassess site for redness, edema, or pain.	*Checks for problems related to positioning, local infiltration, or phlebitis*
15. Discontinue IV lock and restart if unable to get blood return (see Nursing Procedures 7.4 and 7.5).	*Prevents injury due to nonfunctional catheter; establishes functional line*
16. If blood returns, insert saline.	*Flushes catheter*

Proceed to Step 17.

For an IV Infusion Line Currently Running (Primary Line)

10. Insert needle of syringe, or needleless syringe with needleless system present, containing sterile saline nearest insertion site.	*Provides access to port near catheter site for easy observation when aspirating into center of port*
11. Pinch IV tubing just above port (Fig. 5.24).	*Allows for one-way flow during aspiration*
12. Pull back on plunger and observe for blood return in the tubing; or lower fluid and tubing below level of extremity for 1 to 2 minutes.	*Aspirates for blood return; verifies catheter placement*

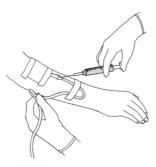

FIGURE 5.24

Action	Rationale
13. If no blood returns, reposition extremity in which catheter is placed.	
14. Reassess site for redness, edema, or pain.	*Checks for problems related to positioning, phlebitis, or infiltration*
15. Discontinue primary IV and restart if unable to get blood return (see Nursing Procedures 7.4 and 7.5).	*Establishes patent IV line*
16. If blood returns, instill saline.	*Flushes blood from catheter*
17. Cleanse rubber port to be used for insertion with alcohol.	*Reduces microorganisms*
18. Insert needle attached to tubing of mixed medication into IV lock port; for piggyback method, insert needle into port closest to top of primary tubing.	*Connects to main infusion line*
19. Secure needle with tape.	*Prevents needle dislodgment*
20. For piggyback/bolus method, lower primary bag to about 6 inches below secondary bag (mixed medication bag; Fig. 5.25).	*Provides more gravitational pull for secondary bag than for primary infusion*

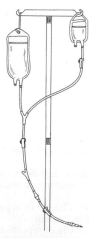

FIGURE 5.25

Action	Rationale
21. Slowly open tubing roller clamp and adjust drip rate (see Nursing Procedure 7.7).	*Prevents adverse reactions from too rapid an infusion rate*
22. Periodically assess client every 10 to 15 minutes during infusion.	*Monitors for adverse reactions and effectiveness of infusion*
23. When infusion is complete, disconnect tubing from infusion and leave medication and tubing on pole if tubing is not expired (and when administering several different piggyback medications).	*Provides greater mobility for client while maintaining cleanliness of IV tubing for future use*
24. Carefully remove needle from primary tubing and recap; for piggyback/bolus method, leave connected to port.	*Decreases destruction of primary tubing port*
25. If tubing has expired, disconnect and discard medication and tubing.	*Reduces contamination of system*
26. Insert needle of second syringe of sterile saline and inject into IV lock; then insert heparin or saline flush or readjust drip rate for primary infusion.	*Clears catheter and tubing*
27. Discard or restore all equipment appropriately.	*Promotes clean environment*
28. Remove gloves and perform hand hygiene.	*Reduces microorganism transfer*
29. Document administration on medication record.	*Serves as legal record of administration; prevents accidental remediation*

Evaluation

Were desired outcomes achieved? Examples of evaluation include:

● Desired outcomes met: Client demonstrates decreasing signs of infection and states that upper abdominal pain has stopped.
● Desired outcome met: Client's IV is patent and site free of of redness, inflammation, or pain.
● Desired outcome met: Client reports a decrease in pain rating 30 minutes after administration of IV medication.

Documentation

The following should be noted on the client's chart:
- Name, amount, and route of drug given
- Purpose of administration, if given on a when-needed (p.r.n) basis or one-time order
- Assessment data relevant to purpose of medication
- Assessment findings related to IV site
- Effects of medication on client
- Teaching of information about drug

Sample Documentation
Date: 2/17/05
Time: 2100

Client received initial dose of IV tobramycin, 80 mg via IV piggyback. Client tolerated medication with no untoward reaction. IV site remains intact. No redness or drainage from abdominal wound. Client denies abdominal pain. Temp 99.8°F, other vital signs within normal limits. Client verbalizes understanding of medication and procedure for administration.

Administering Medication by Nasogastric Tube

Purpose

Delivers medication for absorption through the gastrointestinal tract when client cannot take medication orally

Equipment

- Medication record or electronic medication record
- Pen
- Disposable gloves
- Plastic medicine cup
- Medication to be administered (liquid, capsule, powder, tablet; no enteric-coated or time-release tablets or capsules)
- Water (4 oz at room temperature)

- 30-mL syringe (cone-tipped)
- Disposable protective pad or small towel
- Tube clamp (on client's tubing)

Assessment

Assessment should focus on the following:
- Condition of nasal mucosa
- Placement of nasogastric tube
- Patency of nasogastric tube
- Form of drug (tablet, capsule, liquid suspension) and appropriateness to be crushed or diluted (and proper solution)

Nursing Diagnoses

Nursing diagnoses may include the following:
- Anxiety related to dysphagia and change in health status
- Risk for injury related to aspiration of oral medication secondary to dysphagia

Outcome Identification and Planning

Desired Outcome

Sample desired outcomes include the following:
- Client demonstrates no signs of anxiety within 1 hour of administration of sedative by nasogastric tube.
- Client tolerates medications administered by nasogastric tube without complications.

Special Considerations in Planning and Implementation

Delegation

As a basic standard, medication preparation, teaching, and administration are done by a licensed registered or vocational nurse. Some drugs may be given by registered nurses only. Policies vary by agency and state. BE SURE TO NOTE SPECIFIC AGENCY POLICIES FOR A GIVEN ROUTE AND DRUG BEFORE DELEGATING ADMINISTRATION!

Implementation

Action	Rationale
1. Perform hand hygiene.	*Reduces microorganism transfer*
2. Prepare medication, adhering to the five rights of drug administration (see Nursing Procedure 5.1).	*Ensures safe drug preparation; decreases chance of drug error*

Action	Rationale
3. Identify client by reading identification bracelet and addressing client by name.	*Confirms identity of client*
4. Explain procedure and purpose of drug.	*Decreases anxiety; promotes cooperation*
5. Verify allergies listed on medication record or electronic medication record.	*Alerts nurse to possibility of allergic reaction*
6. Prepare medication: • For a tablet: Crush tablet with a pill crusher or mortar and pestle, or between two spoons (Fig. 5.26). Mix with 10 to 20 mL lukewarm tap water. • For a capsule: Empty contents of capsule in medicine cup. Mix with 10 to 20 mL lukewarm tap water. Check medication resource or procedure manual to make sure guidelines for drug administration are being followed.	*Allows medication to go down nasogastric tube; prevents clogging the tube*
7. Assist client into proper position: semi-Fowler's in bed or sitting up in wheelchair.	*Promotes flow of fluid and medication into nasogastric tube and stomach*
8. Don gloves.	*Decreases exposure to client's body secretions*
9. Place towel or disposable pad over client's chest.	*Promotes cleanliness*
10. Release clamp on client's tube or disconnect from tube feeding.	*Provides access to open tubing system to give medication*

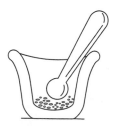 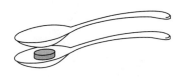

FIGURE 5.26

Action	Rationale
11. Check tube placement medications. • Attach syringe to free end of tube. • Place stethoscope on left upper quadrant below sternum (Fig. 5.27). • Instill 20 mL air into tube while listening for a "swishing" sound. • Aspirate small amount of gastric fluid and check acidity with pH indicator strip	*Prevents aspirations of secretions into tracheobronchial tree; identifies air moving into stomach*
12. Flush tube with 30 to 60 mL water.	*Lubricates inner tube to facilitate movement of medication*
13. Pull medication into syringe, attach syringe to nasogastric tube, and then gently push through tube.	*Delivers medication to stomach with minimal trauma to tissues*

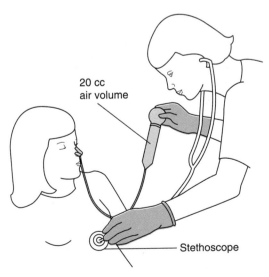

20 cc air volume

Stethoscope

FIGURE 5.27

Action	Rationale
14. Follow medication with instillation of 30 to 60 mL water.	*Prevents obstruction of tubing*
15. Clamp nasogastric tube for 30 minutes or more.	*Closes system and promotes medication passage into stomach*
16. Keep client in upright position for 30 to 45 minutes.	*Decreases risk of aspiration; facilitates movement of medication in gastrointestinal system*
17. Remove gloves and perform hand hygiene.	*Reduces microorganism transfer*
18. Discard disposable equipment and supplies and store reusable supplies.	
19. Document administration on medication record.	*Serves as legal record of administration; prevents accidental remedication*

Evaluation

Were desired outcomes achieved? Examples of evaluation include:
- Desired outcome met: Client verbalizes decreased anxiety 30 minutes after medication administered.
- Desired outcome met: Client tolerated Valium administered in 30 mL water by nasogastric tube without complications.

Documentation

The following should be noted on the client's chart:
- Name, dosage, and route of medication
- Assessment data relevant to verification of tube placement and patency
- Assessment data relevant to purpose of medication
- Client's response to medication and procedure

Sample Documentation
Date: 2/17/05
Time: 2100

NG tube patency checked and placement verified with pH paper. Medication given by NG tube. Valium 10 mg, crushed and combined with 30 mL water for NG administration. NG tube in place; currently clamped. Tubing flushed with 50 mL water after medication. Client resting comfortably in semi-Fowler's position in bed. Denies anxiety.

Administering Rectal Medication

Purpose

Delivers medication for absorption through mucous membranes of rectum

Equipment

- Medication record or electronic medication record
- Pen
- Disposable gloves
- Suppository to be administered
- Packet of water-soluble lubricant

Assessment

Assessment should focus on the following:
- Complete medication order
- Condition of anus and buttocks (ulcerations, tears, hemorrhoids, excoriation, abnormal discharge, foul odor)
- Abdominal girth, if distention present
- Client's knowledge regarding use of suppositories

Nursing Diagnoses

Nursing diagnoses may include the following:
- Risk for constipation related to insufficient fiber intake
- Pain related to gastrointestinal infection

Outcome Identification and Planning

Desired Outcomes

Sample desired outcomes include the following:
- Client has normal bowel movement within 24 hours.
- Abdominal girth decreases to 36 inches in 24 hours.
- Client verbalizes absence of abdominal pain.

Special Considerations in Planning and Implementation

Home Health

Instruct client and caregiver, when applicable, in rectal medication administration before discharge; observe return demonstration of administration procedure by client and caregiver.

Delegation

As a basic standard medication preparation, teaching, and administration are done by a licensed registered or vocational nurse. Some drugs may be given by registered nurses only. Policies vary by agency and state. BE SURE TO NOTE SPECIFIC AGENCY POLICIES FOR A GIVEN ROUTE AND DRUG BEFORE DELEGATING ADMINISTRATION!

Implementation

Action	Rationale
1. Perform hand hygiene.	*Reduces microorganism transfer*
2. Prepare medication, adhering to the five rights of drug administration (see Nursing Procedure 5.1).	*Ensures safe drug preparation; decreases chance of drug error*
3. Identify client by reading identification bracelet and addressing client by name.	*Confirms identity of client*
4. Explain procedure and purpose of drug.	*Decreases anxiety; promotes cooperation*
5. Verify allergies listed on medication record or electronic medication record.	*Alerts nurse to possible allergic reaction*
6. Don gloves.	*Decreases exposure to client's body secretions*
7. Position client in prone or side-lying position.	*Permits good exposure of anal opening*
8. Place towel or linen saver under buttocks.	*Protects sheets*
9. Remove suppository from wrapper and inspect tip.	*Reduces risk of injury from sharp tip*
10. If pointed end of suppository is sharp, gently rub tip until slightly rounded.	*Decreases chance of tearing rectal membranes*
11. Lubricate rounded tip with lubricating jelly.	*Decreases chance of tearing membranes; eases insertion*
12. Gently spread buttocks with nondominant hand.	*Exposes anal opening*
13. Instruct client to take slow, deep breaths through mouth.	*Relaxes sphincter muscles, facilitating insertion*
14. Insert suppository into rectum with index finger of dominant hand until closure of anal ring is felt (Fig. 5.28).	*Minimizes chance that suppository will be expelled*
15. Remove finger, wipe away excess lubricant from skin, and allow buttocks to fall back.	*Promotes client comfort*

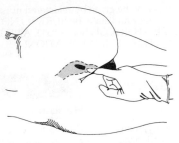

FIGURE 5.28

Action	Rationale
16. Instruct client to squeeze buttocks together for 3 to 4 minutes and to remain in position for 15 to 20 minutes. (Suppositories given to expel gas may be released at any time.)	*Decreases urge to release suppository*
17. Remove and discard gloves and paper wrapper.	*Promotes clean environment*
18. Raise side rails.	*Promotes safety*
19. Place call light and bedpan within reach.	*Facilitates communication; anticipates premature expulsion of suppository or feces*
20. Perform hand hygiene.	*Reduces microorganism transfer*
21. Document administration on medication record.	*Serves as legal record of administration; prevents accidental remediation*

Evaluation

Were desired outcomes achieved? Examples of evaluation include:
- Desired outcome not met: Client has not had a normal bowel movement over the past 24 hours since medication administration.
- Desired outcome not met: Abdominal girth remains 42 inches.
- Desired outcome not met: Client continues to complain of abdominal pain.

Documentation

The following should be noted on the client's chart:
- Name, dosage, and route of drug
- Condition of anus and surrounding area, if abnormal
- Assessment data relevant to purpose of medication

- Client's response to rectal medication and effectiveness of medication
- Teaching of knowledge about drug and self-administration of medication

---

Sample Documentation
Date: 2/17/05
Time: 2100

Acetaminophen, gr. XX suppository given for rectal temperature of 103.4°F. Slight protrusion of hemorrhoids noted. Client denies discomfort in anal area. Decrease in temperature to 101.6°F noted 1 hour after suppository administered.

● Nursing Procedure 5.20

Administering Vaginal Medication

Purpose

Delivers medication for absorption through vaginal membranes for such therapeutic effects as resolving infections and treating inflammation

Equipment

- Medication record or electronic medication record
- Pen
- Basin of warm water
- Disposable gloves
- Washcloth
- Soap
- Towel
- Sanitary pad
- Vaginal applicator
- Vaginal suppository or cream to be administered

Assessment

Assessment should focus on the following:
- Complete medication order
- Condition of vaginal area (presence of lesions, tears, bleeding, tenderness, discharge, or odor)
- Client's or caregiver's understanding of medication and procedure for administration

Nursing Diagnoses

Nursing diagnoses may include the following:
- Ineffective therapeutic regimen management related to deficient knowledge of follow-up care
- Pain related to vaginal irritation

Outcome Identification and Planning

Desired Outcomes

Sample desired outcomes include the following:
- Client has no redness, heat, swelling, abnormal drainage, or pain in vaginal area.
- Client verbalizes understanding of purpose of medication and procedure for administration.

Special Considerations in Planning and Implementation

Pediatric

Mucous membranes are thin in children; therefore, insert suppositories carefully to avoid injury to tissue.

Geriatric

Mucous membranes are thin in older clients; therefore, insert suppositories carefully to avoid injury to tissue.

Delegation

As a basic standard, medication preparation, teaching, and administration are done by a licensed registered or vocational nurse. Some drugs may be given by registered nurses only. Policies vary by agency and state. BE SURE TO NOTE SPECIFIC AGENCY POLICIES FOR A GIVEN ROUTE AND DRUG BEFORE DELEGATING ADMINISTRATION!

Implementation

Action	Rationale
1. Perform hand hygiene.	*Reduces microorganism transfer*
2. Prepare medication, adhering to the five rights of drug administration (see Nursing Procedure 5.1).	*Ensures safe drug preparation; decreases chance of drug error*
3. Identify client by reading identification bracelet and addressing client by name.	*Confirms identity of client*

Action	Rationale
4. Explain procedure and purpose of drug.	*Decreases anxiety; promotes cooperation*
5. Verify allergies listed on medication record or electronic medication record.	*Alerts nurse to possibility of allergic reaction*
6. Provide privacy.	*Decreases embarrassment*
7. Don gloves.	*Decreases exposure to client's body secretions*
8. Assist client into dorsal recumbent or Sims' position.	*Places client in appropriate position for drug placement*
9. Wash and dry perineum if discharge or odor noted.	*Promotes cleanliness; facilitates drug absorption; removes excess secretions*
10. Insert medication into vaginal applicator:	
• For a vaginal cream, place applicator over top of open medication tube, invert applicator/tube combination, and squeeze tube.	*Forces medication into applicator*
• For a vaginal suppository, remove from package and insert suppository into applicator (suppository can be inserted without applicator, if desired).	*Assists with insertion of drug into vagina at depth necessary to facilitate absorption*
11. Spread labia if vagina is not easily visible.	*Exposes vaginal opening*
12. Insert applicator into vagina about 2.5 to 3.0 inches and press applicator top down (Fig. 5.29); if using finger to insert suppository, also insert 2.5 to 3.0 inches.	
13. Remove applicator or finger.	*Completes process*
14. Instruct client to remain in bed in a flat position for 15 to 20 minutes.	*Allows time for medication to be absorbed*
15. Apply sanitary pad.	*Contains discharge*
16. Discard gloves.	*Decreases transfer of microorganisms*
17. Raise side rails.	*Prevents falls*

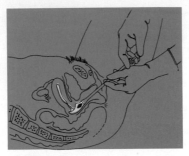

FIGURE 5.29

Action	Rationale
18. Place call light within reach.	*Provides client with means to communicate*
19. Discard or restore equipment properly (applicators may be washed with soap and water and stored in plastic wrapping, box, or washcloth).	*Promotes cleanliness; allows for future use of equipment*
20. Perform hand hygiene.	*Reduces microorganism transfer*
21. Document administration on medication record.	*Provides legal record of administration; prevents accidental remedication*

Evaluation

Were desired outcomes achieved? Examples of evaluation include:
- Desired outcome met: Client has no redness, heat, swelling, abnormal drainage, or pain in vaginal area.
- Desired outcome met: Client verbalized understanding of medication and procedure for administration.

Documentation

The following should be noted on the client's chart:
- Name, dosage, and route of medication
- Assessment data relevant to purpose of medication
- Client's response to medication
- Teaching of information about medication and techniques of self-administration

Sample Documentation
Date: 2/17/05
Time: 2100

Client received final dose of Monistat cream vaginally.
States pain and itching relieved. Verbalized understanding
of medication. Tolerated procedure with minimal
discomfort. No redness, edema, or drainage in vaginal area.

● **Nursing Procedure 5.21**

Applying Topical Medications

Purpose

Delivers medication to skin for local or systemic effects, such as
skin lubrication and reduction of inflammation

Equipment

- Medication to be applied
  (cream, ointment, gel,
  medicated disk, spray)
- Medication record or
  electronic medication
  record
- Pen
- Alcohol swabs
- Washcloth and soap
  (optional)
- Nonsterile gloves or
  sterile gloves
- Medication label or
  small piece of tape
- Dressing (if ordered)
- Medication tray

Assessment

Assessment should focus on the following:
- Complete medication order
- Checking of medication label for expiration date of drug
- Condition of last treatment area and intended site of this
  application
- Client allergy

Nursing Diagnoses

Nursing diagnoses may include the following:
- Impaired skin integrity related to local inflammation
- Deficient knowledge related to use of topical ointment

Outcome Identification and Planning

Desired Outcomes

Sample desired outcomes include the following:
● Client displays no redness, swelling, drainage, pain, or open skin areas.
● Client exhibits signs and symptoms of healing.

Special Considerations in Planning and Implementation

General

Only the specified amount should be administered to avoid overdose.

Pediatric

To promote cooperation, allow the child to apply the medication under your supervision, if possible. Keep ointment out of reach of young children to avoid oral ingestion.

Geriatric

For older clients who have memory problems, use devices that remind them that medication is to be applied (e.g., calendars, body diagrams). Older clients' skin may be sensitive, so apply medications gently to avoid damage to skin.

Home Health

Instruct client and family to monitor for side effects and possible reactions to medications.

Delegation

As a basic standard, medication preparation, teaching, and administration are done by a licensed registered or vocational nurse. Some drugs may be given by registered nurses only. Policies vary by agency and state. BE SURE TO NOTE SPECIFIC AGENCY POLICIES FOR A GIVEN ROUTE AND DRUG BEFORE DELEGATING ADMINISTRATION!

Implementation

Action	Rationale
1. Perform hand hygiene.	*Reduces microorganism transfer*
2. Prepare medication, adhering to the five rights of drug administration (see Nursing Procedure 5.1).	*Ensures safe drug preparation; decreases chance of drug error*

Action	Rationale
3. Identify client by reading identification bracelet and addressing client by name.	*Confirms identity of client*
4. Explain procedure and purpose of drug.	*Promotes cooperation; decreases anxiety*
5. Verify allergies listed on medication record or electronic medication record.	*Alerts nurse to possibility of an allergic reaction*
6. Don disposable gloves if applying gel, cream, ointment, or lotion; apply sterile gloves if applying medication to open wound or incision, and use sterile technique throughout procedure.	*Decreases exposure to client's body secretions; prevents nurse from being affected by the drug*
7. Wash application site with warm, soapy water, rinse, and pat dry (unless contraindicated). If applying drug to open skin area, use sterile cleaning solution and gauze to clean area.	*Removes surface skin debris; facilitates absorption*
8. Perform hand hygiene and change gloves.	*Maintains asepsis*
9. Apply drug to treatment area, using appropriate application method:	*Delivers medication with appropriate technique*
For ointments, creams, lotions, gels:	
• Pour or squeeze ordered amount onto palmar surface of fingers; use tongue blade to obtain if removing from multiple-dose container or jar.	*Removes drug from container*
• Lightly spread with fingers of other hand.	*Thins texture of substance; warms cold gels and creams*
• Gently apply to treatment area, lightly massaging until absorbed or as per package directions.	*Spreads drug for intended effect*
For nitroglycerin ointment:	*Prevents overdose*
• Remove previous ointment pad and wash area.	

Action	Rationale
• Squeeze ordered number of inches of drug onto paper measuring rule that comes with ointment. DO NOT TOUCH PAPER AREA CONTAINING DRUG.	*Obtains accurate dosage of drug; prevents absorption of medication*
• Apply to skin surface that has very little to no hair (e.g., upper chest, upper arm). DO NOT apply to areas where there is a heavy skinfold (abdomen) or heavy muscle mass (gluteal muscles) or to axilla or groin.	*Facilitates absorption for dilation of coronary vessels*
• Secure with adhesive application pad (comes with ointment) or plastic wrap and tape.	*Prevents premature removal of pad; ensures an occlusive dressing*
For medication disks such as nitroglycerin or clonidine [Catapres] patches:	
• Remove outer package.	
• Carefully remove protective back (usually a plastic shield).	*Permits access to disk containing premeasured drug*
• Place patch on skin surface that has little to no hair (such as upper chest, upper arm). DO NOT apply to areas where there is a heavy skinfold (abdomen) or heavy muscle mass (gluteal muscles) or to axilla or groin.	*Facilitates absorption*
• Gently press around edges with fingers. Do not touch disk.	*Provides stability during long-term use; prevents accidental absorption of medication*
For sprays:	
• Instruct client to close eyes or turn head if spray is being applied to upper chest and above.	*Protects against inhaling aerosol particles*
• Apply a light coat of spray onto treatment	

Action	Rationale
area (usually 2 to 10 seconds, depending on size of treatment area).	
10. Discard or restore all equipment properly.	*Promotes cleanliness*
11. Remove gloves and perform hand hygiene.	*Prevents spread of infection*
12. Document administration on medication administration record.	*Serves as legal record of administration; prevents accidental remedication*

Evaluation

Were desired outcomes achieved? An example of evaluation is:
- Desired outcomes partially met: Client displays no swelling, open skin area, or drainage but continues to complain of pain, and redness is present on lower left leg. Treatment continues.

Documentation

The following should be noted on the client's chart:
- Name, dosage, and route of medication
- Assessment data relevant to purpose of medication
- Condition of treatment area
- Client's response to medication
- Teaching of information about medication and techniques of self-administration

Sample Documentation
Date: 2/17/05
Time: 2100

Mentax cream applied to left foot for treatment of tinea pedis. Client still has dry, flaky skin from the web area onto the dorsum of the foot. States no itching. No other skin abnormalities noted.

Oxygenation

OVERVIEW

- Increasing restlessness or a decreased level of
  consciousness is a characteristic sign of hypoxia. Note
  associated signs or symptoms, including elevated
  respiratory rate, tachycardia, or dysrhythmia.
- One key to successful chest drainage and oxygen therapy
  is tube patency. Tubing must remain free of clots, kinks, or
  other obstructions to ensure proper equipment function.
- Agency policy and physician protocols vary regarding milking
  or stripping of chest tubes. Consult policy before intervening.
- High oxygen levels can be lethal to certain clients.
- Remember "No Smoking" signs—OXYGEN IS HIGHLY
  COMBUSTIBLE.

- When suctioning, instilling normal saline is no longer an acceptable practice because research has shown that it causes hypoxia.
- Improper maintenance of an artificial airway or tube cuff can cause trauma to mucous membranes, edema, and obstruction.
- Some major nursing diagnostic labels related to oxygenation include ineffective airway clearance, ineffective breathing pattern, impaired gas exchange, and anxiety.
- The assessment of skin color is subjective and depends on the sensitivity of the observer to color.
- For clients of African, Mediterranean, Native American, Spanish, or Indian descent:
  - The nurse must first establish the baseline skin color when caring for clients with highly pigmented skin.
  - Daylight is the best light source for this assessment; if not available, a lamp with at least a 60-watt bulb should be used.
  - Observation of skin surfaces with the least amount of pigmentation may be helpful. These include the palms of the hands, the soles of the feet, the abdomen and buttocks, and the volar (flexor surface) of the forearm.
  - The nurse should look for an underlying red tone, which is typical of all skin regardless of how dark or light its pigment. An absence of this red tone may indicate pallor.
  - Nailbeds may be highly pigmented, thick, or lined and may contain melanin deposits. Nonetheless, for baseline assessment, it is important to evaluate how rapidly the color returns to the nailbed after pressure has been released from the nail.
  - Pulmonary function is influenced by the size of the thoracic cavity. The largest chest volumes are found in whites and blacks. Asians and Native Americans have smaller chest volumes.

● Nursing Procedures 6.1, 6.2

Chest Drainage System Preparation (6.1)

Maintaining a Chest Tube (6.2)

Purpose

Removes fluid or air from chest cavity
Restores negative pressure, facilitating lung reexpansion

Equipment

- Disposable chest
- Suction source and setup
- Nonsterile gloves
- Sterile irrigation solution, saline or sterile water (500-mL bottle)
- Funnel (optional)
- 2-inch tape
- Sterile gauze sponges

Assessment

Assessment should focus on the following:
- Doctor's orders for type of drainage system (water-seal or suction) and amount of suction
- Purpose and location of chest tube(s)
- Type of drainage systems available
- Agency policy regarding use of saline or water in drainage system
- Baseline data, including level of consciousness; breath sounds; use of accessory muscles; respiratory rate, depth, and character; skin color; pulse rate and rhythm; temperature; pulse oximetry reading; arterial blood gas results
- Ongoing data, including comparison to baseline data and chest drainage type and amount

Nursing Diagnoses

Nursing diagnoses may include the following:
- Ineffective breathing pattern related to decreased lung expansion

Outcome Identification and Planning

Desired Outcomes

Sample desired outcomes include the following:
- Client ventilates effectively, as evidenced by smooth, non-labored respirations and a respiratory rate within client's normal limits.
- Client demonstrates lung reexpansion by breath sounds audible in all lobes.

Special Considerations in Planning and Implementation

General

Rules regarding clamping or not clamping chest tubes vary greatly among facilities and doctors. Investigate your agency's policy BEFORE an emergency occurs. Encourage client to ambulate with assistance as soon as it is allowed.

Pediatric

Prolonged immobility can result in frustration and restlessness in children.

Geriatric

Prolonged immobility can result in joint stiffening in older clients. Encourage ambulation with assistance as soon as it is allowed.

Delegation

The chest drainage system should be maintained by licensed personnel and should not be delegated to unlicensed assistive personnel.

Implementation

Action	Rationale
Preparing a Chest Drainage System	
1. Perform hand hygiene and organize equipment.	*Decreases microorganism transfer; promotes efficiency*
2. Open saline or water container. Unwrap drainage system and stand it upright.	*Prepares equipment*
3. Fill chambers to appropriate level: • Place funnel in tubing or port leading to suction control chamber.	*Establishes proper amount of water-seal pressure* *Prevents spillage of water*
• Pour fluid into suction control port until designated amount is reached per doctor's orders, or to specific line marked on bottle, usually indicating the 20-cm water pressure level.	*Controls amount of suction pressure*
• Fill water-seal chamber of drainage system to the 2-cm level.	*Allows air to escape chest while preventing air reflux into chest*
4. Don gloves, and connect drainage system to chest tube and suction source, if suction is indicated. • Connect tubing from client to tubing entering drainage collection chamber. MAINTAIN STERILITY OF CONNECTOR ENDS.	

Action	Rationale
• If changing drainage systems, ask client to take a deep breath, hold it, and bear down slightly while tubing is being changed quickly. Some systems have an easy snap-out and snap-in connection for system tubing changes; others require disconnecting tubing nearer chest tube insertion site.	*Prevents air influx into chest while water seal is broken*
• If indicated, connect tubing from suction control chamber to suction source.	
5. Adjust suction flow regulator until quiet bubbling is noted in suction control chamber.	*Regulates flow of suction, not pressure; vigorous flow is unnecessary unless large air leak is present*
6. Discard gloves and disposable materials.	*Reduces transmission of microorganisms*
7. Position client for comfort, with call button within reach.	*Promotes comfort and safety*

Maintaining a Chest Tube

Action	Rationale
1. Observe water-seal chamber for bubbling. Suspect an air leak if bubbling is present and client has no known pneumothorax. Also suspect an air leak if bubbling is noted and chest tube is clamped or if bubbling is excessive. Check tube connections.	*Bubbling indicates air entering system (from client or air leak); determines if air is entering system through loose tube connections*
2. Every 1 to 2 hours (depending on amount of drainage or orders):	
• Mark drainage in collection chamber.	*Detects hemorrhage or increased or decreased drainage*
• Monitor drainage system for bubbling in suction control chamber.	*Indicates that suction is intact*
• Check for fluctuation in water-seal chamber with respirations.	*Indicates patent tubing (may not fluctuate if lung reexpanded)*
3. If drainage slows or stops, consult agency policy and, if	*Reestablishes clear flow of drainage by breaking clots that*

Action	Rationale
allowed, gently milk chest tube (or strip as a last resort unless against agency policy). To milk the tubing (Fig. 6.1A):	*may be clogging tubing. Stripping tubes causes extreme pain and can cause hemorrhage.*
• Perform hand hygiene and don gloves.	*Reduces transmission of micro-organisms*
• Grasp tube close to chest and squeeze tube be-tween fingers and palm of hand.	*Pushes clotted blood toward drainage system*
• Move other hand to next lower portion of tube and squeeze.	
• Release first hand, and move to next portion of tube.	*Exerts gentle increased suction to facilitate drainage*
• Continue toward drainage container.	
• When finished, remove gloves and perform hand hygiene.	*Reduces transmission of micro-organisms*
To strip the tubing (see Fig. 6.1B):	

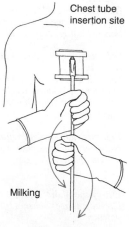

Chest tube insertion site

Milking

To drainage

A

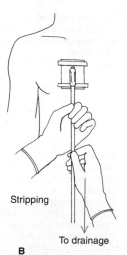

Stripping

To drainage

B

FIGURE 6.1

Action	Rationale
• Perform hand hygiene and don gloves.	*Reduces transmission of micro-organisms*
• Place lubricant on fingers of one hand and pinch chest tube with fingers of other hand.	
• Squeeze tubing below pinched portion with lubricated fingers and slide fingers down tube toward drainage system.	*Decreases pulling on tube while stripping; stabilizes tube to prevent dislodging*
• Slowly release pinch of nonlubricated fingers, then release lubricated fingers.	*Exerts increased suction to facilitate drainage (may disrupt tissue healing and cause hemorrhage, so perform with caution)*
• Repeat one or two times. Notify doctor if unable to clear clots from tubing. Monitor for tension pneumothorax/ hemothorax.	
• When finished, remove gloves and perform hand hygiene.	*Reduces transmission of micro-organisms*
4. Every 2 hours (more frequently if changes are noted):	*Facilitates prompt detection and early intervention should problems arise*
• Monitor chest tube dressing for adequacy of tape seal and amount and type of soiling.	*Determines possible source of air leak, hemorrhage, or tube obstruction and leakage at tube insertion site*
• Assess breath sounds.	*Indicates progress toward lung reinflation*
5. Every 2 to 4 hours, monitor vital signs and temperature. Use the following troubleshooting tips in maintaining chest tube drainage.	*Facilitates detection of such complications as hemorrhage, tension pneumothorax/hemothorax, and infection*
• If drainage system is turned over and water seal is disrupted, reestablish water seal and assess client.	*Prevents additional air reflux and determines presence of pneumothorax*
• If drainage decreases suddenly, assess for tube obstructions (i.e., clots or kinks), and milk tubing.	*Determines if drainage has been blocked and reestablishes tube patency*
• Check that gravity drainage systems and	*Ensures proper gravitational pull and negative water seal*

Action	Rationale
suction systems are below level of client's chest.	
• WATCH FOR TENSION PNEUMOTHORAX AND HEMOTHORAX.	*Indicates air or blood is entering chest cavity, increasing pressure on structures in chest cavity*
• If drainage increases suddenly or becomes bright red, take vital signs, observe respiratory status, and notify doctor.	*May indicate hemorrhage*
• If dressing becomes saturated, reinforce with gauze and tape securely. If permitted, remove soiled dressings without disturbing petroleum jelly gauze seal and apply new gauze pads.	*Retains original seal around chest tube*
• If drainage system becomes broken, clamp tube with Kelly clamp or hemostat and replace system immediately OR place end of tube in sterile bottle of saline solution, place bottle below level of chest, and replace drainage system immediately.	*Prevents air from entering chest; establishes temporary water seal*
NOTE: CLAMP CHEST TUBES FOR NO MORE THAN A FEW MINUTES (SUCH AS DURING SYSTEM CHANGE).	*Air can enter pleural cavity with inspiration; if it cannot escape, it will cause tension pneumothorax.*

Evaluation

Were desired outcomes achieved? Examples of evaluation include the following:
• Desired outcome achieved: Client respirations decreased from 36 breaths per minute to 18 breaths per minute.
• Desired outcome achieved: Client breath sounds heard throughout all lung fields.

Documentation

The following should be noted on the client's chart:
• System function (type and amount of drainage)
• Time suction was initiated or system changed

- Client status (respiratory rate, breath sounds, pulse oximetry, pulse, blood pressure, skin color and temperature, mental status, and core body temperature)
- Chest dressing status and care done
- Drainage characteristics and amount

Sample Documentation
Date: 1/7/05
Time: 2100

Client alert and oriented; skin warm and dry. Size 36
French chest tube intact on left 7th-8th intercostal space
anterior axillary line, with dressing dry and intact.
Disposable drainage system changed, with no signs of air leak
noted. Suction maintained at 20 cm. Drainage scant, with
10 ml serous fluid this hour. Respirations, 12; nonlabored,
with breath sounds in all lobes. Pulse oximetry at 95%.
Pulse and blood pressure within client's normal range.

● **Nursing Procedure 6.3**

Performing Autotransfusion/ Reinfusion of Chest Tube Drainage

Purpose

Reinfuses blood lost during trauma or surgery back into the client

Equipment

- Clean gloves
- Chest drainage system
- Autotransfusion collection bag or system
- Normal saline solution
- Blood tubing with microemboli filter
- Anticoagulant as prescribed

Assessment

Assessment should focus on the following:
- Physician's orders and client's response to previous treatment, if applicable

- Patent IV site, IV fluids, type and rate of administration
- Chest drainage system, including type, amount of blood in collection chamber, and amount of water in water seal
- Temperature, respiratory rate, breath sounds, blood pressure, pulse, level of consciousness

Nursing Diagnoses

Nursing diagnoses may include the following:
- Risk for imbalanced fluid volume related to sustained loss or excess fluid administration
- Risk for infection related to contamination of blood by aspiration of enteric contents

Outcome Identification and Planning

Desired Outcomes

Sample desired outcomes include the following:
- Client maintains balanced intake and output, and blood pressure and pulse are within normal or acceptable limits (as specified by physician).
- Client exhibits no signs and symptoms of respiratory infection.

Special Considerations in Planning and Implementation

General

Before beginning autotransfusion, review agency's policies and procedures for handling and transfusing blood and administering anticoagulants. Familiarize yourself with the agency's equipment. Autotransfusion systems may vary among facilities. The procedure noted in this text is a procedure with references to the Sahara Pleur-evac Autotransfusion system (Teleflex Medical).

Geriatric

Older adults are at high risk for fluid-related problems. Due to decreased heart and kidney function, they cannot compensate as easily for fluid volume excess.

 Transcultural

Assess religious beliefs regarding blood administration. Clients belonging to the Jehovah's Witness religion may believe that receiving blood has eternal consequences. Explain that the use of autotransfusion does not violate those beliefs.

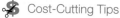 Cost-Cutting Tips

Autotransfusion/reinfusion is considered to be a cost-saving procedure because of the costs of allogenic blood collection, preparation, storage, and transport.

Delegation

This procedure must be performed by a registered nurse and cannot be delegated to unlicensed assistive personnel.

Implementation

Action	Rationale
1. Perform hand hygiene, don gloves, and organize equipment.	*Reduces microorganism transfer; promotes efficiency*
2. Explain procedure to client.	*Reduces anxiety*
3. Connect autotransfusion device to chest drainage system (always review manufacturer's guidelines):	*Allows proper function of equipment to collect blood drainage*
• Close the two clamps on top of the unit.	*Decreases risk of exposure to blood and bloody drainage of open tubing*
• Align and connect chest drainage system to autotransfusion system.	*Provides connection between the two systems, enhancing stability of the drainage systems*
• Drain remaining blood from chest tube into drainage system.	*Decreases chance of blood exposure and blood drainage from open tube; provides accurate record of drainage output*
• Clamp chest tube and disconnect from drainage set tube.	*Minimizes effects of open system on lung*
• Connect chest tube to red tube of autotransfusion set (red to red).	*Permits drainage to enter the autotransfusion set instead of chest drainage system*
• Connect the blue tube of the chest drainage system to the blue tube of the autotransfusion set (blue to blue).	*Allows use of suction from the chest drainage system by the autotransfusion system*
• Open all clamps.	*Allows for drainage*
4. As prescribed, add anticoagulants through the needleless port of the autotransfusion connector device. Remember to reinfuse within 6 hours of collection and always refer to agency policy.	*Prevents blood coagulation; prevents administration of coagulated blood to client.*
5. When ready to reinfuse, press excessive negative pressure valve on chest drainage set.	*Prevents excessive negative pressure from being administered to client*
6. Clamp the chest tube and both clamps on the autotransfusion collection device.	*Minimizes effects of open system on lung*
7. Reconnect the chest tube to the chest drainage system and unclamp the chest tube.	*Resumes standard chest drainage*

Action	Rationale
8. Connect the red and blue connectors on the auto-transfusion bag.	*Prevents leakage of blood from bag during administration*
9. Disconnect the autotrans-fusion system from the chest drainage system setup.	*Allows for blood administration*
10. Invert collection bag so that spike is exposed.	*Allows access to spike for connection of tubes*
11. Remove cap and insert a microaggregate filter into the spiked port using a constant twisting motion.	*Provides a means to administer filtered autotransfusion*
12. Attach an infusion set according to manufacturer's recommendations.	*Creates a system for administration of autotransfusion*
13. Open infusion set clamp and squeeze all air from bag until the filter and drip chamber assembly are primed with blood.	*Removes all air from bag and administration set tubing*
14. Close clamp on infusion line.	*Prevents air from being mixed with blood in tubing during priming procedure*
15. Invert bag and suspend from IV pole.	*Positions bag properly for blood administration*
16. Open infusion clamp and carefully flush line.	*Removes air from line*
17. Administer blood according to agency policy. If using a pressure cuff for blood administration, do not exceed 150 mm Hg.	*Excessive pressure may damage blood products during administration.*
18. Remove gloves, perform hand hygiene, and discard equipment.	*Reduces microorganism transfer*
19. Monitor vital signs as ordered.	*Assesses client's tolerance of procedure*

Evaluation

Were desired outcomes achieved? Examples of evaluation include:

- Desired outcome met: Client demonstrates balanced input and output.
- Desired outcome not met: Client demonstrates elevated temperature and other signs of infection.

Documentation

The following should be noted on the client's chart:
- Blood pressure, pulse, respiration, and temperature before, during, and after autotransfusion
- Client's level of consciousness and general tolerance of autotransfusion
- Amount of blood drained in chest tube and amount reinfused to client
- Amount of anticoagulant used for reinfusion of blood
- Type of system used for autotransfusion
- Patency and site of IV catheter; size of IV catheter; type of fluids (normal saline) hung with blood administration

---

Sample Documentation
Date 1/7/05
Time 2100

Size 36 French chest tube intact in left 7th-8th intercostal space anterior axillary line, with dressing dry and intact. Autotransfusion drainage system present, with no signs of air leak noted. Suction maintained at 20 cm. Drainage of 200 mL bright red blood this hour. Reinfusion of blood begun at rate of 100 mL/hour in right subclavian central IV line. Respirations, 12; nonlabored, with breath sounds in all lobes. Pulse oximetry at 95%. Pulse and blood pressure within client's normal range.

● Nursing Procedure 6.4

Performing Chest Physiotherapy: Postural Drainage, Chest Percussion, and Chest Vibration

Purpose

Loosens secretions in airways
Drains and removes excessive secretions
Decreases accumulation of secretions in unconscious or weakened clients

Equipment

- Large towel (optional)
- Suctioning equipment
- Emesis basin or tissues and paper bag
- Pillows, as needed

Assessment

Assessment should focus on the following:
- Bilateral breath sounds
- Respiratory rate and character
- Physician's orders regarding activity and position restrictions
- Ability to tolerate position changes
- Tolerance of previous physiotherapy
- Current chest radiographs
- Vital signs

Nursing Diagnoses

Nursing diagnoses may include the following:
- Ineffective airway clearance related to excessive secretions
- Risk for infection related to retained secretions
- Deficient knowledge related to purpose and techniques

Outcome Identification and Planning

Desired Outcomes

Sample desired outcomes include the following:
- The client's respirations are 14 to 20, of normal depth, smooth, and symmetric.
- Breath sounds are clear in target areas; chest radiograph reveals clear lung fields.
- Arterial blood gases are within normal limits for client.
- Client remains free of signs and symptoms of infection.
- Client verbalizes purpose of and states steps associated with the techniques.

Special Considerations in Planning and Implementation

General

Avoid performing postural drainage in clients with poor tolerance to lying flat (i.e., clients with increased intracranial pressure or extreme respiratory distress). Expect to alter the length of therapy time or degree of head elevation based on the client's tolerance. Avoid initiating therapy until 2 or more hours after solid food intake (1 hour after liquid intake). Perform therapy before meals and at bedtime to open airways for easier breathing during meals and at night. Do not percuss or vibrate over areas of skin irritation or breakdown, soft tissue, the spine, or wherever there is pain. Always have suction equipment available.

Pediatric

With children, ensure that suction equipment is functioning and readily available in case of aspiration. Use less pressure during percussion or vibration to prevent fractures.

Geriatric

Modify pressure used in percussion or vibration to prevent fracturing the brittle bones of elderly clients.

End-of-Life Care

Postural drainage, chest percussion, and chest vibration are helpful in clearing secretions and maintaining comfortable breathing for dying clients. Many dying clients have excessive secretions, and even with these techniques lung fields may not be clear.

Home Health

Use pillows and rolled linens to achieve the necessary positions. Teach procedure to family caregivers.

Delegation

Generally, this procedure may be delegated to unlicensed assistive personnel after appropriate training.

Implementation

Action	Rationale
1. Explain and demonstrate procedure to client and family.	*Facilitates relaxation and cooperation*
2. Perform hand hygiene and organize equipment.	*Reduces microorganism transfer; promotes efficiency*
3. Administer bronchodilators, expectorants, or warm liquids, if ordered or as desired.	*Loosens and liquefies secretions*
4. Encourage client to void.	*Prevents interruption of therapy*
5. Position client to drain specific lung area (Fig. 6.2). **To drain upper lung segments/lobes:**	
• Have client sit upright in bed or chair; perform therapy to right and left anterior chest (see Fig. 6.2A)	*Drains anterior right and left apical segments*
• With client leaning forward in sitting position, perform therapy to posterior chest (see Fig. 6.2B).	*Drains posterior right and left apical segments*

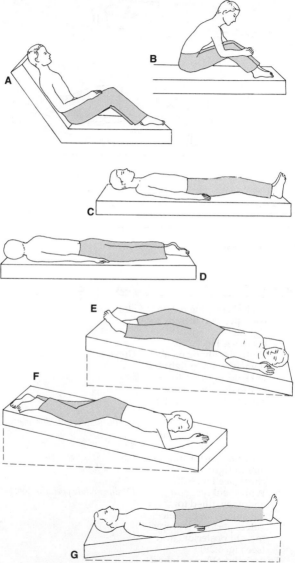

FIGURE 6.2

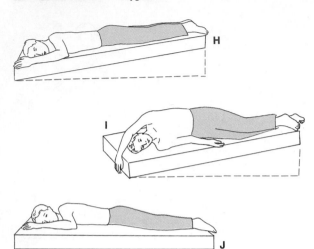

FIGURE 6.2 (continued)

Action	Rationale
• With client lying flat on back, perform therapy to right and left anterior chest (see Fig. 6.2C).	*Drains anterior segments*
• With client lying on abdomen, tilted to right or left side, perform therapy to right or left posterior chest (see Fig. 6.2D).	*Drains posterior segments*
To drain middle lobe:	
• With client lying on back, tilted to left side in Trendelenburg's position, perform therapy to right anterior chest (see Fig. 6.2E).	*Drains middle anterior lobe*
• With client lying on abdomen, tilted to left side, with hips elevated, perform therapy to right posterior chest (see Fig. 6.2F).	*Drains middle posterior lobe*
To drain basal/lower lobes:	
• With client lying in Trendelenburg's position	*Drains anterior basal lobes*

Action	Rationale
on back, perform therapy to right and left anterior chest (see Fig. 6.2G).	
• With client lying in Trendelenburg's position on abdomen, perform therapy to right and left posterior chest (see Fig. 6.2H).	*Drains posterior basal lobes*
• With client lying on right or left side, in Trendelenburg's position, perform therapy to posterior chest (see Fig. 6.2I).	*Drains lateral basal lobes*
• With client lying on abdomen, perform therapy to right and left posterior chest (see Fig. 6.2J).	*Drains superior basal lobes*
6. Maintain client in position and perform chest percussion:	*Loosens secretions in target area*
• Place towel over skin, if desired.	*Decreases friction against skin*
• Close fingers and thumb together and flex them slightly, making shallow cups of your palms (Fig. 6.3).	*Allows palms to be used to trap air and cushion blows to chest*
• Strike target area using palm cups, holding wrists stiff, and alternating hands (a hollow sound should be produced).	*Delivers cushioned blows and prevents "slapping" of skin with flat palm or fingertips*

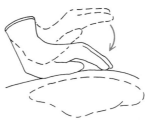

FIGURE 6.3

Action	Rationale
• Percuss entire target area, using a systematic pattern and rhythmic hand alternation.	*Ensures loosening of secretions in entire target area*
• Continue percussion for 1 to 2 minutes per target area, if tolerated.	*Maximizes loosening of secretions from airway*
7. Perform chest vibration:	
• Instruct client to breathe in deeply and exhale slowly (may use pursed-lip breathing).	*Uses air movement to push secretions from airways*
• With each respiration, perform vibration techniques as follows:	
○ Place hands on top of one another over target area (Fig. 6.4).	
○ Instruct client to take deep breath.	
○ As client exhales slowly, deliver a gentle tremor or shaking by tensing your arms and hands and making hands shake slightly.	*Provides gentle vibration to shake secretions loose*
○ Continue tremor throughout exhalation phase.	*Moves secretions from lobes of lungs and bronchi into trachea*
○ Relax arms and hands as client inhales.	
○ Repeat vibration process for five to eight breaths, moving hands to different sections of target area.	*Loosens secretions over entire target area*

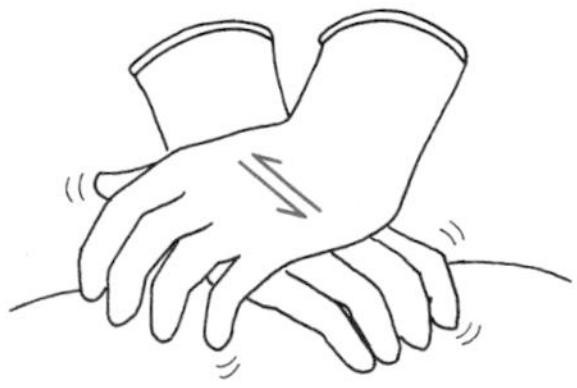

FIGURE 6.4

Action	Rationale
8. Assist client into position for coughing or position client for suctioning of trachea.	*Removes secretions from lungs accumulating in trachea*
9. Position client to drain next target area and repeat percussion and vibration.	
10. Continue sequence, repeating percussion, vibration, and cough/suction until identified target areas have been drained.	*Completes drainage of congested lung fields; clears secretions from obstructed lung fields and prevents obstruction of airways*
11. Assess breath sounds in targeted lung fields.	*Evaluates effectiveness of therapy and need for additional treatment*
12. Assist client with mouth care.	*Removes residual secretions from oral cavity and freshens mouth*
13. Position client in bed with head of bed elevated 45 degrees or more.	*Facilitates lung expansion and deep breathing*
14. Turn client on his or her side with pillow at back.	*Facilitates movement of secretions*
15. Raise side rails and place call light within reach.	*Promotes safety; allows communication*
16. Perform hand hygiene and document procedure.	*Reduces microorganism transfer; facilitates client care*

Evaluation

Were desired outcomes achieved? Examples of evaluation include:
- Desired outcome met: Breath sounds clear to auscultation in all lung fields.
- Desired outcome met: Respiratory rate 14 breaths per minute and without retractions.
- Desired outcome met: Productive cough with expectoration of moderate amount of white sputum.

Documentation

The following should be noted on the client's chart:
- Breath sounds before and after procedure
- Character of respirations
- Significant changes in vital signs
- Color, amount, and consistency of secretions
- Ability to expectorate sputum or need to suction secretions
- Tolerance to treatment (e.g., state of incisions, drains)
- Replacement of oxygen source, if applicable

Sample Documentation
Date: 1/7/05
Time: 2100

Postural drainage with chest percussion and vibration performed to right upper, middle, and lower lung lobes. Cough productive with thick, yellow sputum. Positioned on left side with oxygen at 2 L per cannula.

● **Nursing Procedure 6.5**

Applying a Nasal Cannula/ Face Mask 🖑

Purpose

Provides client with additional concentration of oxygen to promote tissue oxygenation

Equipment

- Oxygen humidifier (and distilled water, if needed for humidifier)
- Oxygen source wall or cylinder)
- Oxygen flow meter
- Nasal cannula or appropriate face mask

- Nonsterile gloves
- "No Smoking" sign
- Cotton balls
- Washcloth
- Petroleum jelly

Assessment

Assessment should focus on the following:
- Doctor's order for oxygen concentration, method of delivery, and parameters for regulation (blood gas levels, pulse oximetry values)
- Baseline data: level of consciousness, respiratory status (rate, depth, signs of distress), blood pressure, and pulse
- Color of skin and mucous membranes

Nursing Diagnoses

Nursing diagnoses may include the following:
- Ineffective breathing pattern related to neuromuscular impairment
- Anxiety related to inability to breathe
- Ineffective tissue perfusion (cardiopulmonary) related to poor oxygen distribution

Outcome Identification and Planning

Desired Outcomes

Sample desired outcomes include the following:
- Respiratory rate ranges from 14 to 20 breaths per minute; breaths of normal depth, smooth, and symmetric; lung fields are clear; no cyanosis.
- Client demonstrates no anxiety about breathing.

Special Considerations in Planning and Implementation

General

Check agency policy about the need for a physician's order to initiate oxygen therapy. In most acute situations, placing the client on oxygen is a nursing decision and does not require a doctor's order. Once oxygen is applied, notify the doctor for further orders. Use a face mask rather than a nasal cannula to provide better control of inspired oxygen concentration. If high oxygen percentages are needed, the nasal cannula may be unsuitable for emergency oxygen delivery. If the client has a history of chronic lung disease or extensive tobacco abuse, DO NOT USE MORE THAN 2 TO 3 L OF NASAL OXYGEN (30% FACE MASK) WITHOUT A DOCTOR'S ORDER.

Pediatric

An oxygen tent or canopy is the most suitable oxygen delivery method for infants and very young children. Young children are very sensitive to high levels of oxygen. Be careful not to expose them to a high percentage of oxygen for extended periods unless ordered.

Geriatric

Monitor for signs of chronic lung disease and take appropriate precautions.

End-of-Life Care

Administer supplemental oxygen as ordered, even though oxygen does not relieve the classic air hunger that occurs during the dying process. A fan that circulates cool air or opening the windows can make the client more comfortable. Keep the bed away from the wall so that air can circulate freely. If the client experiences dyspnea and tachypnea, expect to administer morphine as prescribed. Morphine reduces anxiety and the feeling of breathlessness.

Home Health

Contact the medical equipment supplier for assistance with problems. Place "No Smoking" signs on the door of the client's home if oxygen is in use. Use extra-long tubing to permit the client to move from room to room without moving the oxygen cylinder. Expect to use pulse oximetry in place of arterial blood gas sampling to assess oxygenation.

▼▼▼ Transcultural

Clients from certain ethnic/cultural backgrounds consider touching the head a taboo. Discuss alternatives (e.g., have client or family member apply the cannula or mask). With clients of African or Mediterranean descent, use caution when assessing for cyanosis, particularly around the mouth, because this area normally appears dark blue. Evaluate each client individually because coloration varies from person to person.

Cost-Cutting Tips

Use humidification only for long-term oxygen therapy via nasal cannula, for rates over 3 to 4 L/min, or if the client is dehydrated.

Delegation

This procedure may be performed by respiratory therapy personnel. The registered nurse should carefully monitor oxygen administration. Unlicensed assistive personnel may reapply oxygen therapy (e.g., after assisting a client to the bathroom), but the assistant should not initiate therapy.

Implementation

Action	Rationale
1. Perform hand hygiene and organize equipment.	*Decreases microorganism transfer; promotes efficiency*
2. Explain equipment and procedure to client.	*Decreases anxiety and facilitates cooperation*
3. Insert flow meter into outlet on wall, or place oxygen cylinder near client.	*Allows for control of oxygen flow*
4. Prepare humidifier. Add distilled water, if needed, or remove prefilled bottle from package and screw enclosed spiked cap to bottle (Fig. 6.5A).	*Delivers moistened oxygen to mucous membranes of airway*
5. Connect humidifier to flow meter (see Fig. 6.5B).	*Provides moisture to oxygen*

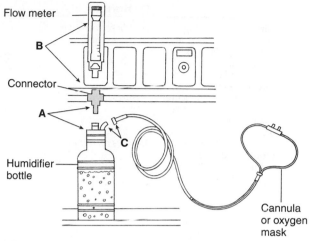

Flow meter

B

Connector

A

C

Humidifier
bottle

Cannula
or oxygen
mask

FIGURE 6.5

Action	Rationale
6. Connect humidifier to tubing attached to cannula or mask (see Fig. 6.5C).	*Connects humidification to delivery mechanism*
7. Turn on oxygen flow meter until bubbling is noted in humidifier. If no bubbling is noted, check that flow meter is securely inserted, ports of humidifier are patent, and connections are tight. Contact respiratory therapist or supervisor if you cannot correct the problem.	*Determines if oxygen flow is adequate and connections are intact*
8. Regulate flow meter as ordered.	*Permits delivery of correct oxygen concentration*
9. Don clean gloves.	*Prevents contact with secretions*
10. Have client blow nose or clear nares of secretions with moist cotton balls.	*Removes secretions*
11. Apply nasal cannula or face mask: **For nasal cannula:** • Place cannula prongs into client's nares.	

Action	Rationale
• Slip attached tubing around client's ears and under chin (Fig. 6.6). Place cotton between tubing and ear for comfort, as needed.	*Aids in securing cannula; provides comfort*
• Tighten tubing to secure cannula, but make sure client is comfortable.	*Ensures proper fit*
For face mask:	
• Place mask over nose, mouth, and chin.	*Ensures correct fit*
• Adjust metal strip at nose bridge of mask to fit securely over bridge of client's nose.	*Individualizes fit*
• Pull elastic band around back of head or neck.	*Secures mask*
• Pull band at sides of mask to tighten (Fig. 6.7).	*Ensures secure fit*
• If appropriate, place cotton or gauze pad under bridge of face mask.	*Decreases pressure on nasal area*
12. Check oxygen flow rate and doctor's orders every 8 hours.	*Ensures correct level of oxygen administration*
13. Remove cannula each shift or every 4 hours to assess skin, apply petroleum jelly to nares, and clean accumulated secretions. Remove mask every 2 to 4 hours, wipe	*Provides opportunity to assess skin condition; promotes comfort; prevents infection*

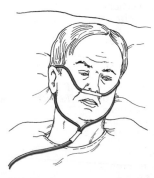

FIGURE 6.6

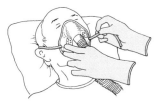

FIGURE 6.7

Action	Rationale
away accumulated mist, and assess underlying skin.	
14. Position client for comfort with head of bed elevated.	*Facilitates lung expansion for gas exchange*
15. Dispose of or store equipment appropriately.	*Decreases spread of micro-organisms*
16. Discard gloves and perform hand hygiene.	*Reduces transfer of micro-organisms*
17. Place "No Smoking" signs on door and over bed.	*Prevents fire (oxygen is combustible)*
18. Evaluate respirations.	*Aids in determining effectiveness of oxygen administration*

Evaluation

Were desired outcomes achieved? Examples of evaluation include:

- Desired outcome met: Pulse oximetry 95%.
- Desired outcome met: Client does not display restlessness or other signs of anxiety.
- Desired outcome met: Mucous membranes pink and capillary fill time less than 3 seconds.

Documentation

The following should be noted on the client's chart:

- Time of initiation of oxygen therapy
- Amount of oxygen and delivery method
- Respiratory status before and after initiation
- Color of skin and mucous membranes
- Teaching performed regarding therapy, and client's understanding of teaching
- Blood gas results
- Pulse oximetry levels
- Pulse rate
- Signs of anxiety
- Capillary fill time

Sample Documentation
Date: 1/7/05
Time: 2100

Client complained of chest pain and shortness of breath.
Rated pain as 6 on scale of 1 to 10 (1 no pain, 10 worst
pain ever experienced). Three liters O_2 begun per nasal
cannula. Respiratory rate, 32/min before oxygen
administration, decreased to 24/min within 10 min.
Resting comfortably.

● **Nursing Procedure 6.6**

Inserting an Oral Airway

Purpose

Holds tongue forward to maintain open airway
Facilitates removal of secretions

Equipment

- Oral airway
- Equipment for suctioning
- Tape strips—one approximately 20 inches, one 16 inches
  (may use commercially manufactured airway holder)
- Tongue depressor
- Petroleum jelly
- Mouth moistener or swabs with mouthwash
- Nonsterile gloves

Assessment

Assessment should focus on the following:
- Level of consciousness, agitation, and ability to push airway
  from mouth
- Respiratory status (respiratory rate, congestion in upper
  airways), blood pressure, pulse
- Presence of cyanosis
- Color, amount, and consistency of secretions
- Condition of oral mucous membranes
- Alternative methods of maintaining airway
- Use of dentures/dentition aids

Nursing Diagnoses

Nursing diagnoses may include the following:
- Ineffective breathing pattern related to airway blockage by tongue

Outcome Identification and Planning

Desired Outcomes

Sample desired outcomes include the following:
- Client will attain and maintain clear airway passage, evidenced by nonlabored respirations and clear breath sounds.
- Airway is patent and free of secretions.

Special Considerations in Planning and Implementation

General

If client is alert and agitated enough to push airway out or resist it, DO NOT INSERT. Airway could stimulate gag reflex and cause client to aspirate. Use another method of maintaining airway, if needed. If goal is to prevent client from biting on endotracheal tube, use a bite block, preferably a dental bite block, and secure it well to prevent block from sliding to back of throat.

Pediatric

Check for appropriate airway size before insertion because pediatric-sized oral airways are available. Use the Broselow pediatric kit or place the airway on the outside of the child's face in the appropriate position to approximate size.

Geriatric

Remove dentures, if present, before insertion.

End-of-Life Care

If desired, use oral airways to maintain an open airway and provide access for suctioning in clients who are not alert. Do not use them in clients who are alert, as they are uncomfortable and unnatural.

Home Health

Teach family how to insert airway and perform maintenance between nurse's visits.

Transcultural

Clients from some ethnic/cultural backgrounds consider touching the head a taboo. Discuss alternatives, such as having a family member assist with insertion. With clients of African or Mediterranean descent, use caution when assessing for cyanosis, particularly around the mouth, because this area may be dark blue normally. Coloration varies from person to person and should be carefully evaluated on an individual basis.

Delegation

Insertion of oral airways should not be delegated to unlicensed assistive personnel. Respiratory therapy personnel often perform the procedure.

Implementation

Action	Rationale
1. Explain procedure to client and family.	*Decreases anxiety and facilitates cooperation*
2. Perform hand hygiene and organize equipment.	*Reduces microorganism transfer; promotes efficiency*
3. Lay long strip of tape down with sticky side up and place short strip of tape over it with sticky side down, leaving equal length of sticky tape exposed on either end of long strip. Split either end of tape 2 inches (Fig. 6.8). A commercial holder may also be used.	*Prepares tape to hold airway*
4. Don gloves.	*Avoids contact with secretions*
5. Rinse airway in cool water.	*Facilitates insertion*
6. Open mouth and place tongue blade on front half of tongue.	*Flattens tongue, making insertion easier*
7. Turn airway on side and insert tip on top of tongue (Fig. 6.9).	*Promotes deeper insertion of airway without stimulating gag reflex*
8. Slide airway in until tip is at lower half of tongue.	*Follows groove of oral passage*
9. Remove tongue blade.	
10. Turn airway so tip points toward tongue; outer ends of airway should be vertical.	*Ensures accurate placement*
11. Place tape under client's neck with ends lying on either side.	*Places tongue under curve of airway, holding tongue forward and away from pharynx*
12. Pull one end of tape across client's mouth with splits taped across upper and lower ends of airway (Fig. 6.10).	*Secures airway in mouth*
13. Repeat with other end of tape.	*Places nonsticky portion under neck*
14. Suction mouth and throat if needed.	*Removes pooled secretions*

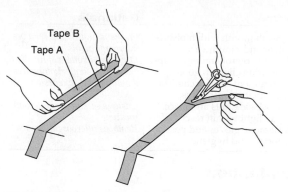

FIGURE 6.8

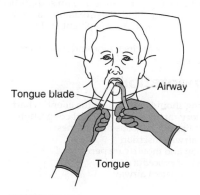

FIGURE 6.9

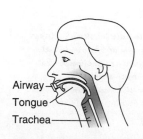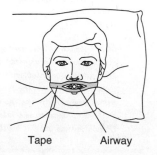

FIGURE 6.10

Action	Rationale
15. Swab mouth with moisturizer and mouthwash.	*Freshens mouth and removes microorganisms*
16. Apply petroleum jelly to lips.	*Decreases dryness of lips*
17. Position client in good alignment and for comfort.	*Facilitates comfort; enhances diaphragmatic excursion*
18. Evaluate respirations.	
19. Raise side rails and place call light within reach.	*Ensures safety; permits communication*
20. Remove gloves and perform hand hygiene.	*Removes microorganisms*

Evaluation

Were desired outcomes achieved? Examples of evaluation include:
- Desired outcome met: Respirations even and unlabored with a rate of 12 breaths per minute. Breath sounds heard bilaterally clear to auscultation. Pulse oximetry at 98%.
- Desired outcome met: Airway patent and free of excess secretions.
- Desired outcome not met: Lips and mucous membranes dry and cracked.

Documentation

The following should be noted on the client's chart:
- Respiratory rate, quality, degree of congestion
- Status of lips and mucous membranes
- Time of airway insertion
- Suctioning and mouth care performed
- Tolerance of procedure
- Evidence of patent airway

Sample Documentation

Date: 1/7/05
Time: 2100

Client semicomatose, moves arms to painful stimuli. Upper airway congestion noted, with tongue at back of throat. Oral airway inserted, with no resistance. Suctioned clear secretions from mouth. Mouth swabs to oral area, petroleum jelly to lips. No broken skin noted on lips or in oral area. Respirations rate at 14 breaths per minute. Breath sounds present bilaterally.

Inserting and Maintaining a Nasal Airway 🖐

Purpose

Facilitates removal of secretions
Maintains airway patency

Equipment

- Nasal airway
- Equipment for suctioning
- Water-soluble lubricant
- Petroleum jelly
- Moist tissue/cotton balls
- Cotton-tipped swabs
- Nonsterile gloves
- Washcloth

Assessment

Assessment should focus on the following:
- Level of consciousness, agitation, and inability to tolerate oral airway
- Alternative methods of maintaining airway
- Respiratory status (respiratory rate, congestion in upper airways)
- Blood pressure, pulse
- Color, amount, and consistency of secretions
- Nasal patency and condition of nares

Nursing Diagnoses

Nursing diagnoses may include the following:
- Ineffective airway clearance related to excessive secretions
- Impaired skin integrity (nares) related to use of nasal airway

Outcome Identification and Planning

Desired Outcomes

Sample desired outcomes include the following:
- Client attains and maintains clear airway passage.
- Client exhibits smooth, nonlabored respirations.
- Breath sounds are clear.
- Skin integrity of the nose is maintained; nasal mucous membranes are intact and without dryness or irritation.

Special Considerations in Planning and Implementation

General

Base the decision to use a continuous or intermittent nasal air-way on the client's needs and the circulation to the underlying tissue. If circulation is poor, anticipate the need to move the airway between nares frequently or consider an alternate method of airway maintenance. If airway is difficult to insert, expect to maintain it continuously; check the airway and pro-vide care frequently.

Pediatric

Inspect the airway every 1 to 2 hours. The small airway diame-ter can easily become obstructed by blood, mucus, vomitus, or the soft tissue of the pharynx.

Geriatric

Check the nasal area and provide skin care frequently because the older client's tissue is often thin and fragile and easily traumatized.

End-of-Life Care

Nasal airways are useful in end-of-life care to maintain an open airway.

Home Health

Teach family members how to insert the airway and perform maintenance between the nurse's visits.

Transcultural

With clients of African or Mediterranean descent, use caution when assessing for cyanosis, particularly around the mouth, because this area may be dark blue normally. Coloration varies from person to person and should be evaluated on an individ-ual basis.

Cost-Cutting Tips

For home use, instruct the family to purchase an extra nasal airway so the airways can be alternated. The nasal airway can be washed with soap and water and reused.

Delegation

Insertion of a nasal airway should not be delegated to unli-censed assistive personnel. Respiratory therapy personnel often perform this procedure.

Implementation

Action	Rationale
Inserting the Airway	
1. Explain procedure to client and family.	*Decreases anxiety; promotes cooperation*
2. Perform hand hygiene and organize equipment.	*Reduces microorganism transfer; promotes efficiency*
3. Don gloves.	*Avoids contact with secretions*
4. Ask client to breathe through one naris while the other is occluded; repeat with other naris.	*Determines patency of nasal passage*
5. Have client blow nose with both nares open (if client cannot assist, proceed to next step).	*Removes excess mucus and dried secretions*
6. Clean mucus and dried secretions from nares with wet tissue or cotton-tipped swab.	*Clears nasal passage*
7. Lubricate airway with water-soluble lubricant.	*Facilitates insertion*
8. Insert airway into naris in a smooth downward arch (Fig. 6.11).	*Decreases trauma to nasal tissue*
9. Roll airway from side to side while gently pushing down.	*Promotes deeper insertion of airway without tissue damage*
10. Slide airway in until horn of airway fits against outer naris.	*Ensures accurate placement*

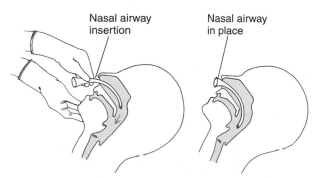

Nasal airway insertion

Nasal airway in place

FIGURE 6.11

Action	Rationale
11. Remove excess lubricant.	*Promotes comfort*
12. Suction pharynx and mouth if needed (see Nursing Procedure 6.10).	*Removes pooled secretions*
13. Apply petroleum jelly to nares.	*Decreases dryness*
14. Reposition client.	
15. Evaluate respirations.	*Determines if airway is patent*
16. Discard gloves.	*Decreases spread of organisms*
17. Raise side rails and place call light within reach.	*Prevents falls; permits communication*

Maintaining the Airway

Action	Rationale
18. At least once each shift, don gloves, slide airway slightly outward, and inspect underlying tissue.	*Assesses condition of nasal mucosa and tissues*
19. Lubricate naris with petroleum jelly and massage gently.	*Keeps tissue moist; promotes skin circulation*
20. Alternate nares (if both are unobstructed) if airway is to be maintained for extended periods or inserted and removed for each suctioning episode.	*Maintains integrity of nasal mucosa*
21. Clean and store the airway:	
• Don gloves and gently pull airway out using a side-to-side twisting motion.	*Prevents transfer of microorganism and reduces risk of trauma to mucous membranes*
• Cover tube with washcloth as it is withdrawn.	*Prevents client from seeing dirty tube*
• If client cannot maintain airway while cleaning takes place, insert another nasal airway.	
• Clean nares with moist cotton ball, and apply petroleum jelly to nares.	*Decreases dryness*
• Place tube in warm, soapy water and soak for 5 to 10 minutes; pass water through tube several times.	*Loosens thick and dried secretions*
• Use cotton and cotton-tipped swabs to clean lumen of tube.	*Removes secretions*

Action	Rationale
• Rinse tube with clear water.	Removes soap and secretions
• Dry lumen with cotton-tipped swabs.	Removes remaining water
• Cover airway in clean, dry cloth and store at bedside.	Keeps airway clean and dry for future use
• Discard soiled equipment appropriately and remove gloves.	Removes microorganisms

Evaluation

Were desired outcomes achieved? Examples of evaluation include:
- Desired outcome met: Respiratory rate 12 with nonlabored respirations.
- Desired outcome met: Airway is patent.
- Desired outcome met: Nasal mucosa intact without dryness or tears.

Documentation

The following should be noted on the client's chart:
- Purpose for insertion
- Time of airway insertion
- Client's tolerance of procedure
- Suctioning and skin care performed
- Respiratory rate, quality, degree of congestion
- Status of nares

Sample Documentation
Date: 1/7/05
Time: 2100

Client alert, restless, moves arms to painful stimuli. Upper airway congestion noted with tongue at back of throat. Nasal airway inserted with no resistance. Suctioned clear secretions from pharynx. Oral moisturizer swabs to oral area, petroleum jelly to nasal entrance. No broken skin on nares. Respiratory rate 14 breaths per minute and nonlabored; lungs clear to auscultation.

Suctioning an Oral Airway

Purpose

Clears oral airway of secretions
Facilitates breathing
Decreases halitosis and anorexia by removing excess pooling of
secretions on the mouth

Equipment

- Suction source (wall suction or portable suction machine)
- Large towel
- Nonsterile gloves
- Irrigation saline or sterile water
- Cup
- Oral moisturizer swabs
- Mouthwash (optional)
- Petroleum jelly
- Suction catheter (adult, size 14 to 16 French; pediatric, 8 to 12)
  or oral suction tool (Yankauer)

Assessment

Assessment should focus on the following:
- Respiratory status (respirations, breath sounds, respiratory
  character)
- Lips and mucous membranes (dryness, color, amount and
  consistency of secretions)
- Circulatory indicators (skin color and temperature, capillary
  fill, blood pressure, pulse)
- Ability or desire of client to perform own suctioning
- Evidence of secretions (color, amount, consistency)

Nursing Diagnoses

Nursing diagnoses may include the following:
- Ineffective airway clearance related to weak cough
- Altered nutrition: less than body requirements related to
  excess oral secretions

Outcome Identification and Planning

Desired Outcomes

Sample desired outcomes include the following:
- Client's upper airway patency is attained and maintained.

- Client's respiratory rate ranges between 12 and 20 breaths per minute (or within normal limits for client).
- Client exhibits a clear upper airway and no pooling of oral secretions.

Special Considerations in Planning and Implementation

General

If a client, adult or child, is capable and wishes to manage suctioning independently, provide instruction in the use of the suction catheter or Yankauer catheter.

Pediatric

Suctioning of infants may require two people. Enlist the help of parents in assisting and in soothing the infant.

Geriatric

Remove dentures before suctioning.

Home Health

Client and caregivers may use a bulb syringe for oral suctioning at home. These can be purchased at a pharmacy. Oral Yankauer suction catheters may be reused after being cleaned with soap and water.

 Cost-Cutting Tips

Oral Yankauer suction catheters can be reused after being cleaned.

Delegation

Unlicensed assistive personnel may perform oral suctioning.

Implementation

Action	Rationale
1. Explain procedure to client.	*Reduces anxiety*
2. Perform hand hygiene and organize equipment.	*Reduces microorganism transfer; promotes efficiency*
3. Check suction apparatus for appropriate functioning.	*Maintains safety*
4. Position client in semi-Fowler's or Fowler's position.	*Promotes forward draining of secretions in mouth*
5. Turn suction source on and place finger over end of attached tubing. Use 50 to 120 mm Hg pressure.	*Tests suction apparatus*
6. Open sterile irrigation solution and pour into cup.	*Allows for sterile rinsing of catheter*

Action	Rationale
7. Open mouthwash and dilute with water (optional).	*Freshens mouth and decreases oral microorganisms*
8. Don gloves.	*Prevents contact with secretions*
9. Open suction catheter package.	*Provides access to equipment*
10. Place towel under client's chin.	*Prevents soiling of clothing*
11. Attach suction control port of suction catheter to tubing of suction source.	*Promotes suction through catheter*
12. Lubricate 3 to 4 inches of catheter tip with irrigating solution.	*Prevents mucosal trauma when catheter is inserted*
13. Ask client to push secretions to front of mouth.	*Makes secretion removal easier*
14. Insert catheter into mouth along jawline and slide to oropharynx until client coughs or resistance is felt. BE SURE FINGER IS NOT COVERING OPENING OF SUCTION PORT.	*Promotes removal of pooled secretions*
15. Withdraw catheter slowly while applying suction by covering suction port.	*Removes secretions from oropharynx*
16. AVOID DIRECT CONTACT OF CATHETER WITH IRRITATED OR TORN MUCOUS MEMBRANES.	*Prevents additional trauma to oral tissue*
17. Place tip of suction catheter in sterile solution and apply suction for 1 to 2 seconds.	*Clears secretions from tubing*
18. Ask client to take three or four breaths while you auscultate for bronchial breath sounds and assess status of secretions.	*Permits reoxygenation; determines need for repeat suctioning*
19. Repeat steps 13 to 17 once or twice if secretions are still present.	*Promotes clearing of airway*
20. When secretions are removed, irrigate mouth with 5 to 10 mL mouthwash and ask client to rinse out mouth.	*Removes microorganisms and thick secretions; freshens breath and improves taste sensation*
21. Suction mouth; repeat irrigation and suctioning.	*Removes secretions and residual mouthwash*
22. Disconnect suction catheter from machine tubing, turn off suction source, and discard catheter.	

Action	Rationale
23. Apply petroleum jelly to lips and mouth moistener to inner lips and tongue, if desired.	*Prevents cracking of lips and maintains moist membranes*
24. Dispose of or store equipment properly.	*Decreases spread of microorganisms; promotes organization for future use*
25. Discard gloves.	
26. Position client for comfort with head of bed elevated 45 degrees.	*Lowers diaphragm and promotes lung expansion*
27. Raise side rails and leave call light within reach.	*Prevents falls; permits communication*

Evaluation

Were desired outcomes achieved? Examples of evaluation include:
- Desired outcome not met: Client still displays pooling of secretions.
- Desired outcome met: Client maintains normal respiratory rate.

Documentation

The following should be noted on the client's chart:
- Breath sounds after suctioning
- Character of respirations after suctioning
- Color, amount, and consistency of secretions
- Type of suctioning performed
- Tolerance to treatment
- Replacement of oxygen equipment on client after treatment
- Condition of mouth and oral mucous membranes

Sample Documentation
Date: 1/7/05
Time: 2100

Suctioned moderate amount of thick, cream-colored secretions from mouth and oropharynx. Mouth care given. Upper airway clear; respirations nonlabored. Ventimask reapplied at 40% FiO_2.

Performing Nasopharyngeal/ Nasotracheal Suctioning 🧤

Purpose

Clears airway of secretions
Makes breathing easier

Equipment

- Suction machine or wall suction setup
- Large towel or linen saver
- Sterile saline or water
- Cup
- Suction catheter (adults, size 14 to 16 French; children, 8 to 12 French) or sterile suction kit
- Sterile gloves
- Cotton-tipped swabs
- Moist tissue/cotton swabs
- Goggles and mask or face shield

Assessment

Assessment should focus on the following:
- Physician's order for area to be suctioned
- Respiratory status (respiratory character, breath sounds)
- Circulatory indicators (skin color and temperature, capillary refill, blood pressure, pulse)
- Nasal skin and mucous membranes
- Mucous membranes in the throat
- Color, amount, and consistency of secretions
- Facility policy regarding use of irrigation in suctioning

Nursing Diagnoses

Nursing diagnoses may include the following:
- Ineffective airway clearance related to weak cough
- Anxiety related to inability to breathe effectively

Outcome Identification and Planning

Desired Outcomes

Sample desired outcomes include the following:
- Client's respirations are 14 to 20 breaths per minute, of normal depth, smooth, and symmetric.

- Upper lung fields are clear.
- Client does not display restlessness or other indicators of anxiety.

Special Considerations in Planning and Implementation

General

In clients sensitive to decreased oxygen levels, suction for shorter durations but more frequently to ensure adequate airway clearance without hypoxia. Whenever possible, secure the help of another person to minimize tube manipulation and to perform bagging with less risk of contamination. Suction only when necessary: question any routine order for suctioning at regular intervals. Regular suctioning is appropriate if the client has excessive secretions, but suctioning causes trauma to the mucosa and should be performed only as needed.

Pediatric

Two people may be required to suction infants and children to minimize trauma. Measure from the tip of the child's nose to the ear lobe, then to the midsternum to determine the proper length for insertion of suction catheter. That length should be used to prevent tracheal trauma.

End-of-Life Care

Dying clients often experience pulmonary congestion and hypoxia and need suctioning.

Home Health

Teach caregivers how to suction using clean, not sterile, technique. Advise caregivers that suction catheters may be cleaned and reused.

Cost-Cutting Tips

If possible, use prepackaged suction catheter kits. Depending on the brand used, these kits usually are less expensive than the items gathered individually.

Delegation

This skill can be delegated to specially trained and certified personnel.

Implementation

Action	Rationale
1. Explain procedure to client.	*Reduces anxiety*
2. Perform hand hygiene and organize equipment.	*Reduces microorganism transfer; promotes efficiency*
3. Position client in semi-Fowler's position.	*Allows maximal breathing during procedure*

Action	Rationale
4. Turn suction machine on and place finger over end of tubing attached to suction machine. Use 60 mm Hg for children and up to 120 mm Hg for adults for normal secretions.	*Tests suction pressure*
5. Open sterile irrigation solution and pour into sterile cup.	*Allows for sterile rinsing of catheter*
6. Open sterile gloves and suction catheter package.	*Maintains aseptic procedure*
7. Place towel under client's chin.	*Prevents soiling of clothing*
8. Apply nonsterile gloves.	*Prevents contact with secretions*
9. Ask client to breathe through one naris while the other is occluded. Repeat with other naris.	*Determines patency of nasal passage*
10. Have client blow nose with both nares open.	*Clears nasal passage without pushing microorganisms into inner ear*
11. Clean mucus and dried secretions from nares with moist tissues or cotton-tipped swabs.	*Promotes skin integrity*
12. Don sterile glove on dominant hand (on top of nonsterile glove).	*Maintains sterile technique*
13. Wrap suction tubing partially around dominant hand. Holding suction catheter control port in sterile hand and tubing for suction source in nondominant hand, attach suction catheter port to tubing of suction source.	*Maintains sterility while establishing suction*
14. Slide sterile hand from control port to suction catheter tubing.	*Facilitates control of tubing*
15. Lubricate 3 to 4 inches of catheter tip with irrigating solution.	*Prevents mucosal trauma when catheter is inserted*
16. Ask client to take several deep breaths (make sure there is an oxygen source nearby).	*Provides additional oxygen to body tissues before suctioning*
17. Insert catheter into an unobstructed naris, using slanted downward motion.	*Allows unrestricted insertion of catheter*

Action	Rationale
BE SURE FINGER IS NOT COVERING OPENING OF SUCTION PORT.	*Prevents trauma to membranes due to suction from catheter*
18. As catheter is being inserted, ask client to open mouth.	*Allows nurse to see tip of catheter once inserted*
19. Apply suction: For nasopharyngeal suctioning:	
• Once catheter is visible in back of throat or resistance is felt (Fig. 6.12), place thumb over suction port.	*Applies suction*
• Withdraw catheter in a circular motion, rotating it between thumb and finger.	*Promotes cleaning of large area and sides of lumen*
DO NOT APPLY SUCTION FOR MORE THAN 10 SECONDS.	*Prevents hypoxia*
• Place tip of suction catheter in sterile solution and apply suction for 1 to 2 seconds.	*Clears secretions from tubing*
• Allow client to take about five breaths while you listen to bronchial breath sounds and assess status of secretions.	*Determines if repeat suctioning is needed*
• Repeat steps once or twice if assessment indicates that secretions have not cleared well. Proceed to step 20 for completion of procedure.	*Promotes adequate clearing of airway*

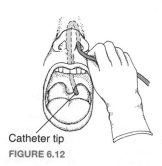

Catheter tip

FIGURE 6.12

Action	Rationale
For nasotracheal suctioning:	
• Once catheter is visible in back of throat or resistance is felt, ask client to pant or cough.	*Opens trachea and facilitates entrance into trachea*
• With each pant or cough, attempt to insert the catheter deeper.	*Decreases resistance to catheter insertion*
• Place thumb over suction port.	*Initiates suction*
• Encourage client to cough.	*Makes loosening and removing secretions easier*
• Withdraw catheter in a circular motion, rotating it between thumb and finger.	*Minimizes adherence of catheter to sides of airway*
DO NOT APPLY SUCTION FOR MORE THAN 10 SECONDS.	*Prevents hypoxia*
• Place tip of suction catheter in sterile solution and apply suction for 1 to 2 seconds.	*Clears clogged tubing*
• Allow client to take about five breaths while you listen to bronchial breath sounds and assess status of secretions.	*Determines if repeat suctioning is needed*
• Repeat steps once or twice if assessment indicates that secretions have not cleared well.	*Promotes adequate clearing of airway*
20. Complete the suctioning procedure:	
• Perform oral airway suctioning.	*Clears secretions from oral airway*
• Disconnect suction catheter from suction tubing and turn off suction machine.	
• Properly dispose of or store all equipment.	*Prevents spread of micro-organisms*
21. Assess incisions and wounds for drainage and approximation.	*Detects complications, such as bleeding or weakened incisions, from coughing and straining*
22. Position client for comfort.	*Promotes slow, deep breathing*
23. Raise side rails and leave call light within reach.	*Prevents falls; permits communication*
24. Remove gloves and perform hand hygiene.	*Reduces transfer of micro-organisms*

Evaluation

Were desired outcomes achieved? Examples of evaluation include:
- Desired outcome met: Breath sounds clear to auscultation.
- Desired outcome met: Client appears calm and rests quietly.

Documentation

The following should be noted on the client's chart:
- Breath sounds before and after suctioning
- Character of respirations before and after suctioning
- Significant changes in vital signs
- Color, amount, and consistency of secretions
- Tolerance to treatment (e.g., state of incisions, drains)
- Replacement of oxygen equipment on client after treatment
- Client's need for oxygen

Sample Documentation
Date: 1/7/05
Time: 2100

Suctioned moderate amount of thick, cream-colored secretions via nasopharynx (nasotrachea). Lungs clear in all fields after suctioning. Client slightly short of breath after procedure. Deep breaths taken. Respirations are 22, smooth and nonlabored. O_2 per nasal cannula reapplied at 3 L/min. Chest dressing dry and intact.

● **Nursing Procedure 6.10**

Suctioning and Maintaining an Endotracheal Tube 🖐

Purpose

Maintains open airway for breathing assistance and continuous positive airway pressure
Promotes clearance of secretions

Equipment

- 5-mL syringe
- Nonsterile gloves
- Suction machine or wall suction setup
- Suction catheter or kit (adult, 14 to 16 French; pediatric, 6.5 to 12 French)
- Sterile gloves (in kit)
- Large towel (or linen saver, possibly in kit)
- Sterile irrigation saline in sterile container
- Saline (prefilled tubes or a filled 3- to 10-mL syringe) for rinsing
- Wrist restraints (optional)
- Goggles or protective glasses
- Gown or protective apron
- Face mask
- Endotracheal tube holder, 1-inch tape, or elastic adhesive dressing
- Benzoin or skin preparation (optional)
- Nasal/oral care items (e.g., oral swabs or moistener, cotton swabs)
- Petroleum jelly
- Sphygmomanometer

Assessment

Assessment should focus on the following:
- Physician's orders
- Airway patency (clear inspiratory and expiratory breath sounds, absence of mucous plugs in tubing, consistency of secretions, absence of triggering of ventilator pressure alarm)
- Ventilation adequacy (respiratory rate of 12 to 16 breaths per minute or within range of baseline rate; respirations even and nonlabored; mucous membranes and nailbeds pink)
- Endotracheal (ET) tube stability (tube placed securely; cuff properly inflated with minimum or no leak audible; pressure in cuff at 14 to 18 mm Hg or 20 to 25 cm H_2O)
- Functioning of oxygen apparatus (chest rises with ventilator cycle, excursion symmetric, breath sounds audible bilaterally to bases, and respiratory rate not less than ventilator rate setting [with mandatory ventilation setting—intermittent mandatory ventilation (IMV)])
- Apparatus settings: oxygen level (FiO_2), type of setting (assist-control or mandatory ventilations), tidal volume, and positive end expiratory pressure (PEEP) or continuous positive airway pressure (CPAP)
- Client's level of consciousness (tendency to pull or disconnect tubing, resist ventilation, or resist suctioning)

Nursing Diagnoses

Nursing diagnoses may include the following:
- Inadequate respiratory pattern related to muscle paralysis
- Ineffective airway clearance related to weak cough
- Anxiety related to inability to breathe effectively

Outcome Identification and Planning

Desired Outcomes

Sample desired outcomes include the following:
- Respirations are 14 to 20 breaths per minute, of normal depth, smooth, and symmetric.
- Lung fields are clear; no cyanosis.
- Client demonstrates no signs of anxiety or shortness of breath.

Special Considerations In Planning and Implementation

General

Before beginning suctioning, ensure that clients sensitive to decreased oxygen levels (e.g., with head injury or with possibly increased intracranial pressure) are well ventilated and oxygenated to prevent carbon dioxide buildup. Suction these clients briefly, and increase the frequency of suctioning. Enlist the aid of another person before beginning the procedure to ensure client safety and maximize oxygenation during suctioning and tracheostomy care. Use soft wrist restraints if necessary for clients who are confused to prevent ET tube dislodgment.

Pediatric

Stabilize the child's head to prevent extubation, if indicated. Use two people when performing suctioning or ET tube care. Use soft wrist restraints if necessary to prevent ET tube dislodgment.

Geriatric

Take special measures to prevent skin breakdown because the elderly client's skin is often thin and sensitive to pressure.

End-of-Life Care

Dying persons often experience pulmonary congestion and hypoxia; suction as needed or desired to promote comfort.

Home Health Care

Use oxygen saturation levels, instead of arterial blood gas results, as a guide for suctioning.

 Cost-Cutting Tips

In-line suction circuits are less expensive than items assembled individually; goggles, mask, and face shields are not needed.

Delegation

Suctioning may be performed by respiratory therapy personnel.
Unlicensed assistive personnel should not perform this procedure.

Implementation

Action	Rationale

Suctioning an Endotracheal Tube

1. Explain procedure to client.
2. Perform hand hygiene and organize equipment.
3. Perform any procedures that loosen secretions (e.g., postural drainage, percussion, nebulization).

Proceed to Step 4 for an open or closed system.

Reduces anxiety
Reduces microorganism transfer; promotes efficiency
Removes secretions from all lobes

Open System

4. If changing ET tube, prepare tape (see Nursing Procedure 6.13).

Determine length of catheter to be inserted:
- For nasal tracheal: Measure distance from tip of nose to earlobe and along side of neck to thyroid cartilage (Adam's apple).
- For oral tracheal: Measure from mouth to midsternum.

Maintains proper tube placement

5. Don gloves, goggles, gown, and mask.
6. Position client on side or back with head of bed elevated.
7. Turn suction machine on and place finger over end of tubing attached to suction machine. Pressure should range from 50 mm Hg in infants to 120 mm Hg in adults.
8. Open sterile irrigation solution and pour into sterile cup. Open sterile gloves

Protects nurse from contact with secretions
Maximizes breathing during procedure

Tests suction pressure

Allows for sterile rinsing of catheter; maintains sterility of procedure

Action	Rationale
and suction catheter package.	
9. Place towel under client's chin.	*Prevents soiling of clothing*
10. Don sterile glove on dominant hand (over nonsterile glove).	*Maintains sterile technique*
11. Wrap suction tubing partially around dominant hand. Holding suction catheter control port in sterile hand and tubing for suction source in nondominant hand, attach suction catheter port to tubing of suction source.	*Maintains sterility; ensures correct attachment of catheter*
12. Slide sterile hand from control port to suction catheter tubing.	*Facilitates control of tubing*
13. Lubricate 3 to 4 inches of catheter tip with irrigating solution.	*Facilitates passage of suction catheter into ET tube*
14. With nonsterile hand, disconnect oxygen supply tubing from ET tube and attach Ambu bag. Set oxygen on Ambu bag to 100% and turn on full flow.	*Provides an additional source for oxygen*
15. Have assistant deliver ventilations, administering three to five deep ventilations, and then remove Ambu bag (Fig. 6.13). If client is able, have him or her take three to five deep breaths.	*Supplies additional oxygen to body tissues before suctioning*
16. Perform suctioning: • Insert catheter into ET tube using a slanted, downward motion (Fig. 6.14). BE SURE FINGER IS NOT COVERING OPENING OF SUCTION PORT. Continue insertion until resistance is met or coughing is stimulated. If catheter meets resistance after being inserted the expected	*Prevents trauma to membranes due to suction from catheter*

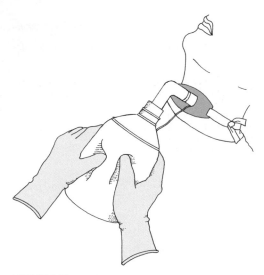

FIGURE 6.13

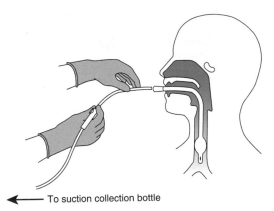

← To suction collection bottle

FIGURE 6.14

Action	Rationale
distance, it may be on the carina. If so, pull back 1 cm before advancing further or suctioning.	
• Place thumb over suction port.	*Applies suction*
• Encourage client to cough.	*Loosens and removes secretions*
• Withdraw catheter in a circular motion, rotating between thumb and finger.	*Promotes cleaning of sides of lumen of ET tube*
DO NOT APPLY SUC-TION FOR MORE THAN 10 SECONDS.	*Prevents hypoxia and mucosal trauma from suction*
17. Place tip of suction catheter in sterile solution and apply suction for 1 to 2 seconds.	*Clears clogged suction catheter and tubing*
18. Repeat Steps 16 and 17 once. Allow client to take about five breaths while you auscultate bronchial breath sounds and assess status of secretions.	*Determines if repeat suctioning is needed*
Repeat suctioning once or twice if assessment indicates that secretions are not cleared.	*Promotes clearing of airway*
19. Deflate ET tube cuff and re-peat suctioning. Reinflate cuff to appropriate pressure.	*Removes secretions pooled above tube cuff; prevents trauma to tracheal tissue from excessive pressure*
Proceed to Step 20.	
Closed System	
4. Position client on side or back with head of bed elevated.	
5. Open sterile package of closed suction device.	*Prepares equipment*
6. Don sterile gloves (or sterile glove on dominant hand and clean glove on non-dominant hand).	*Maintains sterility*
7. Attach 10-mL unit dose syringe of saline.	*Prepares for rinse of line*
8. Attach suction connecting tube to suction port if not already attached.	*Prepares for the suctioning and removal of secretions*

Action	Rationale
9. Turn on suction 15% to 20% higher than usual (120 mm Hg).	*Adjusts for the extra length of the tracheal care catheter*
10. Advance catheter 1 to 2 inches down tracheal tube or 4 to 5 inches down ET tube.	*Moves catheter into position for secretion removal*
11. Turn on thumb port.	*Allows suction*
12. Stabilize the ET tube with the nondominant hand while advancing the catheter 2 inches at a time until the carina is reached (at pre-measured point for child).	*Avoids moving the ET tube while advancing the catheter*
13. Pull back 1 cm and begin withdrawing slowly, using continuous suction and twisting the catheter between your fingers.	*Prevents trauma to membranes due to suction from catheter*
14. Repeat as necessary.	*Ensures that secretions are removed*
15. Withdraw the catheter until the black line can be seen through the bag.	*Ensures that catheter is out of airway*
16. Depress the thumb port and hold it down while gently squeezing in the saline from the unit dose syringe.	*Allows for rinsing of catheter*
17. Lock thumb port.	*Prevents inadvertent application of suction*
18. Close rinse port.	*Closes potential entry port into catheter*
19. Position catheter within storage sleeve.	*Prevents inadvertent displacement of catheter*
20. Suction oral airway and perform oral care (see Nursing Procedure 6.8).	*Removes pooled secretions*
21. Disconnect suction catheter from suction tubing and turn off suction machine.	
22. Assess incisions and wounds for approximation and drainage.	*Promotes early detection of complications or bleeding from wound areas and incisions*
23. Position client with head of bed at 45 degrees, side rails up, and call light within reach (restraints on, if ordered and required).	*Maximizes lung expansion; facilitates communication; prevents falls; prevents tube dislodgment*
24. Discard equipment and gloves appropriately.	*Promotes clean environment; reduces transfer of microorganisms*

Action

Maintaining an Endotracheal Tube

1. Perform hand hygiene and don nonsterile gloves.

2. Every 2 hours, assess client for:
   - Level of consciousness, respiratory status, vital signs, and temperature. IF CLIENT IS CONFUSED, USE SOFT WRIST RESTRAINTS (obtain physician's order, if required).

   - Symmetry of chest excursion with inspiration and presence of breath sounds bilaterally

3. Inspect ET tube every 2 to 4 hours to determine if it is obstructed by kinks, mucous plugs, secretions, or client's bite.

4. Check ventilator, if applicable, for high or increasing ventilation pressures.

5. Check tube holder or tape for severe odor, soiling, and stability.
   IF ET TUBE HOLDER/TAPE REQUIRES REPLACEMENT, ENLIST AN ASSISTANT TO HOLD TUBE STABLE.

6. Replace tape/holder only when needed. To replace holder, see vendor's instructions. To replace tape to secure tube:
   - Tear two long strips of tape (one 14 inches, the other 24 inches; see Fig. 6.8).
   - Lay 24-inch strip of tape down with sticky side up.
   - Place short strip of tape (sticky side down) on center of 24-inch strip.

Rationale

Rea... organis... ...fer of micro-

Determines whethe... quately oxygenated; pr...t is adequate client from dislodging ET...ts ...

Determines correct tube placement (mainstem bronchus)

Indicates need for suctioning, tube repositioning, or bite block to maintain patency

Indicates resistance to flow of air

Indicates need for adjustment or replacement of holder/tape

Maintains placement of tube during manipulation

Prepares non-sticky area of tape for neck

Action	Rationale
• Split each en~~tape~~ ~~24-inch str~~ ~~es.~~	*Allows secure taping of ET tube*
• Place no~~.~~ neck. under ~~.~~e, position	
• For corner of mouth, tub one sticky tape ~~.~~ld, press half of split tape end across upper lip, and wrap other half around tube (Fig. 6.15). Repeat steps with other end of tape.	
• For nasal tube, press half of split tape end across upper lip and wrap other half around tube. DO NOT OCCLUDE NARIS. Repeat steps with other end of tape. (Use of elastic adhesive or application of benzoin may provide a secure hold.)	*Resists perspiration and skin oils*
7. Inspect area around the tube.	
• With nasal ET tube, inspect naris for redness, drainage, ulcer, or pressure area around tube.	

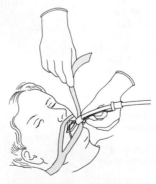

FIGURE 6.15

Action	Rationale
• With oral ET tube, inspect oral cavity and lips for irritation, ulcer, or pressure areas. Rotate tube position to opposite side of mouth every 24 to 48 hours.	*Detects skin breakdown; prevents continuous pressure on one area of lips*
8. Perform oral care every 2 to 4 hours (suctioning, swabs, petroleum jelly to lips).	*Removes pooled secretions and moistens lips and mucous membranes*
9. Assess cuff status (see Nursing Procedure 6.12).	*Prevents tracheal tissue damage from cuff overinflation*
10. Properly dispose of or store supplies or equipment.	*Prevents spread of microorganisms*
11. Position client for comfort with head of bed at 45 degrees, side rails up, call light within reach (and restraint on, if needed).	*Facilitates lung expansion; permits communication; ensures client safety*
12. Perform hand hygiene.	*Decreases spread of organisms*

Evaluation

Were desired outcomes achieved? Examples of evaluation include:
- Desired outcome met: Breath sounds clear to auscultation.
- Desired outcome met: Respirations even and nonlabored with a rate of 14 breaths per minute.
- Desired outcome met: Client appears relaxed and displays no signs of anxiety.

Documentation

The following should be noted on the client's chart:
- Breath sounds before and after suctioning
- Character of respirations before and after suctioning
- Status skin around ET tube
- Significant changes in vital signs
- Color, amount, and consistency of secretions
- Tolerance to treatment (i.e., state of incisions, drains)
- Use of oxygen before treatment and replacement of oxygen equipment after treatment

Sample Documentation
Date: 1/7/05
Time: 2100

Suctioned moderate amount of thick, cream-colored secretions via ET tube. Lungs clear in all fields after suctioning. Tracheostomy care done. Client slightly short of breath after procedure. Respirations smooth and nonlabored. Lips and mucous membranes pink and without irritation.

● Nursing Procedure 6.11

Caring for a Tracheostomy (Suctioning, Cleaning, and Changing the Dressing and Tie)

Purpose

Clears airway of secretions
Promotes tracheostomy healing
Minimizes tracheal trauma or necrosis

Equipment

- Tracheostomy care kit:
    - Sterile bowls or trays (two)
    - Cotton-tipped swabs
    - Pipe cleaners
    - Nonabrasive cleaning brush
    - Tracheostomy ties
    - Gauze pads
- Normal saline (500-mL bottle)
- Hydrogen peroxide
- Suction machine or wall suction setup
- Suction catheter (size should be half of the lumen of the trachea; adult, 14 to 16 French)
- Pair of nonsterile gloves
- Pair of sterile gloves (often in suction catheter kit)
- Towel or waterproof drape

- Goggles or protective glasses
- Gown or protective apron (optional)
- Hemostat

Assessment

Assessment should focus on the following:
- Agency policy regarding tracheostomy care
- Status of tracheostomy (i.e., time since immediate post-operative period)
- Type and size of tracheostomy tube (i.e., metal, plastic, cuffed)
- Respiratory status (respiratory character, breath sounds)
- Color, amount, and consistency of secretions
- Skin around tracheostomy site
- Condition of dressing and ties securing tracheostomy

Nursing Diagnoses

Nursing diagnoses may include the following:
- Ineffective airway clearance related to weak cough
- Risk of infection related to impaired skin integrity

Outcome Identification and Planning

Desired Outcomes

Sample desired outcomes include the following:
- Respirations are 14 to 20 breaths per minute, of normal depth, smooth, and symmetric.
- Upper lung fields are clear.
- Tracheostomy site remains intact without redness or signs of infection.

Special Considerations in Planning and Implementation

General

For safety and to provide maximum oxygenation, enlist the aid of another person before beginning suctioning and tracheostomy care. Clients sensitive to decreased oxygen levels should be suctioned for shorter durations but more frequently to ensure airway clearance without hypoxia or carbon dioxide buildup. If client has a nasogastric (NG) tube and cuffed tracheostomy, monitor closely for signs of pharyngeal trauma. Encourage client to participate in tracheostomy care to provide an opportunity to teach home care.

Pediatric

Ensure that the suction catheter size is appropriate for the child's age and size. Obtain assistance to stabilize the child's position, or use soft wrist restraints.

Geriatric

Anticipate the need for more frequent suctioning in elderly clients because they often have a decreased cough reflex and increased secretions.

End-of-Life Care

Perform suctioning for terminally ill clients to help remove excessive secretions and decrease the workload of breathing. Doing so may help promote comfort and ease dying.

Home Health

Substitute clean technique for sterile technique in home health care, extended care, and care in other facilities. Teach family members how to perform care and assist nurse in care. Tape hemostat to head of bed or wall above bed for emergency use if the tracheostomy tube becomes dislodged. Advise caregivers that suction catheters can be cleaned and reused.

Delegation

Tracheostomy care and suctioning is never delegated to unlicensed assistive personnel.

Implementation

Action	Rationale
Suctioning a Tracheostomy	
1. Explain procedure to client.	*Reduces anxiety*
2. Perform hand hygiene and organize equipment.	*Reduces microorganism transfer; promotes efficiency*
3. Perform any procedure that loosens secretions (e.g., postural drainage, percussion, nebulization).	*Promotes removal of secretions from all lobes of lungs*
4. Position client on side or back with head of bed elevated.	*Promotes maximal breathing during procedure*
5. Turn suction machine on and place finger over end of tubing attached to suction machine.	*Tests suction pressure (should not exceed 120 mm Hg)*
6. Open sterile irrigation solution and pour into sterile cup.	*Allows for sterile rinsing of catheter*
7. If performing tracheostomy care, set up tracheostomy care equipment (Fig. 6.16). (See Step 2 of "Cleaning a Tracheostomy.")	*Provides fluid for irrigation of lungs to loosen secretions during suctioning*

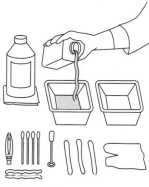

FIGURE 6.16

Action	Rationale
8. Increase oxygen concentration to tracheostomy collar or Ambu bag to 100%.	*Provides hyperoxygenation before suctioning*
9. Open sterile gloves and suction catheter package.	*Ensures asepsis*
10. Place towel or drape on client's chest under tracheostomy.	*Prevents soiling of clothing*
11. Don nonsterile gloves, goggles, gown, and mask.	*Protects nurse from contact with secretions*
12. Place sterile glove on dominant hand (glove-on-glove technique).	*Maintains sterile technique*
13. With sterile hand, pick up suction catheter and attach suction control port to tubing of suction source (held with non-sterile hand).	*Ensures correct attachment of catheter*
14. Slide sterile hand from control port to suction catheter tubing (may wrap tubing around hand).	*Facilitates control of tubing*
15. Lubricate 3 to 4 inches of catheter tip with irrigating solution.	*Prevents mucosal trauma when catheter is inserted*
16. Ask client to take several deep breaths with tracheostomy collar intact (Fig. 6.17) or Ambu bag at tracheostomy tube	*Provides additional oxygen to body tissues before suctioning*

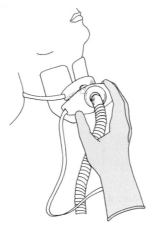

FIGURE 6.17

Action	Rationale
entrance. If necessary, have assistant deliver four or five deep breaths with Ambu bag.	
17. Remove tracheostomy collar or Ambu bag.	*Allows access to tracheostomy*
18. Insert catheter approximately 6 inches into inner cannula (or until resistance is met or cough reflex is stimulated). BE SURE FINGER IS NOT COVERING OPENING OF SUCTION PORT.	*Places catheter in upper airway and promotes clearance; prevents trauma to membranes due to suction from catheter*
19. Encourage client to cough.	*Promotes loosening and removal of secretions*
20. Place thumb over suction port.	*Initiates suction (often catheter stimulates cough)*
21. Withdraw catheter in a circular motion, rotating catheter between thumb and finger. Intermittently release and apply suction during withdrawal. APPLY SUCTION FOR NO MORE THAN 10 SECONDS.	*Removes secretions from sides of the airway* *Prevents hypoxia; minimizes trauma to mucosa*

Action	Rationale
22. Place tip of suction catheter in sterile solution, and apply suction for 1 to 2 seconds.	*Clears clogged tubing*
23. Allow client to take about five breaths while you auscultate bronchial breath sounds and assess status of secretions. If necessary, have assistant deliver four or five deep breaths with Ambu bag.	*Determines whether repeat suctioning is needed; permits reoxygenation*
24. Repeat steps 19 to 23 once or twice if secretions are still present.	*Promotes clearing of airway*
25. If performing tracheostomy cleaning, wrap catheter around sterile hand (do not touch suction port) and proceed to Step 3 below.	*Maintains sterility and control*
If not performing tracheostomy cleaning or dressing/tie change, discard materials.	*Completes procedure*
26. Position client for comfort and place call light within reach.	*Provides for client safety and communication*
27. Remove gloves and perform hand hygiene.	*Prevents spread of micro-organisms*

Cleaning a Tracheostomy and Changing Dressing

Action	Rationale
1. Perform hand hygiene and don nonsterile gloves.	*Reduces transfer of micro-organisms*
2. Set up tracheostomy care equipment (see Fig. 6.16).	
• Open tracheostomy care kit and spread package on bedside table.	*Establishes sterile field*
• Maintaining sterility, place bowls and tray with supplies in separate locations on paper.	*Arranges equipment for easy access without contamination*
• Open sterile saline and peroxide bottles, and fill first bowl with equal parts of peroxide and saline (do not let container touch the bowl).	*Provides half-strength peroxide mixture for tracheostomy cannula cleaning; maintains sterility of supplies*

Action	Rationale
• Fill second bowl with saline.	*Provides rinse for cannula*
• Don sterile gloves (glove-on-glove technique).	*Maintains sterility*
3. Place four cotton-tipped swabs in peroxide mixture, then place across tracheal care tray.	*Provides moist swabs for cleaning skin*
4. Pick up one sterile gauze with fingers of sterile hand.	*Allows touching of nonsterile items while maintaining sterility*
5. Stabilize neck plate with nonsterile hand (or have assistant do so).	*Decreases discomfort and trauma during removal of cannula*
6. With sterile hand, use gauze to turn inner cannula counterclockwise until catch is released (unlocked).	*Separates inner and outer cannulas*
7. Gently slide cannula out using an outward and downward arch (Fig. 6.18).	*Follows curve of tracheostomy tube*
8. Place cannula in bowl of half-strength peroxide.	*Softens secretions*
9. Discard gauze.	*Avoids contaminating sterile items*
10. Unwrap catheter and suction outer cannula of tracheostomy.	*Removes remaining secretions*
11. Have client take deep breaths or use Ambu bag to deliver 100% oxygen.	*Provides oxygenation after suctioning*

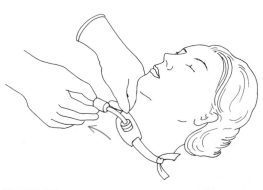

FIGURE 6.18

Action	Rationale
12. Disconnect suction catheter from suction tubing and remove sterile gloves, pulling up and over the suction catheter. Discard.	*Prevents spread of microorganisms*
13. Remove tracheostomy dressing.	*Exposes skin for cleaning*
14. Using gauze pads, wipe secretions and crusts from around tracheostomy tube.	*Removes possible airway obstruction and medium for infection*
15. Use moist swabs to clean area under neck plate at insertion site.	*Decreases risk for infection*
16. Discard gloves.	*Prevents spread of microorganisms*
17. Don sterile gloves.	
18. Pick up inner cannula and scrub gently with cleaning brush.	*Removes crusts and secretions from outside and inside of cannula*
19. Use pipe cleaners to clean lumen of inner cannula thoroughly.	*Decreases accumulation of mucus in lumen*
20. Run inner cannula through peroxide mixture.	*Removes remaining debris*
21. Rinse cannula in bowl containing sterile saline.	*Rinses away peroxide mixture and residual debris*
22. Place cannula in sterile gauze and dry thoroughly; use dry pipe cleaner to remove residual moisture from lumen.	*Prevents introduction of fluid into trachea*
23. Slide inner cannula into outer cannula (keeping inner cannula sterile), using smooth inward and downward arch and rolling inner cannula from side to side with fingers.	*Facilitates insertion and reduces resistance*
24. Hold neck plate stable with other hand and turn inner cannula clockwise until catch (lock) is felt and dots are in alignment.	*Ensures that inner cannula is securely attached to outer cannula*
25. Discard gloves and replace with nonsterile gloves.	
26. Have assistant hold tracheostomy by neck plate while you clip old tracheostomy ties and remove them.	*Prevents accidental dislodgment of tracheostomy during tie replacement*

Action	Rationale
27. Slip end of new tie through tie holder on neck plate, and tie a square knot 2 to 3 inches from neck plate (Fig. 6.19).	*Allows tie to be removed while holding tracheostomy tube firm*
28. Place tie around back of client's neck and repeat above step with other end of tie, cutting away excess tie.	*Places dressing in position to catch secretions from tracheostomy or surrounding insertion site*
29. Apply tracheostomy dressing: • Hold ends of tracheostomy dressing (or open gauze and fold into V shape). • Gently lift neck plate and slide end of dressing under plate and tie. • Pull other end of dressing under neck plate and tie. • Slide both ends up toward neck, using a gentle rocking motion, until middle of dressing (or gauze) rests under neck plate (Fig. 6.20).	

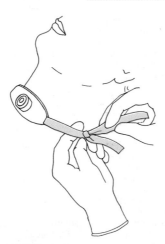

FIGURE 6.19

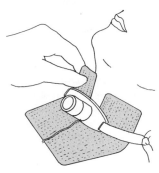

FIGURE 6.20

Action	Rationale
30. Position client for comfort.	
31. Discard materials and perform hand hygiene.	*Reduces spread of infection*
32. Raise side rails and leave call light within reach.	*Prevents falls; permits communication*

Evaluation

Examples of evaluation include the following:
- Desired outcome met: Tracheostomy site dry with no redness or swelling.
- Desired outcome met: Breath sounds clear to auscultation bilaterally.
- Desired outcome met: Respirations are 14 to 20 breaths per minute, of normal depth, smooth, and symmetric.

Documentation

The following should be noted on the client's chart:
- Breath sounds before and after suctioning
- Number of times suctioned
- Character of respirations
- Status of tracheostomy site
- Size of trach cannula
- Cleaning provided and dressing change
- Significant changes in vital signs
- Color, amount, and consistency of secretions
- Tolerance to treatment (i.e., state of incisions, drains)
- Replacement of oxygen equipment after treatment

Sample Documentation
Date: 1/7/05
Time: 2100

Suctioned moderate amount of thick, cream-colored secretions via tracheostomy. Lungs clear in all fields after suctioning. Tracheostomy care done. #__ Inner cannula cleaned and replaced. Ostomy site dry, with no redness or swelling. Client slightly short of breath after procedure. Respirations smooth and nonlabored after deep breaths with 100% O_2 taken. O_2 per tracheostomy collar reapplied at 30% as ordered. Client tolerated procedure with no pain or excess gagging. Client observed procedure with mirror to learn care procedure.

● **Nursing Procedure 6.12**

Managing a Tracheostomy/ Endotracheal Tube Cuff

Purpose

Maintains minimum amount of air in cuff to ensure adequate ventilation without trauma to trachea
Prevents aspiration

Equipment

- 10-mL syringe
- Blood pressure sphygmomanometer
- Three-way stopcock
- Mouth-care swabs, moistener, and mouthwash
- Suctioning equipment
- Nonsterile gloves

Assessment

Assessment should focus on the following:
- Size of cuff
- Maximum cuff inflation pressure (check cuff box)
- Bronchial breath sounds
- Respiratory rate and character
- Agency policy or physician's orders regarding cuff care

Nursing Diagnoses

Nursing diagnoses may include the following:
- Ineffective airway clearance related to thick secretions
- Risk for aspiration related to use of tracheostomy tube

Outcome Identification and Planning

Desired Outcomes

Sample desired outcomes include the following:
- The client's respirations are 14 to 20 breaths per minute, of normal depth, smooth, and symmetric.
- The client's lung fields are clear.
- Minimum occlusive pressure is maintained while cuff is inflated.
- The client experiences no undetected tracheal damage.
- The client does not demonstrate any signs of aspiration.

Special Considerations in Planning and Implementation

General

Some cuffs are low-pressure cuffs and require minimum manipulation, but the client should still be monitored periodically to ensure proper cuff function.

Pediatric

Tracheal tissue is extremely sensitive in children. Smaller cuffs require lower inflation pressures: be very careful not to overinflate them.

Home Health

Clients with permanent tracheostomies typically have a cuffless tracheostomy for home use.

Delegation

Management of cuff pressure should not be delegated to unlicensed assistive personnel. Respiratory therapy personnel often manage endotracheal and tracheal cuff pressure.

Implementation

Action	Rationale
1. Perform hand hygiene, don gloves, and organize equipment.	*Reduces microorganism transfer; promotes efficiency*
2. Check cuff balloon for inflation by compressing between thumb and finger (should feel resistance).	*Indicates cuff is inflated*
3. Attach 10-mL syringe to one end of three-way stopcock. Attach manometer to another stopcock port. Close remaining stopcock port.	*Establishes connection between syringe and manometer*
4. Attach pilot balloon port to closed port of three-way stopcock (Fig. 6.21).	
5. Instill air from syringe into manometer until 10-mm Hg reading is obtained.	*Prevents rapid loss of air from cuff*
6. Auscultate tracheal breath sounds, noting presence of smooth breath sounds or gurgling (cuff leak).	*Determines if cuff leak evidenced by gurgling is present*
7. If smooth breath sounds are noted:	

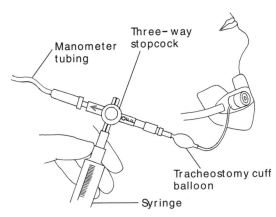

Manometer tubing

Three-way stopcock

Tracheostomy cuff balloon

Syringe

FIGURE 6.21

Action	Rationale
• Turn stopcock off to manometer. • Withdraw air from cuff until gurgling is noted with respirations. Once gurgling breath sounds are noted, insert air into cuff until gurgling is noted only on inspiration.	*Provides minimum leak and minimizes pressure on trachea (airway is larger on inspiration)*
8. Turn stopcock off to syringe.	*Reestablishes a closed system*
9. Note manometer reading as client exhales. Record reading (note if pressure exceeds recommended volume; do not exceed 20 mm Hg). Notify physician if excessive leak persists or if excess pressure is needed to inflate cuff.	*Allows reading of pressure in cuff; indicates expiratory cuff pressure identifying minimum occlusive volume (cuff pressure on tracheal wall)*
10. Turn stopcock off to pilot balloon and disconnect. If physician orders intermittent cuff inflation, proceed to Step 11. If not, proceed to Step 12.	*Disconnects from system*
11. To perform intermittent cuff inflation:	
• Auscultate tracheal breath sounds, noting presence of smooth breath sounds (cuff inflated) or vocalization/ hiss (cuff deflated).	*Determines cuff inflation*
• If smooth breath sounds are noted, withdraw air from cuff until faint gurgling is noted with respirations. If vocalization or hiss is noted, insert air into cuff until faint gurgling is noted with respirations.	
• Once gurgling breath sounds are noted, insert air into cuff until gurgling is noted only on inspiration.	*Provides minimum leak and minimizes pressure on trachea (airway is larger on aspiration)*
• Monitor breath sounds every 2 hours until cuff is deflated.	*Determines that minimum leak remains present*

Action	Rationale
12. To maintain cuff:	
• Every 2 to 4 hours, check tracheal breath sounds (more frequently if indicated) and note pressure of pilot balloon between fingers.	*Determines if minimum or excessive cuff leak is present*
• Every 8 to 12 hours or per agency policy, check cuff pressure and note if minimum occlusive volume increases or decreases.	*Indicates if tracheal tissue damage or softening is occurring or if tracheal swelling is present*
• If oral or tube feedings are being given, assess secretions for tube feeding or food particles.	*Indicates possible tracheoesophageal fistula*
13. To perform cuff deflation:	*Prepares for removal of secretions pooled on top of cuff; facilitates oxygenation*
• Obtain and set up suctioning equipment.	
• Enlist assistance and perform oral or nasopharyngeal suctioning.	*Removes secretions pooled in pharyngeal area*
• Set up Ambu bag (if client is not on ventilator and long-term cuff inflation has been used).	*Provides for deep ventilations to remove secretions*
• Have assistant initiate deep sigh with ventilator, or administer deep ventilation with Ambu bag as you remove air from cuff with syringe.	*Pushes pooled secretions into oral cavity as cuff is deflated*
• Suction pharynx and oral cavity again.	*Removes remaining secretions*
14. Perform mouth care with swabs and mouthwash.	*Promotes client comfort*
15. Apply lubricant to lips.	*Promotes comfort*
16. Dispose of supplies appropriately.	*Reduces risk of microorganism transmission*
17. Position client for comfort with call light within reach.	*Promotes comfort and safety; permits communication*

Evaluation

Were desired outcomes met? Examples of evaluation include:
- Desired outcome met: Client's respirations are 14 to 20 breaths per minute, of normal depth, smooth, and symmetric.
- Desired outcome met: Client's lung fields are clear.
- Desired outcome met: Tracheal tube cuff with 15 mm Hg minimum occlusive pressure.
- Desired outcome met: Client experiences no undetected tracheal damage.
- Desired outcome met: Client does not demonstrate any signs of aspiration.

Documentation

The following should be noted in the client's chart:
- Cuff pressures noted and tracheal breath sounds
- Suctioning performed and nature of secretions
- Tolerance to procedure (changes in respiratory status and vital signs)
- Cuff deflation and inflation

Sample Documentation
Date: 1/7/05
Time: 2100

Tracheal tube cuff checked, with 15 mm Hg minimum occlusive pressure noted. Suctioned scant, thin secretions via nasopharynx, then cuff deflated fully. Client remains in bed with head of bed elevated. Respirations even and nonlabored. Breath sounds clear. No complaint of pain after procedure.

● Nursing Procedure 6.13

Capping of a Tracheostomy Tube

Purpose

Assesses client's ability to breathe through natural airway
Prepares client for weaning before decannulation (removal of tracheostomy)

Equipment

- 20-mL syringe
- Tracheostomy cap
- Clean gloves
- Suction kit (including sterile solution and 2 suction catheters)

Assessment

Assessment should focus on the following:
- Breath sounds
- Frequency of suctioning
- Ability to cough and clear secretions
- Vital signs (heart rate, respiratory rate, blood pressure)
- Pulse oximetry results
- Level of consciousness
- Skin color
- Work of breathing
- Tracheal and oral secretion status

Nursing Diagnoses

Nursing diagnoses may include:
- Body image disturbance related to presence of tracheostomy
- Anxiety related to impending removal of tracheostomy

Outcome Identification and Planning

Desired Outcomes

Sample desired outcomes include the following:
- Respirations even and nonlabored with a rate of 12 to 20 breaths per minute.
- Client spontaneously coughing small amounts of white sputum.
- Client speaking short phrases after capping.
- Client verbalizes comfort with use of cap.

Special Considerations in Planning and Implementation

General

ALWAYS DEFLATE THE CUFF OF A CUFFED TRA-
CHEOSTOMY TUBE BEFORE CAPPING. Cuff inflation will
lead to asphyxia and death. If the client has significant edema
of the upper airway or proximal trachea, expect the physician
to order downsizing of the tracheostomy tube to a smaller
tube before capping. Evaluate the client with a cuffed tracheostomy tube for a cuffless tracheostomy tube if medically
appropriate to eliminate the need for cuff deflation when

capping. Optimally, cap the tracheostomy tube no earlier than 24 hours after reinsertion of a tracheostomy tube to a smaller size. Trauma may occur during reinsertion, causing swelling and possibly impairing the client's ability to breathe when the tracheostomy is capped. Use the Passy-Muir valve (PMV) as an alternative for tracheostomy capping for clients who can tolerate capping for only short periods of time. The PMV can be used to assist the client's transition from an open tracheostomy tube to capping by allowing the client to adjust to a more normal breathing pattern through the upper airway on exhalation. Before capping, assess the client for the ability to clear secretions with coughing and the frequency of required suctioning. Label the pilot balloon of cuffed tubes and the wall over the client's bed with a notice or warning label that states, "Do not inflate cuff."

Pediatric

Generally, tracheostomies are not capped in children. The exception to this is the use of the PMV, which provides children a means for speech.

Geriatric

Assess the respiratory status of the geriatric client frequently for his or her response to capping. Older adults may not tolerate capping.

End-of-Life Care

Consider using the PMV during end-of-life care for a client with a tracheostomy to enhance communication between the client and others. This device was developed to allow tracheotomy and ventilator-dependent clients to speak more normally.

Home Health

Teach the family why the cuff on cuffed tracheostomy tubes must not be inflated. If using the PMV, ensure that the client has at least one additional PMV to wear as a backup while the other is being cleaned. Instruct family caregivers to clean the PMV with warm water and fragrance-free soap, air drying it thoroughly. Advise them not to use hot water, peroxide, bleach, vinegar, alcohol, or cleaning brushes.

Cost-Cutting Tips

Clean the PMV properly: it is guaranteed for 2 months if properly cleaned. Contact Passy-Muir for more information at www.passy-muir.com.

Delegation

This procedure should not be delegated to unlicensed assistive personnel.

Implementation

Action	Rationale
1. Check physician's order.	*Verifies accuracy of the procedure*
2. Explain the procedure to the client and family.	*Promotes communication and helps allay fear*
3. Perform hand hygiene and arrange equipment.	*Prevents spread of micro-organisms; promotes efficiency*
4. Check oxygen saturation via pulse oximeter (see Nursing Procedure 6.15.)	*Provides a means to assess oxygen saturation and tolerance of procedure*
5. If cuffed tube in place, suction nasopharynx and tracheostomy (see Nursing Procedures 6.9 and 6.11).	*Clears pooled secretions above cuff of tube and removes excessive secretions from tracheostomy*
6. Tracheostomy tubes with cuffs MUST BE DEFLATED before capping. If present, deflate the tracheostomy tube cuff by:	*Prevents asphyxia with cap application*
• Attach the 20-mL empty syringe to the pilot balloon (Fig. 6.22).	*Ensures that all air is removed from the cuff*
• Aspirate air until no further air can be withdrawn.	*Completes removal of all air from the cuff so that obstruction does not occur when capping*
• Note any change in client's respiratory status. Some clients do not tolerate the capping procedure and may experience respiratory distress. If client becomes short of breath or experiences	*Indicates client's ability to tolerate capping*

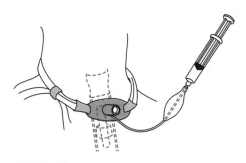

FIGURE 6.22

Action	Rationale
any signs of respiratory distress, or if the pulse oximetry reading drops to less than 90%, do not cap the tracheostomy; reinflate the cuff with air and call the physician.	
7. Don clean gloves.	*Protects nurse from contact with secretions*
8. Suction the tracheostomy again after cuff deflation according to Nursing Procedure 6.11.	*Removes any secretions that may have been dislodged from the deflated cuff*
9. Stabilize the tracheostomy tube with the nondominant hand.	*Prevents accidental dislodgement of the tracheostomy tube*
10. Attach the cap onto the end of the tracheostomy tube with the other hand and twist the cap into place.	*Ensures proper placement of the cap*
11. Assess client's response. Observe for adequate airflow around the capped tracheostomy tube. Decreased airflow and respiratory distress indicate intolerance for tracheostomy capping. If client exhibits signs of respiratory distress, immediately remove the cap and reassess for airway patency.	*Indicates client's ability to adapt to capped tracheostomy*
12. Dispose of or replace supplies appropriately. Remove gloves and perform hand hygiene.	*Reduces microorganism transfer*

Evaluation

Were desired outcomes met? Examples of evaluation include:
- Desired outcome met: Respirations even and nonlabored with a respiratory rate of 16 breaths per minute.
- Desired outcome met: Client coughing spontaneously and infrequently.
- Desired outcome met: Client speaking short phrases after capping.
- Desired outcome met: Client verbalizes comfort with use of cap.

Documentation

The following should be noted on the client's chart:
- Type of cap
- Type or size of tracheostomy
- Position of cuff (deflated)
- Color and amount of secretions suctioned
- Client's tolerance of procedure
- Respiratory status and vital signs before and after procedure
- Pulse oximetry readings before and after procedure

Sample Documentation
Date: 1/7/05
Time: 0800

Respirations even and nonlabored with rate of 16 breaths
per minute. Pulse oximetry 96%. Shiley cuffed
tracheostomy in place with cuff inflated. Suctioned small
amount of clear secretions.

Time: 0830

Cuff deflated. No respiratory distress noted. Pulse oximetry
remains at 95% with even and unlabored respirations at
15 breaths per minute. Suctioned small amount of clear
secretions after cuff deflation.

Time: 0815

Cap applied without difficulty. Client tolerated procedure with
no respiratory distress and pulse oximetry remaining 95% to
95%. Respirations nonlabored at 15 breaths per minute.

● Nursing Procedure 6.14

Collecting a Suctioned Sputum Specimen

Purpose

Gathers a specimen for analysis with minimal risk of contamination

Equipment

- Goggles
- Gown and mask
- Sterile sputum trap
- Suctioning equipment (see procedure for specific type of suctioning)
- Specimen bag and labels
- Gloves, sterile and nonsterile

Assessment

Assessment should focus on the following:
- Physician's orders for test to be done and method of obtaining specimen
- Breath sounds indicating congestion and need for suction
- Previous documentation to determine if secretions are thick or if suction catheter insertion (nasotracheal or nasopharyngeal) was difficult

Nursing Diagnoses

Nursing diagnoses may include the following:
- Risk for infection related to pooled secretions

Outcome Identification and Planning

Desired Outcomes

Sample desired outcomes include the following:
- The client's airway is clear of secretions before discharge.
- An uncontaminated sputum specimen is obtained.

Special Considerations in Planning and Implementation

General

If possible, collect sputum samples in the morning, because sputum collects during the night. Always use new sterile equipment because the procedure is a sterile procedure. However, after the specimen is obtained, the suction catheter can be cleaned and reused if the client is being cared for at home.

Pediatric

Enlist assistance from another person when obtaining a suctioned specimen from a child.

Geriatric

Older clients may experience dyspnea on exertion because their lung bases are less ventilated. The older person also may have a decreased ability to cough, causing increased secretions.

Home Health

Time home visits to coincide with scheduled suctioning and specimen collection. Early-morning sputum collection is best to ensure an adequate amount of sputum. Deliver the specimen to the laboratory immediately.

 Transcultural

Use necessary precautions for preventing tuberculosis (TB) transmission when collecting sputum samples from at-risk clients. The incidence of TB is higher in Asian Americans, primarily in those who have recently immigrated to the United States from countries with a high endemic rate of TB. Newly arrived Vietnamese, Filipinos, Chinese, and Koreans are at the highest risk for TB.

Delegation

This procedure should not be delegated to unlicensed assistive personnel.

Implementation

Action	Rationale
1. Explain procedure to client.	*Reduces anxiety*
2. Perform hand hygiene and organize equipment.	*Reduces microorganism transfer; promotes efficiency*
3. Don clean gloves, goggles, gown, and mask.	*Protects nurse from contact with secretions*
4. Prepare suction equipment for type of suction to be performed (see appropriate procedure in this chapter).	*Promotes efficiency*
5. Open sputum trap package.	
6. Remove sputum trap from package cover and attach suction tubing to short spout of trap.	*Establishes suction for secretion aspiration*
7. Place sterile glove on dominant hand (glove-on-glove technique).	*Maintains sterility of process*
8. Wrap suction catheter around sterile hand.	*Maintains control of catheter*
9. Holding catheter suction port in sterile hand and rubber tube of sputum trap with nonsterile hand, connect suction catheter to sputum trap (Fig. 6.23).	*Maintains sterility of procedure*
10. Suction client until secretions are collected in tubing	*Obtains specimen; allows collection of thick sputum specimen*

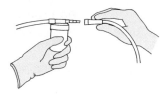

FIGURE 6.23

Action	Rationale
and sputum trap. (If secretions are thick and need to be removed from catheter, suction small amount of sterile saline until specimen is cleared from tubing.)	
11. If insufficient amount of sputum is collected, repeat suction process.	*Ensures adequate specimen*
12. Using nonsterile hand, disconnect suction tubing from sputum trap.	
13. Disconnect suction catheter and sputum trap, maintaining sterility of suction catheter control port, trap tubing, and sterile glove.	*Maintains catheter sterility for further suctioning, if needed*
14. Reconnect suction tubing to catheter and continue suction process, if needed.	*Clears remaining secretions from airway*

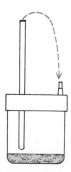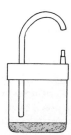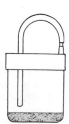

FIGURE 6.24

Action	Rationale
15. Discard suction catheter and sterile glove when suctioning is complete.	*Prevents spread of microorganisms*
16. Connect rubber tubing to sputum trap suction port (Fig. 6.24).	*Seals specimen closed*
17. Place specimen in plastic bag (if agency policy) and label with client's name, date, time, and nurse's initials.	*Ensures proper identification of specimen*
18. Discard equipment.	*Prevents spread of microorganisms*
19. Position client for comfort with side rails up and call light within reach.	*Prevents falls; promotes comfort and communication*
20. Perform hand hygiene.	*Reduces spread of infection*

Evaluation

Were desired outcomes achieved? Examples of evaluation include:
- Desired outcome met: Respirations even and nonlabored with infrequent cough producing thin, white mucus.
- Desired outcome met: Uncontaminated sputum specimen obtained.

Documentation

The following should be noted on the client's chart:
- Date, time, and type of specimen collection
- Type of suction done
- Amount and character of secretions
- Client's tolerance of procedure

Sample Documentation
Date: 1/7/05
Time: 2100

Sputum specimen obtained by nasotracheal suctioning. Large amounts of thick, white mucus obtained; cough reflex stimulated, with strong cough noted. Respirations even and nonlabored; breath sounds clear. Specimen sent to lab.

Obtaining Pulse Oximetry

Purpose

Provides a noninvasive method for monitoring the oxygen saturation of arterial blood

Equipment

- Pulse oximeter
- Sensor (permanent or disposable)
- Alcohol wipe(s)
- Nail polish remover, if indicated

Assessment

Assessment should focus on the following:
- Signs and symptoms of hypoxemia (restlessness; confusion; dusky skin, nailbeds, or mucous membranes)
- Quality of pulse and capillary refill proximal to potential sensor application site
- Respiratory rate and character
- Previous pulse oximetry readings
- Amount and type of oxygen administration, if applicable
- Arterial blood gases, if available

Nursing Diagnoses

Nursing diagnosis may include the following:
- Impaired gas exchange related to excessive secretions
- Ineffective tissue perfusion

Outcome Identification and Planning

Desired Outcomes

Sample desired outcomes include the following:
- Client's arterial oxygen saturation (SaO_2) remains between 95% and 100%.
- Client exhibits signs of adequate gas exchange evidenced by respirations 18 to 20, nailbeds pink, capillary refill less than 3 seconds.
- Client demonstrates knowledge of factors affecting pulse oximeter readings.

Special Considerations in Planning and Implementation

Pediatric

For children, choose an appropriate-sized sensor.

Geriatric

Be sensitive to probe placement in elderly clients: avoid tension on the probe site and be careful when applying tape to dry, thin skin.

Home Health

Pulse oximetry monitoring has mostly replaced home arterial blood gas measurement.

▋▋ Transcultural

Keloids may be present on the earlobes of clients of African descent and may not allow accurate SaO_2 readings. These ropelike scars result from an exaggerated wound-healing process after ear piercing.

Delegation

Pulse oximetry measurement can be performed by unlicensed assistive personnel.

Implementation

Action	Rationale
1. Perform hand hygiene and organize equipment.	*Reduces microorganism transfer; promotes efficiency*
2. Explain procedure to client (if conscious).	*Decreases anxiety; promotes cooperation*
3. Plug in oximeter and choose sensor. Sensor types may vary according to the client's weight and site considerations. If using a disposable sensor, attach sensor to cable.	*Enhances accuracy of results*
4. Prepare site. Use alcohol wipe to cleanse site gently. Remove nail polish or acrylic nails, if needed, if a finger is being used as the monitoring site.	*Ensures site is clean and dry; nail polish and acrylic nails can interfere with pulse oximetry readings*
5. Check capillary refill and pulse proximal to the chosen site.	*Reduces risk of inaccurate readings due to compromised peripheral circulation, caused by a probe that is applied too tightly or by poor circulation due to medications or other conditions*
6. Assess the alignment of the light-emitting diodes (LEDs) and the photo detector (light-receiving	*Ensures proper alignment of sensors to yield an accurate SaO_2 reading*

Action	Rationale
sensor). These sensors should be directly opposite each other (Fig. 6.25).	
7. Turn the pulse oximeter to the ON position. DISPOSABLE SENSORS NEED TO BE ATTACHED TO THE CLIENT CABLE BEFORE TURNING THE PULSE OXIMETER ON.	*Allows emitting sensors (LEDs) to transmit red and infrared light through the tissue so that the receiving sensor (photodetector) will measure the amount of oxygenated hemoglobin (which absorbs more infrared light) and deoxygenated hemoglobin (which absorbs more red light). The pulse oximeter will compute the SaO$_2$ using these data.*
8. Listen for a beep and note waveform or bar of light on front of pulse oximeter.	*Indicates that the pulse oximeter has detected a pulse (beep) and displays the strength of the pulse (light or waveform changes); a weak pulse may not yield an accurate SaO$_2$.*
9. Check alarm limits. Reset if necessary. Make sure that both high and low alarms arc on before leaving the client's room. Alarm limits for both high and low SaO$_2$ and high and low pulse rate are preset by the manufacturer but can be easily reset in response to doctor's orders.	*Identifies the need for possible intervention*
10. Tell the client that common position changes may trigger the alarm, such as bending the elbow or gripping the side rails or other objects.	*Promotes participation in care, thus decreasing anxiety*

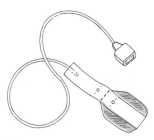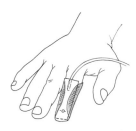

FIGURE 6.25

Action	Rationale
11. Relocate finger sensor at least every 4 hours. Relocate spring tension sensor at least every 2 hours.	*Prevents tissue necrosis*
12. Check adhesive sensors at least every shift.	*Reduces risk of irritation from adhesive*

Evaluation

Were desired outcomes met? Examples of evaluation include:
- Desired outcome met: Pulse oximeter reading 97%.
- Desired outcome met: Client alert and oriented X 3.
- Desired outcome met: Respirations even and nonlabored with rate of 12 breaths per minute.

Documentation

The following should be noted on the client's chart:
- Type and location of sensor
- Presence of pulse proximal to sensor and status of capillary refill
- Percentage of oxygen saturation in arterial blood (SaO_2)
- Rotation of sensor according to guidelines and status of site
- Percentage of oxygen (or room air) client is receiving
- Interventions as a result of deviations from the norm

Sample Documentation
Date: 1/7/05
Time: 1800

Finger sensor (probe) applied to left index finger; capillary refill brisk, radial pulse present. Pulse oximeter yielding SaO_2 of 96% on room air.

Time: 2200

Finger probe applied to right index finger; capillary refill brisk, radial pulse present. Pulse oximeter yielding SaO_2 of 97% on room air.

Maintaining Mechanical Ventilation 🖑

Purpose

Prevents hypoxemia and hypercarbia due to inability of client to maintain ventilatory effort

Improves alveolar ventilation, arterial oxygenation, and lung volumes

Prevents or treats atelectasis

Reduces work of breathing

Equipment

- Mechanical ventilator
- Suction setup and suction catheters
- Stethoscope
- Oxygen source
- Ambu bag (bag-valve mask)
- Clean gloves
- Communication aids
- Pulse oximetry

Assessment

Assessment should focus on the following:
- Type of mechanical ventilator
- Ventilator settings
- Tracheostomy or endotracheal tube (ETT) (type and size)
- Cuff pressure, if appropriate
- Breath sounds
- Respiratory rate and ventilator rate
- Use of accessory muscles
- Arterial blood gas results
- Pulse oximetry readings
- Vital signs
- Amount, color, and consistency of secretions
- Client's response to ventilator
- Oral hygiene supplies, such as lubricant, mouthwash

Nursing Diagnoses

Nursing diagnoses may include the following:
- Impaired gas exchange related to ventilation/perfusion imbalance
- Ineffective airway clearance related to presence of artificial airway
- Impaired spontaneous ventilation related to respiratory muscle fatigue

Outcome Identification and Planning

Desired Outcomes

Sample desired outcomes include the following:
- Client will reestablish/maintain effective respiratory pattern via ventilator with absence of accessory muscle use.
- Arterial blood gases and SaO_2 are within normal range.
- Breath sounds are clear.

Special Considerations in Planning and Implementation

General

Normal ventilation relies on a negative pressure generated when the diaphragm lowers, the thoracic cavity expands, and air enters the lungs. Mechanical ventilation, as most commonly found in acute care settings, relies on a positive pressure from the ventilator forcing air into the lungs. Mechanical ventilation administers oxygen via invasive and noninvasive techniques. Invasive ventilation is administered through an endotracheal tube or tracheostomy. Noninvasive ventilation is administered through a mask that forms a seal over the nose or mouth and nose. An example of this type of ventilation is continuous positive airway pressure (CPAP), which is used to treat clients with sleep apnea.

The amount and pressure of air administered to the client is controlled by the ventilator settings:
- Tidal volume (V_T): the amount of air, in milliliters per breath, delivered during inspiration. Initial setting is 7 to 10 mL/kg; may go as high as 15 mL/kg.
- Rate: the number of breaths per minute administered. Typical initial setting is 10 breaths per minute but will vary based on client's condition.
- Fraction of inspired oxygen (FiO_2): the percentage of oxygen in the air administered. Room air has an FiO_2 of 21%. Initial setting is based on client's condition and usually ranges from 50% to 65%. Up to 100% can be administered, but more than 50% FiO_2 is associated with oxygen toxicity.
- Positive end-expiratory pressure (PEEP): a constant positive pressure in the alveoli that helps keep them open and prevents closing and atelectasis. Typical initial setting of PEEP is 5 cm H_2O. May range as high as 40 cm H_2O in conditions such as adult respiratory distress syndrome (ARDS).

Each change in ventilator settings should be evaluated for effectiveness 20 to 30 minutes later via arterial blood gas analysis, SaO_2 measurement, or end-tidal carbon dioxide reading.

Various modes of ventilation may be used (Table 6.1).

When sounded, ventilator alarms (Table 6.2) require immediate intervention. If you are ever in doubt about a ventilator alarm, assess the pulse oximetry reading quickly to determine the client's oxygenation status. If the SaO_2 reading decreases, dis-

● Table 6.1 Modes of Ventilation

Type	Description
Assist-control (A/C)	Client or ventilator triggers breaths that are either volume or pressure controlled.
Continuous positive airway pressure (CPAP)	Positive pressure is applied during spontaneous breathing and maintained throughout the entire respiratory cycle; decreases intrapulmonary shunting.
Continuous mandatory ventilation (CMV)	Ventilator delivers the breaths at a preset rate and volume or pressure.
Intermittent mandatory ventilation (IMV)	Ventilator delivers breaths at a set rate and volume or pressure. Client can breathe spontaneously between machine breaths.
Mandatory minute ventilation (MMV)	Client breathes spontaneously, yet a minimum level of minute ventilation is ensured.
Pressure-controlled/inverse-ratio ventilation (PC/IRV)	Inspiratory time provided is greater than expiratory time, thereby improving distribution of ventilation and preventing collapse of stiffer alveolar units (auto-PEEP). Client cannot initiate an inspiration.
Positive end-expiratory pressure (PEEP)	Positive pressure is applied during machine breathing and maintained at end-expiration; decreases intrapulmonary shunting.
Pressure support ventilation (PSV)	Client's inspiratory effort is assisted by the ventilator. PSV decreases work of breathing caused by demand flow valve, IMV circuit, and narrow inner diameter of ETT.
Synchronized IMV (SIMV)	Intermittent ventilator breaths are synchronized to spontaneous breaths to reduce competition between ventilator and client. If no inspiratory effort is sensed, the ventilator delivers the breath.

From Stillwell, S. (2002). *Mosby's critical care nursing reference* (3rd ed.). St. Louis: Mosby.

connect the client from the ventilator and attach a bag-valve mask to the ETT and ventilate manually. Call for immediate help.

A chest x-ray should be obtained after initial placement of an ETT. If the physician fails to order the x-ray, question the physician to obtain such an order. Some intensive care units have standing orders to obtain a portable chest x-ray after ETT initiation.

Provide clients with a means of communication, such as a magic slate, dry erase board, Magna Doodle, picture board, or paper and pencil.

● Table 6.2 Ventilator Alarms

Alarm	Possible Causes
High pressure	Secretion buildup, kinked airway tubing, bronchospasm, coughing, fighting the ventilator, decreased lung compliance, biting on endotracheal tubing, condensation in tubing
Low exhaled volume	Disconnection from ventilator, loose ventilator fittings, leaking airway cuff
Low inspiratory pressure	Disconnection from ventilator, loose connections, low ventilating pressure
High respiratory rate	Anxiety, pain, hypoxia, fever
Apnea alarm	No spontaneous breaths within preset time interval

From Stillwell, S. (2002). *Mosby's critical care nursing reference* (3rd ed.). St. Louis: Mosby.

Pediatric

Parents or caregivers should be encouraged to participate in the care of the child. Young children may need alternative methods of communicating (e.g., a picture board rather than a slate).

Geriatric

Older clients may be more susceptible to barotrauma due to the increased rigidity of the thoracic cavity and loss of alveolar elasticity. Clients with chronic obstructive pulmonary disease should be placed on a ventilator as a last resort because weaning is difficult and sometimes impossible for these clients.

End-of-Life Care

Discussion should focus on the client's wishes regarding intubation and ventilator use. Opportunities should be provided for the client or significant other to discuss termination of therapy.

Home Health

As part of the home assessment conducted before the client is discharge from hospital, the nurse should note the layout and size of the rooms, furniture placement, electrical outlets, and doorways. Family members must be taught ventilator management before discharge. Demonstrate procedures and require return demonstrations from caregivers. Practice what to do if alarms sound. The local electric company and fire department should be notified of the presence of a ventilator. Instruct caregivers on the signs and symptoms of complications, such as tension pneumothorax. List names and phone numbers of contact persons and post on wall. Post a "No Smoking" sign plainly on the wall and at the front door. The client should be protected from sources of infection, such as persons with colds and small children. Refer the caregiver to support groups and community resources; encourage "time out" and preventive health practices for the caregiver.

 Cost-Cutting Tips

In the home, reuse of some equipment such as the Ambu bag is acceptable if it is cleaned and sterilized.

Delegation

Unlicensed assistive personnel should not be assigned ventilator management procedures.

Implementation

Action	Rationale
1. Perform hand hygiene.	*Prevents spread of micro-organisms*
2. Gather equipment. Always have stethoscope readily available because it may be needed in emergent situations that require breath sound assessment.	*Ensures efficiency*
3. Assess oxygenation status by doing the following: • Auscultate breath sounds. • Note rate and depth of respirations. • Assess level of consciousness (LOC). • Note any cardiac dysrhythmias. • Note symmetrical chest wall movement.	*Determines efficacy of ventilation; helps identify problems that may require quick intervention or changes in ventilator settings* *Identifies problems due to decreased cardiac perfusion* *Indicates possible barotrauma or possible displacement of ETT*
4. Continuously monitor oxygen saturation with pulse oximetry (see Nursing Procedure 6.15).	*Ensures that changes in oxygen saturation will be quickly identified*
5. Check ventilator settings (V_T, FiO_2, rate, and PEEP) with physician's orders.	*Ensures accuracy of ventilation delivery*
6. Check ventilator alarms for correct function. NEVER TURN OFF ALARMS. Alarms should be heard at the nurses' station.	*Confirms that alarms are set appropriately; allows immediate detection of problems and intervention*
7. Apply gloves.	

Action	Rationale
8. Assess placement of the ETT. If the ETT is in too far, it tends to be displaced in the right mainstem bronchus. The left mainstem bronchus has more of an angle due to the presence of the heart.	*Ensures accurate placement of ETT or allows detection of displacement*
• Note the cm measurement on the ETT at the lips or teeth (Fig. 6.26).	*Establishes a baseline*
• Auscultate breath sounds at least every 2 hours and if respiratory distress occurs. If breath sounds are diminished on one side, the ETT may be inserted too far.	*Assesses lung function and tube placement*
• Obtain chest x-ray (necessary after initial tube placement and as ordered by the physician).	*Confirms proper placement of ETT*
9. Document the cm measurement of ETT entry.	*Enhances communication of findings*
10. Monitor endotracheal or tracheostomy cuff pressure (see Nursing Procedure 6.13). Cuff pressure should not exceed 15 mm Hg.	*Prevents tracheal necrosis*

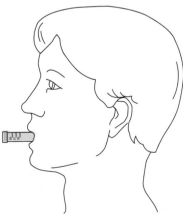

FIGURE 6.26

Action	Rationale
11. Suction client as needed (see Nursing Procedure 6.11).	*Removes secretions*
12. Assess lips and tongue for pressure ulcers.	*Reduces risk of skin breakdown and allows for early intervention*
13. Rotate tube placement from side to side of the mouth.	*Decreases pressure on lips and mouth tissues*
14. Provide oral care and lip care (See Nursing Procedure 4.5).	*Reduces risk of ulceration*
15. Measure PaO_2 and FiO_2 ratio daily.	*Provides an indication of lung status. If PaO_2 decreases while increasing FiO_2, client may be developing adult respiratory distress syndrome (ARDS).*
16. Monitor fluid status every 8 hours: • Weigh daily and compare to previous weights. • Assess skin and mucous membranes. • Monitor intake and output.	*Identifies possible fluid imbalances. Ventilated clients are at risk for fluid volume excess because ventilation stimulates release of antidiuretic hormone, resulting in decreased urine output.*
17. Administer sedation as needed.	*Synchronizes respirations and reduces workload of breathing; reduces risk of client "fighting" the ventilator*
18. Check ventilator tubing for obstruction. Drain tubing of water collected. Do not drain tubing toward client or back in reservoir.	*Prevents impairment of ventilation; prevents client from receiving water in ETT. Draining water back into reservoir would promote bacterial growth.*
19. Communicate with client. Explain procedure as appropriate.	*Reduces anxiety; reduces fear of the unknown*
20. Remove gloves and perform hand hygiene.	*Reduces microorganism transfer*

Evaluation

Were desired outcomes met? Examples of evaluation include:
• Desired outcome met: Respirations symmetric with breath sounds present in all lung fields. No adventitious sounds noted.
• Desired outcome met: Respiratory rate 18 with ventilatory rate of 10. PaO_2 80, pH 7.38, PCO_2 40, HCO_3 26.

Documentation

The following should be noted on the client's chart:
• Ventilator: type, settings, alarms on

- ETT size, cm entry point at mouth, placement in mouth, cuff pressure or tracheostomy status
- Respiratory assessment: breath sounds, presence or absence of adventitious sounds, use of accessory muscles, respiratory pattern, rate, secretions, symmetry of chest wall movements
- Vital signs and level of consciousness (LOC)
- Telemetry: heart rate, rhythm (e.g., normal sinus rhythm, rate 86 with multifocal PVCs at approx. 6 per minute)
- Weight, intake and output, condition of mucous membranes
- ABG results, pulse oximetry readings
- Sedation use, including drug, dosage, time of administration, indications for use, and client's response to administration

---

Sample Documentation
Date: 1/7/05
Time: 2100

Client with #7.5 ETT at 26 cm at lips on right side of mouth. Pressure support ventilation with V_T 500 FiO$_2$ 40%, PEEP of 10. Pulse oximetry 96%. No oral pressure ulcers seen. Oral mucous membranes pink and moist. Respirations even and nonlabored at spontaneous rate of 18 and ventilator rate of 10. Suctioned small amount of yellow, thick secretions. Breath sounds present bilaterally with few crackles in bases. Client sedated with lorazepam (Ativan) 2 mg IV.

● **Nursing Procedure 6.17**

Using Incentive Spirometry

Purpose

Encourages maximal inspirations
Mimics natural sighing or yawning
Promotes lung expansion and prevents atelectasis

Equipment

- Incentive spirometer
- Teaching incentive spirometer for demonstration (optimal, but not required)
- Stethoscope
- Tissues
- Pillow (for surgical clients)

Assessment

Assessment should focus on the following:
- Signs of atelectasis such as decreased breath sounds, shallow respirations, adventitious breath sounds
- Respiratory rate and depth
- Vital signs

Nursing Diagnoses

Nursing diagnoses may include the following:
- Ineffective breathing pattern related to pain
- Ineffective airway clearance related to neuromuscular dysfunction
- Deficient knowledge related to use of spirometer

Outcome Identification and Planning

Desired Outcomes

Sample desired outcomes include the following:
- Breath sounds are clear to auscultation in all lung fields or improvement is noted in previously absent or diminished breath sounds.
- No adventitious breath sounds present.
- Chest x-ray is clear.
- Pulse rate ranges between 60 and 100 beats per minute.
- Temperature is within normal range for client.
- Client states reason for incentive spirometry use.
- Client demonstrates proper technique for use.

Special Considerations in Planning and Implementation

General

Incentive spirometry, also referred to as sustained maximal inspiration (SMI), is contraindicated when clients cannot be instructed or supervised to ensure appropriate use of device, when client is uncooperative, or when hypoxia occurs secondary to interruption of prescribed oxygen therapy. The incentive spirometer should be kept at the bedside within reach of the client to encourage use. Incentive spirometry should be performed for 5 to 10 breaths every hour.

The client must be able to take a deep breath through the mouth only while maintaining a tight seal on the mouthpiece.

Pediatric

Pediatric incentive spirometers are available. Parents should be instructed on use and the child should be encouraged to use the device.

Geriatric

Older clients are at risk for atelectasis due to their decreased lung volume, decreased ability to cough, decreased ventilation to lung bases, increased secretions, and loss of protective airway reflexes. The geriatric client with COPD should be taught pursed-lip breathing to prevent air trapping. There is a potential for barotrauma for clients with emphysema. Dry mouth and dentures may make use of incentive spirometry difficult.

Home Health

The incentive spirometer should be cleaned with soap and water every day.

Cost-Cutting Tips

In a recent literature review, use of incentive spirometry was not shown to decrease the incidence of postoperative pulmonary complications after cardiac or abdominal surgery. Deep-breathing exercises, if performed regularly, are as efficient as incentive spirometry and less expensive.

Delegation

The registered nurse should initiate incentive spirometry therapy and instruct the client in its use. Unlicensed assistive personnel can assist clients with subsequent use.

Implementation

Action	Rationale
1. Explain need for procedure to client.	*Decreases anxiety; facilitates cooperation*
2. Perform hand hygiene and organize equipment.	*Reduces microorganism transfer; promotes efficiency*
3. Assess breath sounds, breathing pattern, and respiratory rate.	*Establishes a baseline for comparison of response before and after procedure*
4. Position the client as erect as possible without causing an increase in pain. Place the spirometer upright in front of the client. Maintain the upright position of the client and device throughout the procedure.	*Lowers the diaphragm and increases thoracic expansion*
5. Describe and demonstrate proper technique of use.	*Teaches client*
6. If the client is preoperative or postoperative, demonstrate splinting of surgical incision with a pillow during technique.	*Reduces pain and provides support to surgical area*

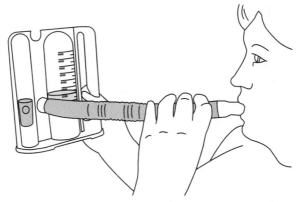

FIGURE 6.27

Action	Rationale
7. Instruct client to exhale normally and completely, then close and seal lips around mouthpiece of the spirometer (Fig. 6.27).	*Prevents air leakage around mouthpiece on inspiration. Incentive spirometry is an inspiratory procedure, and a proper seal must be maintained.*
8. Have client inhale slowly and steadily to full lung capacity.	*Mobilizes secretions and aerates alveoli; may stimulate cough reflex*
9. Hold breath for 3 to 5 seconds with incentive spirometer in place.	*Maintains alveolar aeration*
10. Note the highest level the volume indicator reaches. Make a mark on the incentive spirometer with a pen.	*Establishes a goal for client to reach or exceed on subsequent attempts*
11. Have client remove mouthpiece and breathe normally for a few breaths.	*Allows client to rest and prepare for next inhalation*
12. Repeat steps 7 through 11 between 5 and 10 times. Encourage the client to aim for a higher volume with each attempt.	*Promotes alveolar aeration. Watching the flow indicator motivates clients to take larger inhalations.*
13. Ask the client to cough. Have a tissue available.	*Helps expel secretions mobilized during procedure*
14. Replace the mouthpiece end of the tubing in the notch at the top of the incentive spirometer when finished.	*Keeps mouthpiece clean for next use*

Evaluation

Were desired outcomes met? Examples of evaluation include:
- Desired outcome met: Breath sounds clear to auscultation in all lung fields.
- Desired outcome met: No adventitious breath sounds present.
- Desired outcome met: Chest x-ray is clear.
- Desired outcome met: Pulse rate ranges between 60 and 100 beats per minute.
- Desired outcome met: Temperature is within normal range for client.
- Desired outcome met: Client states reason for incentive spirometry use.
- Desired outcome met: Client demonstrates proper technique for use.

Documentation

The following should be noted on the client's chart:
- Breath sounds before and after procedure
- Inspiratory capacity of best effort with incentive spirometer
- Cough with or without mucous production (including amount, color, and consistency of secretions)
- Demonstration of technique and successful return demonstration by client
- Verbalization of understanding of procedure instructions by client
- Pain assessment and administration of medication, including client's response
- Use of splinting, if appropriate

Sample Documentation
Date: 1/7/05
Time 2100

Crackles in right base before incentive spirometry treatment. Client instructed in use of incentive spirometry. Demonstrated technique on teaching device. Client returned demonstration correctly and verbalized understanding of procedure. Inspiratory capacity of 1 L noted. Respirations even and nonlabored. Productive cough of thick yellow secretions noted. Crackles heard in right base at end of procedure.

Fluids and Nutrition

OVERVIEW

- Initiating intake and output measurements can be done any time the potential for fluid or nutrition imbalance exists. Consider the client's general condition and medical diagnosis in making this determination.
- Aseptic technique is used when administering nutritional support to clients who are malnourished because they are at increased risk for infection. This risk is further increased because nutritional-support substances may provide a medium for microorganism growth.

- Monitoring and regulating fluid administration is crucial to prevent a potentially lethal fluid overload.
- Intake and output and daily weights are used to assess nutritional status and fluid balance.
- Always check the placement of a central line or feeding tube when providing nutritional support. Infusion of hyperosmotic solutions into the thoracic cavity or aspiration into the pulmonary tree could result in major respiratory compromise.
- Appropriate precautions are necessary with infusion procedures to minimize the risk of injury. To prevent exposure to infectious organisms, use standard precautions and wear gloves when contact with body fluids is likely. Safety precautions are also crucial to prevent needlesticks or other injuries. Discard needles and other equipment in proper receptacles. Never reach into a trash can to retrieve an item. Reusable equipment, such as infusion pumps, must be cleaned on a regular basis and in between uses according to agency policy.
- Review the client's medication regimen to determine if there are medications that may contribute to fluid or nutrition imbalances.
- A personal or client history of latex allergy requires appropriate precautions, including the use of hypoallergenic nonlatex gloves.
- Some major nursing diagnostic labels related to fluid and nutrient balance include excess fluid volume, deficient fluid volume, risk for imbalanced fluid volume, decreased cardiac output, and imbalanced nutrition, less than body requirements or more than body requirements.
- Infusion of fluids and nutritional supplements to dying clients is controversial in terms of its palliative versus life-sustaining potential. Consider the desires of the client and family, the physician's orders, and agency policies.

Nursing Procedure 7.1

Managing Intake and Output (I&O)

Purpose

Helps control fluid balance
Provides data to evaluate the effects of therapy, such as diuretics or rehydration

Equipment

- Graduated measuring devices, such as 1,000-mL container, water pitcher, or cups
- Scale
- Nonsterile gloves
- Felt-tipped pen or fine-tip marker

Assessment

Assessment should focus on the following:
- Doctor's orders for frequency of I&O measurements
- Client status indicating need for I&O, such as edema, poor skin turgor, severely low or high blood pressure, heart failure, dyspnea, reduced urinary output, IV infusion therapy
- Client vital signs and weight, including daily weight trends
- Use of medications that can alter fluid status, such as diuretics, antihypertensives, corticosteroids, and laxatives

Nursing Diagnoses

Nursing diagnoses may include the following:
- Deficient fluid volume related to oral fluid restriction
- Risk for fluid imbalance related to medication therapy
- Imbalanced nutrition, less than body requirements related to anorexia

Outcome Identification and Planning

Desired Outcomes

Sample desired outcomes include the following:
- Heart rate, blood pressure, pulse, and respirations are within normal limits.
- Skin returns quickly to position when pinched.
- Client demonstrates non-pitting ankle edema within 48 hours.
- Client demonstrates an output equal to intake (plus or minus insensible loss) in a 24-hour period.
- Client will maintain weight between 130 and 133 pounds.
- Client will gain 1 to 2 pounds within 1 week.

Special Considerations in Planning and Implementation

General

When monitoring strict I&O, account for incontinent urine, emesis, and diaphoresis, if possible. Weigh soiled linens to determine fluid loss, or estimate it. Enlist the aid of family members in obtaining accurate I&O measurements. Explain the rationale and procedure for monitoring I&O. When measuring output, wear gloves to protect against exposure to body fluids.

Pediatric

Weigh diapers to give a rough estimate of output (1 g of weight = 1 mL).

Geriatric

For incontinent clients, weigh linens, waterproof pads, or incontinence briefs as a rough estimate of output (1 g of weight = 1 mL). Anticipate the need for monitoring I&O for older clients who are at risk for dehydration because of poor fluid intake, thin and fragile skin (more prone to environmental insults), and decreased response to thirst, among other factors.

End-of-Life Care

Consider the desires of the client and family, physician's orders, and agency policies related to fluid and nutrition therapy for end-of-life clients; food and drink are associated with health, comfort, and love by many clients and families. Assess dying clients for dehydration, such as from a decreased ability to swallow and a subsequent decrease in blood volume.

Home Health

If the homebound client has difficulty understanding units of measure or seeing calibration lines, make an I&O sheet including columns for common household measurement devices such as drinking glasses, cups of ice, or bowls of jello and soup to represent intake; the client can cross off or check these off. Have client measure output by number of voidings.

Transcultural

In various cultures, health, comfort, and love are associated with food and drink through traditions and rituals. Exercise cultural sensitivity when caring for clients who are on various food and fluid restrictions, and allow the client and family to verbalize concerns.

Delegation

Measuring I&O is often delegated to unlicensed personnel. However, IV intake must be added to intake totals, and the nurse must always check the information gathered and report any evidence of fluid overload or deficit.

Implementation

Action	Rationale
1. Perform hand hygiene and organize equipment.	*Reduces microorganism transfer; promotes efficiency*
2. Post pad on door or in room, and instruct team members to record I&O. Instruct client and family on use of I&O record, with return demonstration. (If calorie count is in progress, list type of food and fluid consumed as well.)	*Ensures complete, accurate record of I&O; allows dietary department to calculate caloric intake correctly based on standard institutional serving sizes*
3. Measure oral intake:	*Takes into account the wide variety of fluids consumed orally*

Action	Rationale
• Place graduated cups in room before consumption.	*Ensures consistency and common units of measurement and minimizes error*
• Record semi-solid substance intake in percentage or fraction of amount based on institution's use of standard portions.	*Provides measurement of foods that would be liquid at room temperature*
• Note volume of water in pitcher at beginning of shift, plus any fluid added, and subtract fluid remaining in pitcher at end of shift.	
• Note amount of ice chips consumed, multiply volume by 0.5 and record amount.	*When melted, the volume of ice is approximately half its previous volume.*
• Measure all liquids such as juices, other beverages, jello, ice cream, sherbet, and broth using graduated devices, package volume, or standard volume measurements from institution's food services.	*Includes all sources of ingested fluids for accurate measurements*
4. Measure nasogastric (NG) or gastric tube feeding:	*Maintains accurate record by including gastrointestinal (GI) intake in addition to oral intake*
• Note volume of feeding hanging at beginning of shift or volume amount on feeding pump readout (amount left from previous shift) plus any amount added during shift; allow prior feeding to infuse almost totally before adding new solution.	*Ensures accuracy of measurement to include all fluids given; indicates volume infusing during current shift; prevents feeding from hanging for more than 8 hours*
• Subtract feeding volume remaining at end of shift (or read infusion total from pump if previous shift has cleared pump total).	

Action	Rationale
• Record amount of fluid used to mix any liquid, oral, or NG medications.	*Maintains complete I&O measurement*
5. Measure all IV intake using same methodology as in Step 4. Volume of each type of intake is often designated on flow sheet (e.g., colloids, blood products).	*Ensures complete and accurate monitoring of all intake regardless of source*
6. If NG irrigation is performed and irrigant is left to drain out with other gastric contents, enter irrigant in intake section of flow sheet (or subtract irrigant amount from total output; see Step 10).	*Ensures accurate accounting of retained fluid*
7. Measure output:	*Ensures measurement of output using standardized measurement units*
• Place one or more graduated containers (size dependent on fluid or drainage being measured) in the room; for small amounts of drainage such as from wounds, place clearly marked graduated cup in room.	*Prevents use of cup for measuring intake*
• For drainage measurement, designate whether urine measurement from urinal will be used or if urine should be poured into graduated containers.	*Helps to maintain standardized measurement units to promote accuracy*
• Measure output, including NG or gastrostomy tube drainage; ostomy drainage or liquid stool; wound drainage; chest tube drainage; urinary catheter drainage or voiding; emesis; blood or serous drainage; and extreme diaphoresis.	*Ensures measurement of all sources of output*
• Weigh soiled pads or linens and subtract dry	*Promotes complete measurement*

Action	Rationale
weight to estimate output.	
8. At end of each shift, or hourly if needed, apply gloves and empty drainage into graduated container. Alternatively, mark the level of drainage on a tape strip on the container with date and time (Fig. 7.1), or calibrate in intervals of desired number of hours. When container is nearly full, empty or dispose of container and replace with new container.	*Minimizes exposure to body fluids during measurement; allows monitoring on a more frequent basis; ensures uninterrupted measurement of output*
9. Record amount and source of drainage, particularly with drains from different sites.	*Identifies drainage amounts from specific sites*
10. If intermittent or ongoing irrigation is performed, calculate true output (urinary or NG) by measuring total output and subtracting total irrigant infused.	*Eliminates double counting of output*
11. At end of 24-hour period, usually at end of evening or night shift, add total intake and total output. Report extreme discrepancy to	*Provides an indication of I&O status over a 24-hour period; identifies possible fluid overload situations; helps determine if third spacing is occurring*

From client

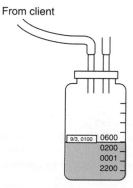

FIGURE 7.1

Action	Rationale
doctor (e.g., if input is 1 to 2 L more than output). Correlate weight gains with fluid intake excesses.	
12. Clean containers, and store in client's room. Discard gloves and perform hand hygiene.	*Prevents infection transmission*

Evaluation

Were desired outcomes achieved? Examples of evaluation include:
- Desired outcome met: Blood pressure, pulse, and respirations were within normal limits (BP 126/74, pulse 72, resp 22).
- Desired outcome met: Skin turgor returns quickly when pinched before client is discharged.
- Desired outcome met: Edema is nonpitting after 48 hours.
- Desired outcome met: Client demonstrates an output equal to intake of 2,200 mL in 24 hours (plus or minus insensible loss).
- Desired outcome met: Weight maintained at 131 pounds.
- Desired outcome met: Client gained 1.5 pounds in past 7 days.

Documentation

The following should be noted on the client's chart:
- Intake from all sources on appropriate graph sheet
- Output from all sources on appropriate graph sheet
- Medication or fluid given to improve fluid balance and immediate response noted (e.g., diuresis, blood pressure increase)
- Vital signs and skin turgor status indicating fluid balance or imbalance, including measurements of edematous areas
- Client weight, as indicated by frequency of orders

Sample Documentation
Date: 2/17/05
Time: 2100

Client excreted 1,200 mL clear yellow urine after furosemide administration. Ankle circumference remains 6 inches with 2+ pitting edema. 500 mL of D₅W infusing into right wrist angiocath at 10 mL/hr by infusion pump.

Testing Capillary Blood Glucose

Purpose

Determines level of glucose in blood
Promotes stricter blood glucose regulation

Equipment

- Blood glucose monitor
- Test strips for blood glucose monitor
- Nonsterile gloves
- Lancets
- Autoclix or lancet injector (optional)
- Cotton balls
- Alcohol wipes
- Watch with second hand or stopwatch
- Sharps biohazard disposal unit

Assessment

Assessment should focus on the following:
- Doctor's orders for frequency and type of glucose testing and sliding scale for insulin coverage
- Client's knowledge of procedure and of diabetic self-care
- Results of and client's response to previous testing

Nursing Diagnoses

Nursing diagnoses may include the following:
- Deficient knowledge regarding diabetes self-care related to lack of understanding of newly diagnosed diabetes
- Risk for injury related to testing procedure and effects of uncontrolled blood glucose levels

Outcome Identification and Planning

Desired Outcomes

Sample desired outcomes include the following:
- Blood glucose elevation is noted and treated promptly per sliding scale.
- Blood glucose level is maintained within acceptable range.
- Client remains free of injury from effects of uncontrolled blood glucose levels.

Special Considerations in Planning and Implementation

General

Plan time for client teaching during the blood glucose testing procedure.

Pediatric

Consider developmental stage and assess the child's ability to understand and perform the procedure. To reinforce teaching, include family members in teaching.

Geriatric

For clients with vision problems, use a glucose-monitoring machine with a large-scale digital readout.

End-of-Life Care

The decision to obtain fingerstick specimens for glucose testing is made on an individual basis by the physician, client, and family. Typically they are done only to support physiologic processes that help the client die in comfort.

Home Health

Suggest using an egg timer to time the test procedure. Have the client test glucose levels as ordered, being consistent with meal times at home.

Delegation

In most areas, this procedure may be delegated to unlicensed assistive personnel; however, the individual must have training on the specific machine being used for glucose testing. Assistive personnel should report all results and indicators of machine malfunction immediately. The nurse must check test results and administer treatment based on the sliding scale, if ordered. Unusually high or low readings should be verified by the nurse.

Implementation

Action	Rationale
1. Perform hand hygiene and organize equipment.	*Reduces microorganism transfer; promotes efficiency*
2. Explain procedure to client and inquire about finger preference and use of lancet injector.	*Promotes cooperation and sense of involvement and control*
3. Calibrate glucose machine: • Turn machine on. • Compare number/ code on machine with	*Ensures that results obtained are accurate*

Action	Rationale
number on bottle of test strips (Fig. 7.2).	
• Prepare machine for operation; consult user's manual for steps and readiness indicator.	
• Validate machine accuracy daily or per laboratory policy with sample low- and high-glucose solutions.	
4. Remove chemical strip from container and place it in the glucose testing machine (according to manufacturer's instructions).	*Prevents delay once sample is obtained*
5. Load lancet in injector, if used, and set trigger.	*Prepares injector for lancet puncture*
6. Don gloves.	*Prevents exposure to blood*
7. Hold chosen finger down and squeeze gently from lower digit to fingertip, or	*Promotes blood flow in area for ease in specimen collection*

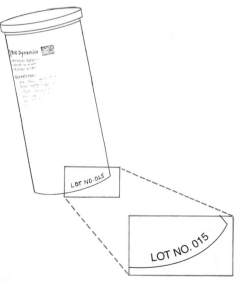

FIGURE 7.2

Action	Rationale
wrap finger in a warm, wet cloth for 30 seconds or longer. (If using arm lancet device, dangle arm for about 1 minute.)	
8. Wipe puncture site with alcohol pad.	*Removes dirt and skin oils and decreases microorganisms*
9. Place injector against side of finger (where there are fewer nerve endings) and release trigger, or stick side of finger with lancet or needle using a darting motion. (If using arm lancet device, puncture site with lancet device.)	*Obtains a large drop of blood with minimal pain*
10. Hold chemical strip under puncture site and squeeze gently until drop of blood is large enough to drop onto strip and cover indicator squares. If using arm lancet device, hold strip close to blood drop after appropriate amount of blood (according to manufacturer's instructions) has formed.	*Ensures that indicator squares are covered with blood; prevents uneven exposure of indicators, which would leading to inaccurate results*
11. If necessary, push timer button on machine as soon as blood has covered indicator squares or area on test strip. Most machines automatically begin timing and require no action to start timing once blood makes contact with strip.	*Activates timing mechanism if necessary*
12. Apply pressure to puncture site until bleeding stops (or have client do so) and place lancet in sharps biohazard disposal unit.	*Reduces risk of needlestick and injury*
13. When timer indicates that appropriate number of seconds has passed, read glucose value on digital readout (Fig. 7.3).	*Ensures accurate reading*
14. Discard soiled materials and gloves in proper container.	*Reduces risk of infection transmission*

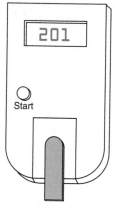

FIGURE 7.3

Action	Rationale
15. Record results on glucose flow sheet and administer insulin if indicated.	*Maintains record of glucose levels*
16. Position client appropriately with call light within reach.	*Promotes comfort and communication*

Evaluation

Were desired outcomes achieved? Examples of evaluation include:

- Desired outcome met: Blood glucose elevation of 215 mg/dL decreased to 154 mg/dL since last 4-hour reading.
- Desired outcome met: Blood glucose is maintained within acceptable range between 80 and 120 mg/dL.
- Desired outcome met: Client remains free of injury from effects of uncontrolled blood glucose levels.

Documentation

The following should be noted on the client's chart:
- Method of glucose testing
- Level of glucose
- Insulin coverage provided and route
- Response to insulin coverage

- Presence or absence of signs of hypo- or hyperglycemia
- Teaching done and demonstration of client understanding, if necessary

---

Sample Documentation
Date: 2/17/05
Time: 2100

Fingerstick blood glucose testing performed by client after teaching and demonstration by nurse. Client's technique good, with good asepsis noted. Results showed 256 mg glucose/dl. No other clinical signs of hyperglycemia noted. Five units regular human insulin given subcutaneously as ordered in abdominal area by client using correct technique.

● Nursing Procedure 7.3

Performing Venipuncture for Blood Specimen 🖐

Purpose

Provides blood specimen for laboratory analysis

Equipment

- Nonsterile gloves
- Alcohol pads or agency-approved antiseptic cleansing agent, such as povidone-iodine
- Tourniquet

For Vacutainer Method

- Blood collecting device or Vacutainer holder with double-point needle
- Appropriately colored test tube or Vacutainer (consult agency laboratory manual) or blood culture bottle(s) (optional)

For Syringe Method

- Sterile needles (20- or 21-gauge or scalp vein [butterfly] device)
- Sterile syringe of appropriate size

Assessment

Assessment should focus on the following:
- Type of lab test ordered
- Time for which test is ordered
- Adequacy of client preparation (e.g., fasting state, medication withheld or given)
- Client's ability to cooperate
- Use of medications that have an anticoagulant effect

Nursing Diagnoses

Nursing diagnoses may include the following:
- Risk for infection related to skin puncture
- Risk for injury related to venipuncture

Outcome Identification and Planning

Desired Outcomes

Sample desired outcomes include the following:
- Client does not demonstrate redness, bruising, or signs of infection at puncture site.

Special Considerations in Planning and Implementation

General

Do not perform venipuncture on arm if client has had a mastectomy on that side or has a dialysis shunt in place. Use opposite arm or location in access site other than that arm. If specimen is being drawn from an extremity with an IV infusion, stop the IV infusion before obtaining the blood sample; draw the specimen distal to the IV insertion site. Specimens for glucose levels drawn from the same extremity as the IV infusion may be inaccurate, even when obtained from a point distal to the IV catheter. When using a tourniquet, release the tourniquet before withdrawing the blood sample to avoid hemoconcentration. Apply pressure for an additional 5 minutes (or more as needed) after blood is drawn on clients who are taking medications with an anticoagulant effect, such as aspirin or warfarin.

Pediatric

To prevent injury, have an assistant restrain the child during venipuncture. Use a butterfly device with syringe to avoid excessive suction on the vein. Document the amount of blood taken in the medical record, as even small amounts may be important for fluid balance measurement and therapy.

Geriatric

Use a blood pressure cuff instead of a tourniquet to prevent excessive stress on the vessel and subsequent collapse or rupture. Elderly clients often have veins that appear large and dilated.

End-of-Life Care

Generally blood drawing is minimized in dying clients. Allow additional time for holding pressure at the site to stop bleeding, as coagulation functions become compromised.

Home Health

Use a blood pressure cuff instead of a tourniquet if necessary, maintaining a pressure greater than the client's diastolic pressure.

Delegation

Typically, blood drawing is not delegated to unlicensed assistive personnel unless they complete specific training. Consult agency policy.

Implementation

Action	Rationale
1. Perform hand hygiene and organize equipment; explain procedure and cooperation required to client.	*Reduces transfer of microorganisms and promotes efficiency; promotes relaxation and fosters compliance*
2. Lower side rail and assist client into a semi-Fowler's position; raise bed to high position.	*Provides access to venipuncture site; promotes comfort; promotes use of proper body mechanics*
3. Open several alcohol and povidone pads.	*Provides easy access to supplies; promotes efficiency*
4. Attach needle to blood collection device, if used, so that needle touches but does not puncture Vacutainer device (Fig. 7.4.).	
5. Place towel under extremity.	*Keeps linens clean*
6. Locate largest, most distal vein (see Nursing Procedure 7.4); place tourniquet on extremity 2 to 6 inches (5 to 15 cm) above venipuncture site.	*Facilitates access; if insertion attempt fails, vein can be entered at a higher point; tourniquet restricts blood flow*
7. Don gloves.	*Reduces microorganism transfer*

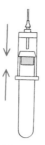

FIGURE 7.4

Action	Rationale
8. Use alcohol to clean area, beginning at the vein and circling outward to a 2-inch diameter. Allow alcohol to dry.	*Maintains asepsis*
9. Encourage client to take slow, deep breaths as you begin.	*Promotes relaxation*
10. Remove cap from needle and hold skin taut with one hand while holding syringe or Vacutainer holder with other hand. If using a butterfly device, pinch "wings" together to hold device.	*Stabilizes vein and prevents skin from moving during needle insertion; helps decrease pain during needle insertion; pinching wings helps stabilize device for insertion*
11. Maintaining needle sterility, insert needle, bevel up, into the straightest section of vein; puncture skin at a 15- to 30-degree angle.	*Promotes puncture into a clear straight vein*
12. When needle has entered skin, lower needle until almost parallel with skin.	*Decreases risk of penetrating opposite wall of vein*
13. Following path of vein, insert needle into wall of vein.	*Ensures proper location for needle insertion*
14. Watch for backflow of blood (not noted with Vacutainer); push needle slightly further into vein.	*Indicates that needle has pierced vein wall and has entered the vein*
15. Gently pull back syringe plunger until an adequate amount of blood is obtained.	

Action	Rationale
16. If using blood collection device, put tube or blood culture bottle into device and push in until needle punctures rubber stopper and blood is pulled into tube by vacuum. Keep tube in device until it is three-fourths full or until culture medium is blood-colored. Remove tube and replace with new tube if additional specimens are needed.	*Establishes suction to allow blood to enter specimen tube; ensures that an adequate amount of blood is obtained for specimen*
17. Place alcohol pad or cotton ball over needle insertion site and remove needle from vein while applying pressure with pad or cotton ball.	*Helps seal vein and decreases bleeding from site*
18. Apply pressure for 2 to 3 minutes (5 to 10 minutes if client is on anticoagulant therapy); check for bleeding and apply pressure until bleeding has stopped.	*Promotes clotting and minimizes risk of hematoma formation*
19. Position client with call light within reach.	*Promotes comfort and communication*
20. Attach properly completed identification label to each tube, affix requisition, and send to lab.	*Reduces risk of errors*
21. Dispose of or store equipment properly (remove needle from Vacutainer device, discarding needle and saving tube holder portion).	*Promotes cost-effectiveness and minimizes risk for injury*
22. Remove gloves and perform hand hygiene.	*Reduces microorganism transfer*

Evaluation

Were desired outcomes achieved? Examples of evaluation include:

- Desired outcome met: Client remains free of injury at insertion site.
- Desired outcome not met: Client verbalizes pain in relation to venipuncture.

Documentation

The following should be noted on the client's chart:
- Time blood is drawn
- Test to be run on specimen
- Client's tolerance of procedure
- Status of skin (e.g., bruising, excessive bleeding)

> *Sample Documentation*
> Date: 2/17/05
> Time: 2100
>
> Blood drawn for complete blood count and electrolytes.
> Specimen sent to laboratory. Needle insertion site intact
> without evidence of bruising or bleeding. Client tolerated
> procedure well.

● Nursing Procedures 7.4, 7.5, 7.6

Selecting a Vein for IV Therapy (7.4) 🧤

Preparing Solutions for IV Therapy (7.5) 🧤

Inserting a Catheter/IV Lock for IV Therapy (7.6) 🧤

Purpose

Provides route for administration of fluids, medications, blood, or nutrients

Provides peripheral venous access route for repetitive blood sampling, thereby minimizing pain associated with repetitive needlesticks

Equipment

- Nonsterile gloves
- Over-the-needle catheter or butterfly device
- IV solution for fluid (if continuous infusion) or infusion plug or cap and flush solution of normal saline 0.9% or diluted heparin solution (as designated by agency policy) for IV lock
- Armboard (optional)
- Infusion tubing
- IV pole (bed or rolling) or IV pump
- IV insertion kit or supplies, including tourniquet (or blood pressure cuff); tape—1-inch wide (or 2-inch tape, cut); alcohol pads [or agency-approved antiseptic, such as povidone]; dressing—2 × 2-inch gauze; transparent dressing (such as Tegaderm or Opsite); adhesive bandage; adhesive labels
- Scissors and soap (optional)
- Towel or linen saver

Assessment

Assessment should focus on the following:
- Reason for initiation of IV therapy for this client
- Orders for type and rate of fluid and/or specified IV site
- Status of skin on hands and arms; presence of hair or abrasions; previous IV sites
- Client's ability to avoid movement of arms or hands during procedure
- Allergy to tape, iodine, or antibiotic solutions
- Client knowledge of IV therapy

Nursing Diagnoses

Nursing diagnoses may include the following:
- Deficient fluid volume related to poor oral intake
- Risk of infection related to invasive procedure

Outcome Identification and Planning

Desired Outcomes

A sample desired outcome is:
- IV insertion site is clean and dry, with no pain, redness, swelling, or drainage.

Special Considerations in Planning and Implementation

General

Wear gloves, because contact with blood is likely. Maintain aseptic technique. Choose tubing and needle appropriate for the solution to provide optimal fluid flow. Viscous solutions require larger needles, but choose the smallest-gauge needle that will meet the need. Small catheters cause less vein wall irritation than large ones. Because venous blood runs upward toward the heart, attempt to enter a vein at its lower (distal) end so that the same vein can be used later at a more proximal site without leakage. If it is difficult to insert a catheter fully, wait until fluid infusion is initiated and then gently advance the catheter. NEVER ATTEMPT TO RETHREAD A CATHETER. (Most devices are now manufactured with a safety feature to prevent rethreading after a needle has been withdrawn from the plastic sheath.) If the client is confused or restless, have an assistant hold the extremity still. For accurate 24-hour management, each shift should report to the oncoming shift the amount of IV fluid remaining and the need for new bottle/bag, tubing or site change, or site care. Check manufacturer's labels and watch medication expiration warnings on labels or drug inserts. Although agencies can use CDC guidelines to determine standard times for fluid bag and tubing changes, some solutions are prepared with medications or products (either by the manufacturer or on site) in such a manner that tubing or bags must be changed more frequently.

Pediatric

Have a parent or an assistant hold the child's extremities still. Use armboards to stabilize an IV in an extremity. Use microdrip tubing with volume control chambers for strict volume control. Infusion devices are often used for additional safety. Provide clear explanations along with a demonstration of the equipment (except needles), using a puppet or game. Explain that a helper is needed to help the child hold the extremity stable during IV insertion. Talk to the child during the procedure. Anticipate using scalp vein needles (butterfly devices) for infants.

Geriatric

The veins of older adults are often fragile. When veins are elevated and clearly visible, perform insertion without a tourniquet, if appropriate.

End-of-Life Care

The infusion of fluids and nutritional supplements to dying clients is controversial in terms of its palliative versus life-sustaining potential. Consider the desires of the client and family, physician's orders, and agency policies for fluid and nutrition therapy for dying clients.

Home Health

If nursing visits are intermittent and IV therapy is continuous, instruct client and family on rate regulation, signs and symptoms of infiltration, and method for discontinuing IV catheter.

Delegation

Unlicensed assistive personnel should not perform IV site care. Although licensed practical nurses (LPNs) do not commonly administer IV medication, they often provide site care to peripheral lines. Delegating site care should be based on agency policy and the skill level of the person providing the care.

Implementation

Action	Rationale
Selecting a Vein for IV Therapy	
1. Perform hand hygiene and organize equipment:	*Reduces microorganisms; promotes efficiency*
• Select the smallest catheter size that meets infusion needs and is appropriate for vein size.	*Prevents irritating the lining of the vein, which could lead to phlebitis and infiltration*
• Include two appropriately sized catheters and one smaller-gauge catheter with other supplies.	*Prevents delay if a second attempt is needed or a smaller vein must be used*
2. Explain procedure, including client assistance needed.	*Decreases anxiety; promotes cooperation*
3. Encourage client to use bedpan or commode before beginning. Help client into gown.	*Promotes easier gown changes during IV therapy; promotes comfort and prevents interruption during IV insertion process*
4. Lower side rail and assist client into a supine or semi-Fowler's position; raise bed to high position. Ask client which hand is dominant.	*Promotes comfort during procedure and use of appropriate body mechanics; placing IV in nondominant hand or arm allows full use of dominant extremity*
5. Apply tourniquet on arm 3 to 5 inches below elbow.	*Distends distal arm and hand veins for assessment*
6. Ask client to open and close hand or hang arm at side of bed.	*Promotes blood flow to the extremity and aids in dilating veins*
7. Inspect the extremity, looking for veins with the largest diameter and fewest curves or junctions:	*Facilitates IV insertion*
• Check anterior and posterior surfaces, selecting a site with 2 inches of skin surface below a vein in the lower arm if possible (Fig. 7.5).	*Promotes use of lower arm as natural splint from radial and ulnar bones; permits taping with greater stability*

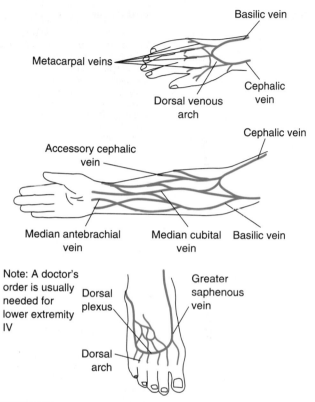

FIGURE 7.5

Action	Rationale
• If lower arm veins are unsuitable, look at hand and wrist veins.	*Provides additional sites for IV insertion*
• If a large vein is needed, remove the tourniquet from below the elbow and apply it just above the antecubital space and search for a suitable upper arm vein.	*Permits use of larger upper extremity veins for larger catheter gauges*

Action	Rationale
• If no suitable site is available, contact the physician about an order for use of lower extremity for IV insertion.	*Ensures that there are no contra-indications for inserting an IV in the lower extremity; reduces risk of thrombophlebitis and other vascular problems. For PICC catheters, the basilic or cephalic veins are most appropriate.*
8. Release tourniquet and allow client to relax.	*Reestablishes blood flow and promotes comfort*
9. If area is hairy, use scissors to clip excessive hair, wash area with soap and water, then dry.	*Helps protective dressing adhere to skin*

Preparing Solutions for IV Therapy

1. Select vein (see Nursing Procedure 7.4).	
2. Open tubing package and check tubing for cracks or flaws. Check ends for covers and verify that regulator/roller clamp is closed (rolled down, clamped off, or screwed closed).	*Ensures that tubing is intact, without defects; maintains steril-ity of tubing; allows for better fluid control and helps minimize air in tubing*
3. Open IV fluid container. Remove outer bag cover-ing; then holding bag by neck in one hand, pull down on plastic tab with other hand to remove tab (Fig. 7.6).	*Prevents squeezing of fluid or air from bag when spike is inserted, increasing accuracy of fluid mea-surement; maintains control of solution; prepares bag for inser-tion of tubing without contami-nating insertion site*
4. Remove protective cover-ing from tubing spike (pointed end) and attach tubing to solution. Push spike into port until flat end of spike and port meet.	*Promotes a closed system for fluid administration; ensures complete connection of bag and tubing*
5. Prime the tubing: • Hang solution con-tainer on an IV pole or wall hook; squeeze and release drip chamber until fluid level reaches ring mark (half- to two-thirds full).	*Removes air from the tubing* *Provides enough fluid to prime tubing*

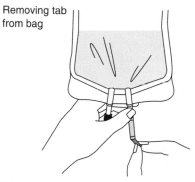

Removing tab
from bag

FIGURE 7.6

Action	Rationale
• Remove cap from end of tubing and open roller clamp, allowing fluid to fill tubing and flow to the end until all air is expelled. During priming, invert medication ports and in-line filters, if present, and tap while fluid is flowing.	*Removes air from tubing; forces air bubbles from ports and filters*
• Close roller clamp and replace cap on end of tubing.	*Reestablishes a closed sterile system*
6. Label the solution container with the client's name, room number, date and time initiated, rate of infusion, and your initials. Apply time strip or attach to infusion pump (see Nursing Procedure 7.8).	*Identifies time of initiating therapy and need for replacement (usually no longer than 24 hours); helps monitor fluid infusion*
7. Label tubing with date and time hung and nurse's initials.	*Indicates time of tubing application and need for replacement (usually every 24 to 72 hours, or according to agency policy)*
8. Proceed to bedside with solution setup. Drape tubing over pole.	*Ensures solution with tubing is readily available for connection once IV catheter is inserted; maintains sterility of tubing*

Action	Rationale
Inserting a Catheter/ IV Lock for IV Therapy	
1. Select vein (see Nursing Procedure 7.4) and prepare solution (see Nursing Procedure 7.5). Place IV tubing on bed beside client.	*Selects most appropriate vein; provides fluid for infusion; places tubing for easy access*
2. Lower side rail and assist client into a supine position. Raise bed to high position.	*Provides easier access to veins; promotes comfort during procedure and use of good body mechanics*
3. Tear three 1-inch tape strips. Cut one piece down the center.	*Allows for quick access to tape to secure catheter once inserted; narrow strip will secure catheter without covering insertion site.*
4. Prepare needle/catheter for insertion. Examine over-the-needle catheter for cracks or flaws, rotating the catheter and holding the needle securely. Check the butterfly needle tip for straight edge without bends or chips.	*Ensures that catheter or needle is intact and will thread smoothly into the vein*
5. Open several alcohol pads or antiseptic agent.	*Provides fast access to cleaning supplies*
6. Place towel under extremity.	*Keeps linens clean*
7. Apply tourniquet on extremity and locate the largest, most distal vein.	*Restricts blood flow, distending vein; permits entrance of vein at higher point so that future punctures can be made without leakage*
8. Place IV tubing on bed beside client, and don clean gloves.	*Permits ready access to tubing; prevents contact with blood*
9. With alcohol pad (or appropriate antiseptic agent), clean site beginning at center and circling outward in a 2-inch diameter. Allow to dry.	*Maintains asepsis*
10. Encourage client to take slow, deep breaths as you begin.	*Promotes relaxation and comfort*
11. Hold skin taut with one hand while holding catheter with other (Fig. 7.7).	*Stabilizes vein and prevents skin movement during insertion*
• For an over-the-needle catheter: Hold the catheter by positioning	*Allows viewing of initial flashback in catheter and reduces risk of additional line contamination*

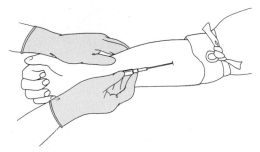

FIGURE 7.7

Action	Rationale
fingers on opposite sides of needle housing, not over catheter hub.	
• For a butterfly: Pinch "wings" of butterfly together to insert needle.	*Provides control of needle*
12. Maintaining sterility, insert catheter into vein parallel to the straightest section of the vein with bevel up. Puncture skin at a 30-degree angle, 1 cm below site where the vein will be entered (Fig. 7.8).	*Allows for full insertion of catheter*
13. Once needle has entered skin, lower it until it is almost flush with the skin (Fig. 7.9).	*Prevents penetration of opposite wall of vein*

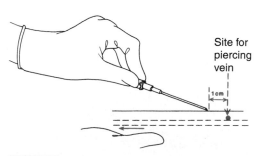

Site for
piercing
vein

|1cm|

FIGURE 7.8

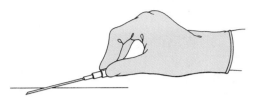

FIGURE 7.9

Action	Rationale
14. Following path of vein, insert catheter moving toward the side of vein wall. (If using an over-the-needle catheter system, insert needle at a 30-degree angle with bevel up and push-off tabs in the up position. Place index finger on the push-off tab and thread the catheter to the desired length.)	
15. Watch for first backflow of blood, then push needle gently into vein.	*Indicates that needle has penetrated vein wall*
• For an over-the-needle catheter, slide needle into vein about a quarter-inch after blood backflow is noted. Then slide catheter over needle and into vein and pull needle out of vein and skin (Fig. 7.10).	*Allows insertion without needle to prevent puncturing of opposite vein wall; facilitates insertion as vein becomes filled with fluid*

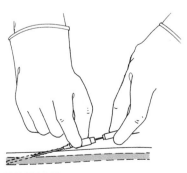

FIGURE 7.10

Action	Rationale
• If unable to insert catheter fully, DO NOT FORCE; WAIT UNTIL FLOW IS INITIATED.	
16. Holding catheter securely, remove cap from IV tubing and insert into hub of catheter or twist on cap for an IV lock (Fig. 7.11A).	*Prevents dislodging of catheter and establishes closed system for administration*
17. Remove tourniquet.	*Prevents vein rupture from infusion of fluid against closed vessel*
18. Open roller clamp and allow fluid to flow freely for a few seconds.	*Establishes fluid flow and helps to determine if catheter is in the vein or wedged against vessel wall; reduces risk of clot formation. Swelling or pain indicates infiltration.*
• For an IV lock, wipe cap with alcohol, attach saline syringe, and flush with saline (see Fig. 7.11B).	

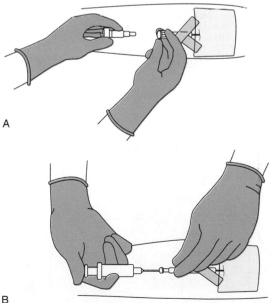

A

B

FIGURE 7.11

Action	Rationale
• Monitor for swelling or pain.	
19. Tape catheter in position that allows free flow of the fluid.	*Reduces risk of positional flow of IV fluids*
• For an over-the-needle catheter or IV lock, put a small piece of tape under hub of catheter and cross over to secure hub to skin. DO NOT PLACE TAPE OVER INSERTION SITE.	*Maintains sterility of insertion site*
• For a butterfly, put smallest pieces of tape across "wings" of butterfly and another piece of tape across the middle to form an H shape. Or put a small piece of tape under wings and tape over to form a V shape; then place piece of tape across the V-shaped tape (Fig. 7.12).	*Stabilizes catheter without covering insertion site*
20. Slow IV solution to a moderate infusion rate.	*Prevents accidental fluid bolus while completing site care*

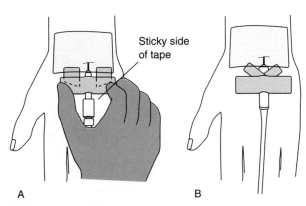

Sticky side of tape

A   B

FIGURE 7.12

Action	Rationale
21. Cover with transparent dressing.	*Reduces risk of contamination and infection of site*
22. Remove gloves and secure tubing:	*Prevents disconnection of tubing from client*
• For an over-the-needle catheter, place tape across top of tubing, just below catheter. Loop tubing and tape to dressing. Secure length of tubing to arm with short piece of tape. Tape the tubing/catheter hub junction.	*Prevents disconnection of tubing from catheter*
• For a butterfly, coil tubing around and on top of IV site and apply tape across coil and hub of needle.	*Prevents dislodgment of needle and disconnection from tubing*
• For an IV lock, if device is made such there is loop tubing with protective cap, apply tape across end of loop tubing near protective cap.	
23. Regulate IV flow manually or set infusion device at appropriate rate (see Nursing Procedure 7.8).	*Ensures flow rate as ordered*
24. On a piece of tape or label, record needle size, type, date and time of insertion, and nurse's initials. Place label over top of dressing.	*Provides information needed for follow-up care*
25. Apply armboard if needed.	*Stabilizes site*
26. Remove towel, discard gloves, and dispose of equipment properly.	*Promotes comfort; prevents spread of microorganisms*
27. Review limitations in range of motion with client. Instruct client in signs and symptoms to report and encourage client to notify nurse immediately of any problems or discomfort.	*Enlists client's assistance in maintaining therapy; promotes feeling of control*
28. Position client appropriately with call light within reach.	*Promotes comfort and safety with ready access to communication*

Action	Rationale
29. Check infusion rate and site after 5 minutes and again after 15 minutes. Check volume every 1 to 2 hours.	*Ensures accurate administration as ordered; detects the need for any adjustments*

Evaluation

Were desired outcomes achieved? An example of evaluation is:
● Desired outcome met: IV insertion site is clean and dry, with no pain, redness, or swelling.

Documentation

The following should be noted on the client's chart:
● Client's tolerance of insertion procedure and fluid infusion
● Site of IV insertion
● Status of IV site, dressing, fluids, and tubing
● Size and type of catheter/needle
● Type and rate of infusion (if continuous infusion)
● Client teaching performed and client's understanding of instructions
● Follow-up assessments of IV site and infusion
● Flush solution used, including type and amount (if IV lock)

Sample Documentation
Date: 2/17/05
Time: 2100

Client has 20-gauge IV catheter inserted in anterior aspect of right lower arm. 1 L D₅W infusing at 125 mL/hr. Site clean, dry, and intact without evidence of redness or infiltration. Client tolerated insertion procedure and fluid infusion without significant changes in vital signs. Teaching done regarding mobility limitations; client voiced understanding.

Calculating Flow Rate (7.7)
Regulating IV Fluid (7.8)

Purpose

Ensures delivery of correct amount of IV fluids

Equipment

- IV pole (bed or rolling) or IV pump
- Calculator (or pencil and pad)
- Watch with second hand

Assessment

Assessment should focus on the following:
- Orders for type and rate of fluid
- Type of infusion control devices available or ordered
- Viscosity of ordered fluids
- Indicators of fluid overload

Nursing Diagnoses

Nursing diagnoses may include the following:
- Risk for fluid imbalance, excess, related to fluctuations in fluid rate

Outcome Identification and Planning

Desired Outcomes

Sample desired outcomes include the following:
- Correct volume of fluid is infused within designated time frame.
- Client remains free of injury from IV infusion.

Special Considerations in Planning and Implementation

General

Check administration of viscous solutions frequently because they may require rate adjustments throughout the infusion process based on actual flow due to accumulation in filter or on sides of tubing. Inspect the IV infusion and calculate the rate. A pump or fluid regulation device does not negate the need for inspection of fluid counts or approximations. Check regularly for signs of malfunction of infusion devices or factors that could interfere with accurate fluid infusion.

Pediatric

Regulate IV infusions carefully because children are often volume-sensitive and prone to fluid overload, particularly with rapid infusion of large volumes. Infusions must be regulated carefully and checked frequently, and clients must be watched closely for tolerance. Use a Volutrol (Buretrol) device as added protection against fluid or medication overinfusion.

Geriatric

Regulate IV infusions carefully because elderly clients are often volume-sensitive and prone to fluid overload, particularly with rapid infusion of large volumes. Infusions must be regulated carefully and checked frequently, and clients must be watched closely for tolerance. Monitor breath sounds carefully in elderly clients with cardiac or pulmonary problems when infusing large volumes of fluid.

End-of-Life Care

Infusion of fluids and nutritional supplements in dying clients is controversial in terms of its palliative versus life-sustaining potential. Consider the desires of the client and family, the physician's orders, and agency policies related to fluid and nutrition therapy for dying clients.

Delegation

Regulation of IV fluid should remain the responsibility of the nurse. However, unlicensed personnel can be enlisted to help monitor the infusion and to report when fluid is nearing completion so the nurse can discontinue or hang an additional infusion.

Implementation

Action	Rationale
Calculating Flow Rate	
1. Check tubing package to determine drop factor of tubing.	*Indicates drops per milliliter for drip rate calculation*
2. Determine the infusion volume in milliliters per hour and flow rate in drops (gtts) per minute using the appropriate formulas (Display 7.1).	*Prevents fluid volume overload*
3. If available, use an infusion chart by looking	*Provides a quick reference for flow rates*

● Display 7.1 IV Calculations

1. Determining the *number of milliliters per hour*

$$\frac{\text{TOTAL VOLUME}}{\text{TOTAL TIME (hours)}} = \boxed{\begin{array}{l}\text{Hourly infusion rate}\\(\text{volume to infuse each hour})\end{array}}$$

Example: 1,000 mL to be infused over 6 hr:

$1,000 / 6 = 167$ mL/hr

2. Determining *flow rate in gtts per minute*

$$\frac{\text{TOTAL FLUID VOLUME}}{\text{TOTAL TIME (minutes)}} \times \frac{\text{DROP FACTOR}}{(\text{drops}/\text{mL})} = \boxed{\begin{array}{l}\text{INFUSION RATE}\\(\text{drops}/\text{min})\end{array}}$$

Example: Volume ordered is 1,000 mL of D_5W over 6 hr; tubing drop factor is 15 drops/mL × 15 drops/mL

$$\frac{1000 \text{ mL}}{6(60) \text{ min.}} \times 15 \text{ drops/mL} = \frac{15,000 \text{ drops}}{360 \text{ min.}} = \begin{array}{l}41.7 \text{ or } 42\\\text{drops/min}\end{array}$$

3. *Or* using hourly infusion rate (see above):

$$\frac{167 \text{ mL} \times 15 \text{ drops}}{60 \text{ min/mL}} = 41.7 \text{ or } 42 \text{ drops/min}$$

- Total fluid volume equals the amount of fluid, expressed in milliliters, to infuse over the ordered period of time (if order is 1 L of D_5W over 12 hr, the total volume is 1 L [1,000 mL]).
- Total time is the number of minutes (hours × 60) over which the fluid should infuse. IF FLUID IS ORDERED PER HOUR OR YOU CALCULATE VOLUME PER HOUR, THE TOTAL TIME WILL EQUAL 60 MINUTES. Total volume will equal hourly infusion rate.
- The drop factor is the number of drops from the chosen tubing that will equal 1 mL. This amount is found on the tubing package and is expressed in drops per milliliter.

Action	Rationale
across chart for drop factor of tubing and counting down chart to line indicating amount of fluid infusing per hour (Table 7.1).	
4. Regulate fluid or set drop rate on fluid regulator.	*Sets accurate flow rate*

● Table 7.1 Flow Rates for Intravenous Infusions

Drop Factor of Tubing (drops/mL)	1000 mL/ 6 hr (drops/ min)	1000 mL/ 8 hr (drops/ min)	1000 mL/ 10 hr (drops/ min)	1000 mL/ 12 hr (drops/ min)	1000 mL/ 24 hr (drops/ min)
10	28	21	17	14	7
15	42	31	25	21	10
20	56	42	34	28	14
60	167	125	100	84	42

Action	**Rationale**
Regulating IV Fluid 1. Calculate or determine appropriate volume per hour or drip rate (drops per minute; see above). 2. If necessary, prepare time tape for fluid based on volume of fluid to infuse over 1 hour (Fig. 7.13). Proceed to Step 3 for appropriate system.	*Allows close monitoring of fluid infusion*

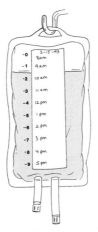

FIGURE 7.13

Action	Rationale
Manual Rate Regulation	
3. Attach appropriate tubing and clear tubing of air.	
4. Adjust pole height and open all clamps except roller clamp/regulator.	*Gravity facilitates flow; limits flow rate control to regulator*
5. Open regulator fully, then slowly close regulator while observing drip chamber—fluid should initially run in a stream. (Table 7.2 lists trouble-shooting tips.)	*Indicates catheter patency*
6. Close roller clamp/regulator until fluid is dropping at slow but steady pace.	
7. Count the number of drops falling in a 15-second interval and multiply by 4.	*Determines the number of drops falling per minute*
8. Adjust the regulator/roller clamp, opening it to increase drop flow if drops per minute rate is less than calculated rate or closing it to decrease drop flow if drops per minute rate is more than calculated rate.	*Regulates rate*
9. Count drops again and continue to adjust flow until desired drip rate is obtained.	*Produces correct rate*
10. Recheck rate after 5 minutes and again after 15 minutes. Proceed to Step 11.	*Detects changes in rate due to expansion or contraction of tubing*
Dial-A-Flo Fluid Regulation	
3. Attach appropriate tubing and clear tubing of air.	
4. At end of IV tubing, attach Dial-A-Flo tubing, if tubing is an add on (Fig. 7.14).	
5. Open all clamps and regulator on IV tubing.	*Prepares equipment*
6. Adjust Dial-A-Flo to open position and clear tubing of air (remove cap if needed).	

● Table 7.2 Troubleshooting Tips for IV Infusion Management

Problem	Actions
Drip chamber is overfilled	Close regulator clamp, turn fluid container upside down, and squeeze fluid from drip chamber until half full or slightly below.
Air is in tubing	Check adequacy of fluid level in drip chamber and security of tubing connections.
	Insert needle and syringe into rubber port distal to air and aspirate to remove air.
Blood is backing up into tubing	Be sure fluid is above the level of the IV catheter site and the level of the heart.
	Check security of tubing connections.
	Check that infusing fluid has not run out and that catheter is in a vein, not an artery (note pulsation of blood in tubing).
Infusion pump alarms indicate flow problem	Check drip chamber for excess or inadequate fluid level.
	Check that clamps and regulators are open, air vent is open (if applicable), and tubing is free of kinks. Check IV catheter site for infiltration, blood clot, kinks, and positional obstruction (open fluid regulator fully and change position of arm to see if fluid flows better in various positions). Insert needle and syringe into medication port and gently flush fluid through catheter. If resistance is met, try to aspirate blood/clot into tubing; if unsuccessful, discontinue IV and restart.
IV is positional (i.e., runs well only when arm or hand is in a certain position)	Stabilize IV site with armboard or handboard, and monitor fluid infusion every 1 to 2 hours.
Fluid is dripping but is also leaking into tissue surrounding puncture site	Discontinue IV and restart in another site. Place warm soak over infiltrated site. Reassess frequently.

Action	Rationale
7. Close fluid regulator roller/screw.	*Prevents fluid flow during connection to IV catheter*
8. Turn Dial-A-Flo regulator until arrow is aligned with	*Regulates fluid to infuse at desired rate*

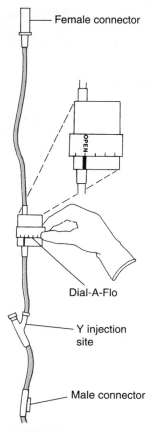

Female connector

OPEN

Dial-A-Flo

Y injection
site

Male connector

FIGURE 7.14

Action	Rationale
desired volume of fluid to infuse over 1 hour.	
9. Check drip rate over 15 seconds and multiply by 4 (should coincide with calculated drip rate).	*Verifies fluid infusion rate*
• Adjust height of pole if necessary.	*Gravity facilitates flow.*

Action	Rationale
10. Recheck drip rate after 5 minutes and again after 15 minutes.	*Detects changes in rate due to expansion/contraction of tubing*
Proceed to Step 11.	
Infusion Pump Regulation	
3. Attach appropriate tubing and clear tubing of air.	
4. Insert tubing into infusion pump according to pump manual (Fig. 7.15).	*Ensures proper functioning of infusion regulator*

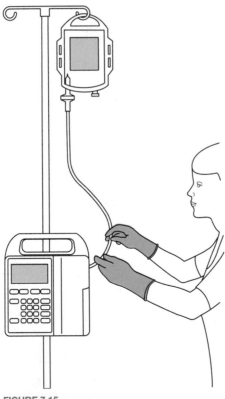

FIGURE 7.15

Action	Rationale
5. Close door to pump and open all tubing clamps and roller/screw.	*Allows pump to regulate fluids*
6. Set volume dials for appropriate volume per hour and volume to be infused.	*Determines amount of fluid pump will deliver*
7. Place electronic eye clamp over drip chamber (optional in some infusion regulators; consult manual).	*Allows pump to monitor fluid flow*
8. Push ON or START button.	*Initiates fluid flow and regulation*
9. Check drip rate over 15 seconds and multiply by 4 (should coincide with calculated drip rate).	*Verifies fluid infusion rate*
10. Set volume infusion alarm. If tubing does not contain a regulator cassette, periodically change the sections of tubing placed inside infusion clamp.	*Notifies nurse when set volume has been infused; prevents tubing collapse due to constant squeezing by pump*

Proceed to Step 11.

Volume Control Chamber (Buretrol) Regulation

Action	Rationale
3. Close off regulator 1 (above chamber) and regulator 2 (below chamber). Insert spike into fluid bag.	*Controls fluids*
4. Open regulator 1 and fill chamber with 10 mL fluid, prime drip chamber, and close regulator 1. Open regulator 2 and clear tubing of air (Fig. 7.16A).	*Helps clear air from tubing*
5. Fill chamber with volume of fluid to infuse in 1 hour (or 2 or 3 hours' worth if volume is small).	*Allows for close monitoring of fluid volume (needed for volume-sensitive or pediatric clients)*
6. Close regulator 1. Make sure air vent is open (see Fig. 7.16B).	*Fluid will not flow if regulator 1 and air vent are closed.*
7. Open regulator 2 and regulate drops to calculated rate (drip rate should equal volume per hour if minidrip tubing system is used [check drop factor]). OR	*Sets volume to infuse over an hour*

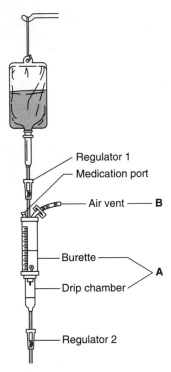

Regulator 1
Medication port
Air vent —— **B**
Burette ——
                    A
Drip chamber ——

Regulator 2

FIGURE 7.16

Action	Rationale
Attach Dial-A-Flo to tubing and leave regulator 2 open. OR Place tubing into infusion pump and leave regulator 2 open.	*Allows infusion pump to regulate fluid*
8. Check drip rate over 15 seconds and multiply by 4 (should coincide with calculated drip rate).	*Verifies fluid infusion rate*
9. Put a time tape on the chamber, if needed (if pump is not used).	*Allows for quick, easy check of fluid infusion progress and the need to add fluid to chamber*
10. Check chamber each hour or two and add 1 to	*Maintains fluid infusion and catheter patency; prevents air*

Action	Rationale
2 hours' more fluid volume as needed. If close fluid monitoring is NOT needed, clamp air vent and open regulator 1.	*from entering tubing; allows fluid to flow directly from bottle/bag into chamber and to client*
11. Mark beginning hour of fluid infusion on time tape.	*Sets times for subsequent checks*
12. Check volume every 1 to 2 hours and compare with fluid remaining in container. • If volume depleted does not coincide with time tape for accuracy, check settings on pump or Dial-A-Flo and readjust if indicated. • Elevate fluid container on pole. • Check catheter site and position for obstruction (see Table 7.2).	*Determines actual volume infused; identifies possible problem; facilitates flow by gravity; identifies malposition of IV catheter or complication at site*
13. Review limitations in range of motion with client. Instruct client to notify nurse of problems or discomfort.	*Allows early detection of problems with catheter or fluid flow*
14. Position client appropriately with call light within reach.	*Promotes client comfort and safety; provides a means of communication*

Evaluation

Were desired outcomes achieved? Examples of evaluation include:

● Desired outcome met: Correct volume of fluid is infused within designated time frame.
● Desired outcome met: Client remains free of complications or injury from IV fluid therapy.

Documentation

The following should be noted on the client's chart:

● Time of initiation of fluid infusion
● Type and volume of fluid infusion
● Infusion device used, if applicable
● Status of catheter insertion site

- Problems with infusion procedure and solutions (e.g., armboard used, catheter repositioned)
- Client tolerance to fluid infusion
- Client teaching and response

Sample Documentation

Date: 2/17/05
Time: 2100

Client receiving D_5W; 1,000-mL bag infusing at 125 mL/hr per Dial-A-Flo. Tolerating fluid infusion well. Catheter site clean and dry, without signs of infiltration or infection. Return demonstration noted regarding arm positions to be avoided during IV fluid infusion.

● **Nursing Procedures 7.9, 7.10**

Changing IV Tubing and Dressing (7.9)

Converting to an IV Lock (7.10)

Purpose

Decreases opportunity for growth of microorganisms by removing possible medium for infection

Equipment

- Alcohol pads or approved antiseptic cleansing agent
- Appropriate infusion tubing
- Towel
- Tape 1 inch wide (may cut 2-inch tape)
- Dressing: 2 × 2-inch gauze or transparent dressing
- IV pole (bed or rolling) or IV pump
- Armboard (optional)
- Adhesive labels
- Nonsterile gloves
- IV infusion cap
- Saline or heparin flush

Assessment

Assessment should focus on the following:
- Doctor's orders for type and rate of fluid
- Date and time of last dressing and/or tubing change
- Appearance of IV site
- Status of skin on hand and arms, presence of hair or abrasions
- Ability to hold arm and hand without movement or resistance for duration of procedure
- Allergy to tape or cleansing agent

Nursing Diagnoses

Nursing diagnoses may include the following:
- Risk for infection related to interruption of skin integrity
- Risk for injury related to complications of IV insertion

Outcome Identification and Planning

Desired Outcomes

Sample desired outcomes include the following:
- No evidence of infection exists around insertion site over the next 72 hours.
- The client will maintain skin integrity around insertion site, as evidenced by lack of pain, redness, or swelling at site.

Special Considerations in Planning and Implementation

General

If possible, replace IV fluid and tubing and change dressing at the same time. This reduces the risk of introducing microorganisms. Many institutions have specified procedures and times for dressing and tubing change. If unsure, consult policy manual. Perform frequent inspection and routine flushing of IV lock sites on a routine schedule and before and after using the lock.

Pediatric

If the child is resistant, confused, or frightened, have an assistant immobilize the child's arm so that the IV line is not accidentally dislodged during the dressing change. Use bio-occlusive dressings, such as Tegaderm, which have been found to be associated with less catheter dislodgment than gauze dressings in children.

Geriatric

If the elderly client is resistant, confused, or frightened, have an assistant immobilize his or her arm to ensure that the IV line is not accidentally dislodged during the dressing change. Paper tape is frequently used for elderly clients because their skin is thin and fragile.

End-of-Life Care

Monitor closely for signs of infection at the IV site. Due to deteriorating circulation, dying clients are more prone to infection.

Home Health

In the homebound client, be constantly alert for subtle signs and symptoms of infection associated with long-term IV therapy. Expect to use control-flow gravity drip infusion devices such as a Dial-a-Flo or manual drip rate setting to administer antibiotic and other infusions in the home setting.

Cost-Cutting Tips

Anticipate using less expensive control-flow gravity drip infusion devices such as a Dial-a-Flo or manual drip rate setting to administer antibiotic and other infusions in the home setting. If a pump is needed for potent drugs, seek out less expensive infusion pumps as an alternative.

Delegation

When delegating IV dressing changes, consider the skill level of the person to whom you are delegating care. Often special training is needed before an LPN or other assistive personnel performs IV dressing changes.

Implementation

Action	Rationale
Changing IV Tubing and Dressing	
1. Perform hand hygiene; organize equipment; explain procedure to client	*Reduces microorganism transfer; promotes efficiency; reduces anxiety*
2. Open new tubing package and check for cracks or flaws. Be sure that caps are on all ports and that the regulator/roller clamp is closed (rolled down, clamped off, or screwed closed).	*Ensures that no defective materials are used and that tubing remains sterile; allows better fluid control, minimizing air in tubing*
3. Check infusing fluid against doctor's orders.	*Validates correct fluid infusion*
4. Remove infusing fluid solution container from IV pole or pump (put pump on hold), invert container, and remove old tubing.	
5. Attach new tubing to solution container, hold container upright, fill drip	*Replaces air in tubing with fluid*

Action	Rationale
chamber, and prime tubing after removing protective cap at end of tubing. Close roller clamp/regulator when tubing is primed.	
6. Loosely cover end of tubing with cap and lay on bed near IV dressing.	*Maintains sterility of tubing*
7. Don gloves.	*Prevents exposure to blood*
8. Turn off flow from old tubing.	*Prevents wetting of dressing and bed*
9. Exchange old tubing for new tubing at catheter hub:	*Establishes new system*
• Place alcohol swab under catheter hub/tubing junction.	*Prevents soiling of dressing or linens*
• Loosen connection at junction of IV catheter and old tubing.	*Prepares catheter for tubing removal*
• Holding catheter firm with one hand, disconnect old tubing and quickly insert new tubing into catheter hub, maintaining sterility of catheter and tip of new tubing (Fig. 7.17).	*Prevents dislodgment of catheter*
• Open roller clamp/regulator and begin flow from new tubing.	*Re-establishes fluid flow and reduces risk of clot formation in catheter*
• Regulate fluid flow or place tubing into pump.	*Promotes accurate infusion rate*
• Tape tubing to dressing and arm unless dressing to be changed.	*Secures tubing and decreases risk of accidental pull on catheter*

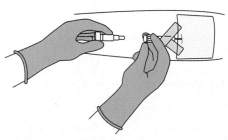

FIGURE 7.17

Action	Rationale
10. Label tubing with date, time hung, and nurse's initials.	*Indicates when tubing replacement is due (every 24 to 72 hours or per agency policy)*
11. Remove gloves.	*Decreases transfer of microorganisms*
12. Tear tape strips 3 inches in length, 1 inch wide. Cut one strip down the center. Hang tape pieces from edge of bedside table.	*Provides a means for securing catheter without covering insertion site; allows for ready access to tape when needed*
13. Open cleansing agent and dressing.	*Promotes efficiency; allows easy access to necessary supplies*
14. Lower side rail and assist client into a supine position.	*Promotes easy access to IV site; promotes comfort and use of good body mechanics*
15. Place towel under extremity.	*Prevents soiling of linens*
16. Don gloves.	*Reduces risk of microorganism transfer*
17. Remove dressing and all tape, except tape holding catheter. If old dressing is transparent, remove it, leaving enough dressing to maintain catheter in place until ready to remove.	*Prevents dislodging of catheter when cleaning site*
18. Clean catheter insertion site beginning at catheter and moving outward in a 2-inch-diameter circle.	*Reduces risk of infection by removing microorganisms from site*
19. Holding catheter secure with one hand, remove remaining tape or transparent dressing and clean under catheter.	*Prevents catheter dislodgment during cleansing*
20. Allow area to dry and secure catheter in position. See Nursing Procedure 7.6 for steps for taping.	
21. Cover site with transparent dressing.	*Protects against microorganisms*
22. Remove gloves and secure tubing.	
23. Apply armboard, if needed.	*Stabilizes site*
24. On a piece of tape or label, record needle size, type, date and time of site care, and nurse's initials; place label over top of dressing.	*Provides information needed for follow-up care*
25. Raise side rails and position client appropriately.	*Promotes client comfort and safety*

Action	Rationale
26. Discard or restore supplies; perform hand hygiene.	*Decreases spread of micro-organisms*
Converting to an IV Lock	
1. Perform Steps 1 to 8 of Nursing Procedure 7.9.	
2. Remove old tubing and apply infusion cap or IV lock.	*Establishes closed system for intermittent use*
3. Flush catheter/IV lock with saline or heparin flush, using twice the amount of solution that fits the capacity of the catheter and its add-on components (check agency policy).	*Maintains catheter/IV lock patency*
4. Tape infusion cap/IV lock securely in place or perform dressing change, if indicated.	*Secures device, preventing dislodgment*
5. Label with date, time, and nurse's initials.	*Indicates when lock was changed*
6. Discard old tubing and other trash.	*Promotes clean environment; reduces risk of infection transmission*
7. If performing dressing change, see above. If not, place tape across junction of tubing and secure catheter.	*Prevents lock from dislodging from catheter*
8. Raise side rails and position client appropriately with call light readily accessible.	*Promotes client comfort and safety; provides a means of communication*
9. Discard gloves and perform hand hygiene.	*Reduces microorganism transfer*

Evaluation

Were desired outcomes achieved? Examples of evaluation include:
- Desired outcome met: No evidence of infection around insertion site over 72 hours.
- Desired outcome met: Client maintained skin integrity around insertion site, with no pain, redness, or swelling at site.

Documentation

The following should be noted on the client's chart:
- Location and status of IV site, dressing, fluids, and tubing
- Size and type of catheter/needle

- Reports of pain at site
- IV site care rendered and client tolerance to care
- Client teaching

Sample Documentation
Date: 2/17/05
Time: 2100

Tubing changed on IV of D₅W infusing at 125 mL/hr in right lower arm. Site care done, #20 angio IV catheter present, site clean without swelling or pain. Client tolerated procedure well. Reinforced teaching regarding mobility limitations; client demonstrated understanding.

Nursing Procedure 7.11

Assisting With Inserting and Maintaining a Central Venous Line/ Peripherally Inserted Central Catheter (PICC)

Purpose

Permits administration of medications and nutritional support that should not be given via a peripheral route or when standard peripheral routes cannot be used

Equipment

- Sterile gloves
- Sterile gauze pads (2 × 2 inches) and transparent dressing
- Face masks
- 1-inch tape (optional)
- Steri-strips
- Approved antiseptic cleansing agent
- IV fluids and tubing or heparin flush or saline flush
- Prep razor

- Suture with needle holder
- Central line (PICC) insertion kit containing:
  Sterile gloves (multiple sizes)
  Antiseptic swabs or solution and gauze
  Sterile towels/drapes
  10-mL syringe (slip-tip)
  $\frac{5}{8}$-, 1-, and 1.5-inch needles
- Lidocaine/Xylocaine (without epinephrine) 1% or 2%
- Central line with introducer (e.g., single-lumen or multi-lumen catheter, Hickman catheter, angiocath)
- Tape measure (PICC only)
- Dressing change label

Assessment

Assessment should focus on the following:
- Type of catheter
- Location of catheter tip
- Type of infusion(s)
- Agency policy regarding central line care

Nursing Diagnoses

Nursing diagnoses may include the following:
- Deficient fluid volume related to nausea and vomiting
- Nutrition imbalance, less than body requirements, related to anorexia
- Risk for infection related to central line insertion
- Risk for injury related to complications of central venous therapy

Outcome Identification and Planning

Desired Outcomes

Sample desired outcomes include the following:
- Client maintains adequate skin turgor during total parenteral nutrition (TPN) administration.
- Client gains 1 to 2 lb per week.
- Client remains free of embolism, pleural effusion, and infection, both systemically and at catheter site.
- Central line remains patent.

Special Considerations in Planning and Implementation

General

If central line was inserted for infusion of TPN, infuse only $D_{10}W$ or D_5W until TPN is available. If multilumen catheter is used, select and mark a catheter port for TPN only. Use strict aseptic technique when performing procedure, as location of site, larger size of insertion opening, and fluids with high glucose content increase client vulnerability to infection. Consult agency policy manual because policies vary greatly regarding use of saline or heparin solution for flushing catheter.

Pediatric

Anticipate the use of PICC lines for critically ill neonates requiring long-term venous access. Use strict aseptic technique, especially with critically ill neonates who are at high risk for sepsis.

End-of-Life Care

Consider the desires of the client and family, the physician's orders, and agency policy when administering fluid and nutrition therapy to dying clients. Use is controversial in terms of its palliative versus life-sustaining potential.

Home Health

Vigilantly assess the homebound client with a central line for signs and symptoms of infection. This line is likely to be in place for a long time.

Delegation

Consult hospital policy for specific central venous and PICC insertion and maintenance procedures. PICCs are inserted only by physicians, physician's assistants, advanced care nurses, or registered nurses specially certified by the hospital. These procedures are not delegated to unlicensed assistive personnel.

Implementation

Action	Rationale
Assisting With Central Venous Line or PICC Insertion	
1. Perform hand hygiene and organize equipment.	*Reduces microorganism transfer and promotes efficiency*
2. Arrange supplies on tray, using appropriate-size gloves for physician.	*Promotes efficiency*
3. Reinforce explanation of procedure to client. Clarify that his/her face will be covered with towels or drapes but that you will be nearby.	*Reduces client anxiety*
4. For central line insertion, put bed and client in Trendelenburg's position. If client has respiratory distress, place in supine	*Dilates vessels in upper trunk and neck; puts less pressure on diaphragm and facilitates breathing*

Action	Rationale
position with feet elevated 45 to 60 degrees (modified Trendelenburg's).	
5. For PICC insertion, position the arm for ease of access to the upper arm or antecubital vein sites—basilic or cephalic—with arm extended at a 45- to 60-degree angle from the body.	*Facilitates access to insertion site*
6. Hold client's hand; obtain assistant and restrain both hands if client is resistant or confused.	*Provides comfort; prevents disruption of procedure or contamination of sterile field*
7. Don face mask and apply mask to client (optional).	*Reduces risk of insertion site contamination*
8. Inform client of progression of the procedure, particularly when needlestick is to occur.	*Prepares client for discomfort; helps to decreases startle reaction*
9. Monitor client for respiratory distress, complaints of chest pain, dysrhythmias, or other problems.	*Allows for early detection of complications such as pneumothorax or air or catheter embolism*
10. After the vein has been punctured and the physician has removed the syringe from the insertion needle and inserted a guidewire through the needle (central line), instruct the client to take a deep breath and to bear down (Valsalva's maneuver) while the guidewire is inserted.	*Prevents air from being sucked into the vein by the increasing intrathoracic pressure*
11. As the multilumen central catheter or a PICC is inserted over the guidewire into the vein and the guidewire is withdrawn, observe for blood backing up into the catheter lumen(s). Aseptically aspirate air from and then flush saline through each catheter lumen.	*Indicates the presence of the catheter in the vein and removes air from the catheter tubing before infusion of fluid*

Action	Rationale
12. Apply IV lock and cap to catheter lumen(s), if needed.	*Maintains sterility of lumen and establishes a closed system to minimize blood loss and air entry*
13. Once the catheter is in place and sutured, apply sterile gauze or transparent dressing and, if needed, tape dressing down securely.	*Protects IV site from air leak, debris, and organisms while allowing visualization of catheter tubing and insertion site*
14. Arrange for chest x-ray and then begin regular infusion rate after catheter position has been confirmed.	*Verifies that catheter tip is in vena cava or right atrium before large amounts of fluid are infused*
15. Position client appropriately with call light within reach; instruct client to report any respiratory distress or pain.	*Promotes client safety; allows early detection of complications*

Monitoring and Performing Maintenance

1. Perform hand hygiene.	*Prevents transfer of micro-organisms*
2. Label each lumen of multi-lumen catheter with name of fluid/medication infusing.	*Prevents mixing of medications*
3. Flush lumens without continuous fluid infusions and capped every 8 hours with heparin solution (usually 1:100 dilution) or normal saline.	*Prevents obstruction of catheter lumen with blood clot*
• Depending on length of tubing and size of catheter, use 1 to 3 mL of flush solution.	*Minimizes leakage via cap or damage to catheter; prevents rupture of PICC tubing due to excess syringe pressure*
• Use 6 mL or ordered amount of flush for Hickman catheter and short small needle ($\frac{5}{8}$ inch, 25 gauge).	
• For PICC lines, use a 10-cc syringe or larger for flushing.	
4. Flush tubing between infusion of medications and drawing of blood, first using saline and then heparin.	*Prevents medication interaction or lumen obstruction*
5. ALWAYS aspirate before infusing medications or flushing.	*Ensures patency of line and validates presence in vessel*

Action	Rationale
6. Monitor for clot formation in lumen. If resistance is met when flushing tubing, DO NOT FORCE. Aspirate and remove clot, if possible; if not, notify physician.	*Reduces risk of embolism; prevents dislodging of clot*
7. Monitor respirations and breath sounds every 4 hours.	*Promotes early detection of fluid entering chest cavity or of pulmonary embolism*
8. Maintain IV fluids above heart level. Do not allow fluid to run out and air to enter tubing (see Table 7.2 and Nursing Procedure 7.8).	*Prevents blood reflux into tubing; prevents infusion of air, which could result in air embolism*

Tubing Change

Action	Rationale
1. Prepare fluid and tubing (review Nursing Procedures 7.5 and 7.9).	*Minimizes exposure to microorganisms*
2. Don mask and sterile gloves.	*Protects against contamination*
3. Expose catheter hub or rubber port of multilumen catheter.	*Precedes connection of tubing*
4. For centrally inserted lines: • Ask client to gently turn head to opposite side, take a deep breath, and bear down (Valsalva's maneuver). • Disconnect old tubing and quickly connect new tubing. • Open fluid and adjust to appropriate infusion rate.	*Increases intrathoracic pressure; prevents air from entering vein; reduces risk of air entering lumen*
5. Proceed to dressing change if needed; if not needed, remove gloves, discard equipment, and position client appropriately.	*Reduces risk of contamination of insertion site; reduces risk of infection transmission; promotes client comfort*

Dressing Change

Action	Rationale
1. Explain procedure to client.	*Reduces anxiety*
2. Perform hand hygiene and gather equipment.	*Reduces microorganism transfer and promotes efficiency*
3. Open packages, keeping supplies sterile.	*Prevents contamination of catheter site*
4. Don clean gloves and mask.	

Action	Rationale
5. Remove tape and previous dressing and inspect site. Discard dressing and gloves.	*Provides access to insertion site; reduces risk of infection transmission; inspection determines status of site in terms of infection or other problems, such as bleeding at site.*
6. Don sterile gloves.	*Prevents site contamination*
7. Beginning at catheter insertion site and wiping outward to the surrounding skin, clean insertion site with alcohol three times, allow it to dry, then clean with an antiseptic agent.	*Decreases contamination and removes microorganisms from site*
8. Cover gauze with tape or transparent dressing; wrap tubing on top and cover tubing with tape.	*Secures dressing; prevents pull on catheter*
9. Remove gloves and mask.	
10. On a piece of tape or label, record date and time of site care and nurse's initials. Place label on dressing.	*Determines time for next site care (usually required every 48 to 72 hours)*
11. Raise side rails and position client for comfort.	*Promotes client safety and comfort*

Evaluation

Were desired outcomes achieved? Examples of evaluation include:
- Desired outcome met: Client remained free of signs and symptoms of embolism, pleural effusion, and infection, both systemically and at catheter site.
- Desired outcome met: Client maintained skin turgor during TPN administration.
- Desired outcome met: Central line remained patent.
- Desired outcome met: Client gained 1 to 2 lb each week.

Documentation

The following should be noted on the client's chart:
- Date and time of catheter insertion
- Type and location of catheter, including the number of lumens
- Care and maintenance procedures performed
- Equipment used with catheter, including any flushing
- Appearance of insertion site
- Problems noted, such as resistance to flushing
- Client tolerance of procedures

Sample Documentation
Date: 2/17/05
Time: 2100

Dressing changed at right subclavian triple-lumen catheter site. No redness, edema, or drainage at site. IV solution and tubing changed. D_5W infusing via infusion pump at 50 mL/hr.

● Nursing Procedure 7.12

Managing Total Parenteral Nutrition 🧤

Purpose

Permits administration of nutritional support when gastro-intestinal tract is traumatized or nonfunctional

Equipment

- IV tubing with filter (for total parenteral nutrition [TPN])
- IV tubing without filter for lipids, if ordered
- Infusion pump
- Sterile gloves

Assessment

Assessment should focus on the following:
- Physician's orders for TPN contents and rate
- Physician's orders for lipid infusion frequency and rate
- Current nutritional status (weight, height, skin turgor, evidence of edema)
- Vital signs
- Laboratory values, particularly albumin level, glucose, and potassium

Nursing Diagnoses

Nursing diagnoses may include the following:
- Nutrition imbalance, less than body requirements, related to anorexia

- Risk for infection related to use of concentrated glucose solutions

Outcome Identification and Planning

Desired Outcomes

Sample desired outcomes include the following:
- Client maintains elastic skin turgor during TPN administration.
- Client gains 1 to 2 lb per week.
- Client has no edema present.
- Client demonstrates serum albumin and potassium levels within normal range and blood glucose level within acceptable range.

Special Considerations in Planning and Implementation

General

Adhere to strict aseptic technique to prevent septicemia. High glucose levels in TPN provide a good medium for bacterial growth. Some facilities use a 3-in-1 total parenteral solution that contains lipids, so no additional lipids are needed. If central line was inserted for infusion of TPN, infuse only $D_{10}W$ or D_5W until TPN is available. If multilumen catheter is used, select and mark a catheter port for TPN use only. Consult agency policy manual.

Pediatric

Infuse TPN volumes cautiously because children tend to be very sensitive to volume changes. Frequently assess children for signs and symptoms of infection, including elevations in temperature, because children are highly susceptible to infection.

Geriatric

Infuse TPN volumes cautiously because elderly clients tend to be very sensitive to volume changes. Frequently assess the older adult for signs and symptoms of infection, including elevations in temperature, because the elderly are highly susceptible to infection.

End-of-Life Care

The infusion of fluids and nutritional supplements in dying clients is controversial in terms of its palliative versus life-sustaining potential. Consider the desires of the client and family, the physician's orders, and agency policy regarding fluid and nutrition therapy for dying clients.

Delegation

Do not delegate central line care to non-RN personnel unless hospital policy dictates and you have assessed that the person to whom you will delegate has been properly instructed and certified.

Implementation

Action	Rationale
1. Perform hand hygiene and organize equipment.	*Reduces microorganism transfer; promotes efficiency*
2. Identify port intended for TPN. DO NOT infuse medications or other solutions through this port.	*Preserves integrity of the port and catheter lumen*
3. Prepare TPN solution and tubing:	
• If refrigerated, allow bag/bottle to stand at room temperature for 15 to 30 minutes.	*Prevents infusion of cold fluid, with resulting discomfort and chilling*
• Put time tape on bag/bottle.	*Aids in monitoring flow rate*
• Close roller clamp/ drip regulator on filtered tubing. Remove cap from filtered tubing to expose spike. Remove tab/cover from TPN bag/bottle.	*Minimizes risk of solution leaking*
• Spike the TPN solution container and prime drip chamber; open roller clamp/regulator and prime tubing. Attach primed tubing to infusion pump.	*Reduces the risk of air embolism; helps to ensure solution is administered at proper rate*
4. Prepare lipid solution if ordered to be given simultaneously by spiking lipid solution container with appropriate tubing and priming drip chamber and tubing.	*Aids in minimizing fatty acid deficiency; reduces the risk of air embolism; permits infusion of lipids simultaneously with TPN without filter causing separation of the lipids*
5. Compare TPN and lipid solution labels with physician's orders.	*Verifies correct dosage of nutrients*
6. Check client's name band with label on TPN and lipid solutions and medication administration record.	*Verifies identity of client*
7. Attach TPN tubing to port on central line and regulate infusion as ordered (Fig. 7.18). Set pump to deliver appropriate volumes per hour.	*Provides a closed system for administration at the proper rate*

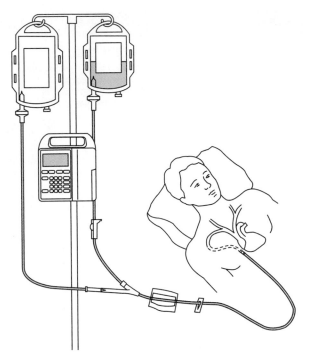

FIGURE 7.18

Action	Rationale
8. Discard gloves and disposable materials; reposition client with call light within reach.	*Reduces risk of microorganism transfer; promotes communication and safety*
9. Monitor flow rate and infusion. If infusion is behind schedule, DO NOT speed up infusion rate. Adjust infusion to prescribed rate and resume proper administration.	*Verifies correct infusion rate; prevents volume overload or glucose bolus*
10. Instruct client to keep solution higher than chest, to avoid manipulating catheter, and to report any pain, respiratory distress, warmth, or flushing.	*Facilitates proper flow of solution; indicates possible catheter dislodgment or infection*

Action	Rationale
11. Monitor client parameters: • Vital signs with temperature every 4 to 8 hours (depending on orders) • Blood glucose levels every 12 to 24 hours (more frequently if client is diabetic) • Urine glucose and electrolytes (watch for signs of hyperglycemia)	*Allows early detection of complications; identifies glucose intolerance*
12. Assess central line site every shift; provide care every 72 hours or per policy.	*Aids in identifying complications early on and reduces the risk for infection*
13. Obtain daily weights and monitor total protein and albumin levels.	*Provides information to evaluate effectiveness of therapy*
14. Encourage client to ambulate if possible.	*Promotes muscle development and a sense of well-being; helps prevent respiratory complications associated with bed rest*

Evaluation

Were desired outcomes achieved? Examples of evaluation include the following:
• Desired outcome met: Client maintained elastic skin turgor during TPN administration.
• Desired outcome met: Client gained 1 to 2 lb each week.
• Desired outcome met: Client has no edema present.
• Desired outcome met: Client maintained serum albumin and potassium levels within normal range and glucose level within acceptable range.

Documentation

The following should be noted on the client's chart:
• Time TPN bottle/bag is hung, number of bottles/bags, and rate of infusion
• Site of IV catheter and verification of patency
• Status of dressing and site, if visible
• Laboratory results
• Vital signs and weights
• Client tolerance to TPN
• Client response to therapy and understanding of instructions given

Sample Documentation
Date: 2/17/05
Time: 2100

Bag #3 of TPN infusing at 80 mL/hr into middle port of
right subclavian triple-lumen catheter. Catheter insertion
site intact with good blood return. No redness, bruising, or
swelling at insertion site. Weight 86 pounds with net 0
change in last 24 hours. Fingerstick blood sugar 110 mg/dL.

● **Nursing Procedure 7.13**

Managing a Pulmonary Artery Catheter

Purpose

Facilitates monitoring of hemodynamic status, providing information about right- and left-sided intracardiac pressures, cardiac output, and mixed venous oxygen saturation

Obtains hemodynamic data necessary for regulating vasoactive medications and fluid administration

Equipment

- Pulmonary artery (PA) line with 3-mL Luer-lok syringe
- Leveler
- Pressure transducer system (including flush solution of heparinized normal saline IV [500- to 1,000-mL bag], pressure bag, pressure tubing with flush device)
- Pressure monitoring system and cardiac output monitor
- Cardiac output set and injectate solution (injectate of 250 mL of D_5W or as determined by manufacturer)
- Cooling coil with ice bucket (optional depending on agency protocol and manufacturer)
- Data records/flow sheets
- Equipment for site care (see Nursing Procedure 7.11)

Assessment

Assessment should focus on the following:
- Client's medical history (particularly pulmonary and ventilatory status)

- Client/family knowledge regarding procedure
- Client ability to tolerate supine position
- Physician's orders regarding PA pressure monitoring
- Previous values for right- and left-sided heart pressures, cardiac output, or other data being collected
- Clinical indicators of peripheral vascular, neurovascular, cardiac, and respiratory status
- Presence and appearance of waveforms
- Insertion site and markings indicating length and position of catheter
- Vital signs
- Heparin allergy or history of heparin-induced thrombocytopenia
- Current anticoagulant medication use
- Agency policy regarding PA catheter management

Nursing Diagnoses

Nursing diagnoses may include the following:
- Decreased cardiac output related to increased preload
- Ineffective tissue perfusion, cardiopulmonary, related to mismatch of ventilation with blood flow
- Impaired gas exchange related to pulmonary artery obstruction
- Risk for infection related to invasive monitoring device
- Risk for injury related to complications of PA catheter insertion

Outcome Identification and Planning

Desired Outcomes

A sample desired outcome is:
- Cardiac output increases as evidenced by pink mucous membranes, warm skin, normal blood pressure, normal cardiac output.

Special Considerations in Planning and Implementation

General

Inspect the PA catheter. The standard PA catheter is 7.5 French and 110 cm long. There are black marks every 10 cm to indicate catheter position. Check the physician's orders about obtaining wedge pressures. Wedge pressures are not performed for all clients, since the risk of PA blockage or rupture may outweigh the benefit of the information. Check physician's orders for determining cardiac output. Cardiac outputs may need to be modified to use minimum fluids with clients who have volume overload concerns. Closely monitor clients with coagulopathies or who are taking anticoagulants for bleeding from insertion sites. Do not use heparin with clients who have heparin-induced thrombocytopenia or allergy to heparin. Consult agency policy manual for recommendations for maintaining PA catheter patency. Research and institutional policies vary greatly regarding the use of saline or heparin solution to maintain PA line patency. For PA catheter site and tubing maintenance, provide care similar to that for a central venous catheter (see Nursing Procedure 7.11); change hemodynamic monitoring sets, including all add-on devices, every 72 hours (depending on agency policy).

Pediatric

Follow agency policy. For cardiac output measurement, injectate volume will be determined by weight.

Geriatric

Take special care when obtaining wedge pressures in elderly clients, since their vessels are less pliable and thus may rupture with excessive balloon inflation pressure. Use digital readings of right atrial pressure if ventilation does not affect the pressure waveform.

End-of-Life Care

The use of aggressive diagnostic and monitoring procedures is limited for dying clients if there has been time for planning and discussion with the client and family. It is generally used only in a critical situation, often requiring quick decisions on the part of family members. Provide frequent and sensitive communication with the client and family to help them to cope, as often they are torn about using aggressive therapy when death is imminent.

Delegation

Only RNs may perform hemodynamic monitoring procedures. Special training or certification may be required.

Implementation

Action	Rationale
1. Explain procedure to client.	*Reduces anxiety*
2. Perform hand hygiene and organize equipment.	*Reduces microorganism transfer; promotes efficiency*
Performing PA Catheter System Calibration	
3. Check amount of flush solution and amount of pressure on flush solution bag to be sure pressure is 300 mm Hg; inflate to increase or maintain pressure as needed. If new bag of he-	*Maintains adequate flow of heparinized solution through tubing to avoid blood backup, clotting at tip of catheter, and unnecessary air in line, which could cause air embolism*

Action	Rationale
parinized flush solution is needed (1,000 U heparin), prepare bag of medicated solution (2 U/mL mixed in 500 mL of normal saline or dextrose 5% and water) or obtain from pharmacy, place in pressure bag, apply 300 mm Hg pressure, and prime tubing system.	
4. Place client in supine position	*Allows leveling of transducer at appropriate point*
5. Level the right atrial and pulmonary artery reference ports (stopcock) of the transducer at the phlebostatic axis (intersection of fourth intercostal space and midchest) (Fig. 7.19).	*Levels the transducer with the tip of the catheter (approximately at the level of the right atrium)*
6. Secure the system to a pole mount or to the client's chest or arm.	*Ensures that air-filled interface zeroing stopcock is maintained at the level of the phlebostatic axis*
• Mark the phlebostatic axis on client's skin with indelible marker if pole mount is used.	*Reduces erroneous readings*
• Keep the transducer at the level of the phlebostatic axis for all future readings.	*Readings will be falsely elevated if stopcock is below the axis and falsely low if stopcock is above the axis.*
7. Zero the right atrial and PA stopcocks to establish a circuit between the transducer and the air:	
• Zero stopcock off to client and open to air and then push the "Zero" button on the hemodynamic monitor.	*Zeroes system for calibration*
• Wait for the reading to register zero (and the waveform to reach the zero level).	*Ensures accuracy of the system with the correct reference point*
• Return the stopcock position off to air and open to client.	*Re-establishes the circuit between the transducer and the client*
8. While observing waveform, rapidly flush solution through the line to perform	*Indicates whether system is correctly dampened*

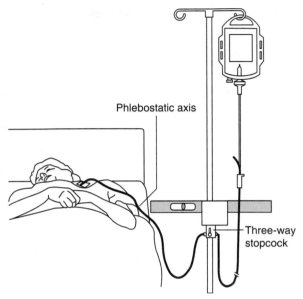

Phlebostatic axis

Three-way stopcock

FIGURE 7.19

Action	Rationale
the dynamic response (square wave test).	
9. Set upper and lower alarm limits.	*Activates bedside and central alarm system*
10. For initial assessment and each time the transducer or client is manipulated (positioned) away from phlebostatic axis, level the transducer.	*Ensures accuracy of subsequent readings*
Measuring Pressure	
11. Position client in supine position with head of bed elevated from 0 to 45 degrees	*Validates that pressures obtained in this position are accurate*
12. Run a dual-channel strip of the ECG and specific wave-	*Accurately determines pressures in varying anatomic areas be-*

Action	Rationale
form of the parameter to be measured (right atrial, PA systolic, PA diastolic, pulmonary artery capillary wedge pressure [PAWP]) off the monitor and mark point of alignment with ECG for appropriate measurement being obtained.	*cause the effects of ventilation can be identified from the graphic*
13. Measure pressures at end expiration; interpret waveforms.	*Obtains accurate reading at point at which effects of pulmonary pressures are minimized*
14. Note the numeric measurement on the monitor and record it on the document flowsheet.	*Establishes a record and provides a means of communication with other health care professionals*

Measuring Pulmonary Capillary Wedge Pressure (PCWP)

Action	Rationale
15. Prefill syringe with 1.5 mL of air and attach to balloon port of PA catheter at the stopcock or the lock valve port.	
16. Open the stopcock or lock the valve port if not using a stopcock.	*Provides open access in line for measurement*
17. While watching the monitor oscilloscope, slowly inflate the catheter balloon with 0.8 to 1.5 mL of air, inflating ONLY to the point that a change in waveform to that of a wedge waveform is noted. Slight resistance will be felt as the balloon floats out into the artery, but it should not be difficult to inflate (Table 7.3).	*Helps determine when catheter balloon has floated and "wedged" for measurement of left ventricular filling pressure; avoids potentially lethal complications*
18. Note the status of the waveform and the numeric measurement of the wedge pressure at end expiration.	*Obtains accurate reading at point at which effects of pulmonary pressures are minimized*
19. Release thumb from plunger and allow balloon to deflate, noting return of PA systolic and diastolic waveforms.	*Deflates balloon*

● **Table 7.3** Troubleshooting PA Catheter Problems

Potential Problem	Procedural Cautions	Indications of Complication	Appropriate Action
Pulmonary Capillary Wedge Pressure			
Potential balloon over-inflation or damage and subsequent balloon rupture	– Do not overinflate balloon. – Do not inflate balloon to obtain wedge reading more than 10 seconds. – Do not pull back to withdraw the instilled air from the syringe, but allow balloon to deflate passively.	– No resistance is sensed as the balloon is advanced for wedging. – Blood backs up into the insertion port. – The inflation syringe has to be manually retracted rather than floating back on its own.	– STOP! – Lock the port (close the port valve or the stopcock mechanism). – Remove the syringe. – Label the port with tape and indicate port is no longer usable. – Assess client's PA systolic and diastolic pressures, pulse and respiratory rates, respiratory character, mental status, skin color and temperature, and breath sounds. – Notify the physician of problem and accompanying data.
Blood flow occluded or blocked, causing infarction or hemorrhage of pulmonary artery	– Always use the syringe that comes with the PA catheter set to avoid overinflation. – Always use the syringe that comes with the PA catheter set to avoid overinflation.	– Continual appearance of wedge waveform when PCWP measurement procedure not being performed.	Do not perform wedge procedure. Label port as unusable and notify physician. Notify physician for follow-up.

Action	Rationale
Measuring Cardiac Output	
20. Obtain client height and weight (in kg), catheter size, and injectate volume to be instilled into proximal port of PA catheter.	*Ensures accuracy of measurement by obtaining correct parameters of height, weight, size of catheter, and injectate volume (see manufacturer's recommendation) based on specific system, thereby enabling accurate calculation of cardiac index*
21. Ascertain that monitor oscilloscope displays normal PA waveform.	*Indicates correct location of PA catheter before obtaining measurement*
22. Prepare injectate fluid, tubing, and monitor: • Prepare closed system tubing and injectate as instructed in manufacturer's guide for the specific system, taking care to prime the tubing of air. • Turn on cardiac output monitor or set monitor setting to cardiac output. • Based on manufacturer's computation scale, set the computation constant as directed.	*Facilitates accurate readings and prevents air from entering system, which would place client at risk for air embolism*
23. Clear the proximal line of any medications in the proximal port. • Discontinue infusions running through the proximal port of the PA catheter. • Flush the line with saline at appropriate rate based on the medication.	*Prevents accidental bolus administration of medications*
24. Attach appropriate-sized syringe to stopcock of prepared injectate tubing line, then open stopcock to the injectate solution to withdraw appropriate volume of injectate (5 or 10 mL) into syringe.	*Withdraws appropriate volume of injectate*

Action	Rationale
25. Instill 10 mL of injectate and record cardiac output for three consecutive instillation cycles of the injectate solution as follows: within a 2- to 4-second period, and with a smooth motion, inject the solution.	*Provides a more realistic reading based on an average of three; rapid injection helps obtain accurate readings*
26. Record measurements immediately after each reading.	*Ensures accuracy*
27. Record injectate volume on intake and output record.	*Accounts for accuracy of fluid intake*
28. Turn stopcock off to the injectate solution and open to the continuous IV infusion line.	*Re-establishes infusion of regular IV fluid and/or medication infusion*
29. Reposition client.	*Promotes comfort*
30. Check position of all lines in client's bed and raise side rails.	*Avoids dislodgment or tension on lines; promotes safety*
31. Discard or replace equipment appropriately.	*Reduces the risk of infection transmission*

Evaluation

Were desired outcomes achieved? An example of evaluation is:
● Client demonstrates improved cardiac output.

Documentation

The following should be noted on the client's chart:
● Pressure readings
● Cardiac output
● Presence or absence of clinical signs associated with monitor readings (e.g., breath sounds, shortness of breath, skin color, level of consciousness, heart rate and rhythm)
● Date and time of PA catheter insertion
● Type and location of catheter, length indicator marking
● Care and maintenance procedures performed
● Equipment used with catheter
● Client tolerance of procedures
● Teaching performed

Sample Documentation
Date: 2/17/05
Time: 2100

Dressing changed at right pulmonary artery catheter insertion site. No redness, edema, or drainage at site. Monitor waveforms indicate continued correct placement of catheter. Clinical parameters as per flow sheet. IV fluids resumed as per flow sheet.

● **Nursing Procedure 7.14**

Managing an Arterial Line

Purpose

Facilitates monitoring of hemodynamic status by providing
   information about arterial blood pressure readings
Obtains hemodynamic data necessary for regulating vasoactive
   medications and fluid administration

Equipment

For Monitoring and Data Collection

- Arterial line with 3-mL Luer-lok syringe
- Normal saline IV solution (500- to 1,000-mL bag)
- Leveler
- Pressure transducer system (including flush solution,
   pressure bag or device, pressure tubing with flush device)

For Drawing Blood Specimens

- Syringes
- Appropriate blood specimen collection tubes
- Gauze pads (2 × 2 or 4 × 4)
- Alcohol or appropriate antiseptic cleansing agent
- Replacement stopcock covers
- Data records/flow sheets

For Changing Dressing

- Alcohol wipes or appropriate antiseptic cleansing agent
- Sterile occlusive dressing
- Strip of tape or label with nurse's initials, date and time of
   site care/dressing change

Assessment

Assessment should focus on the following:
- Client's medical history (particularly pulmonary and ventilatory status)
- Client/family knowledge regarding procedure
- History of heparin allergy or heparin-induced thrombocytopenia
- Current anticoagulant medication use
- Physician's orders regarding arterial pressure monitoring
- Previous values for arterial pressures or other data being collected
- Presence and appearance of waveforms
- Vital signs
- Agency policy regarding arterial catheter management

Nursing Diagnoses

Nursing diagnoses may include the following:
- Ineffective tissue perfusion related to decreased arterial elasticity and increased pressure on arterial walls
- Ineffective tissue perfusion related to decreased blood volume

Outcome Identification and Planning

Desired Outcomes

Sample desired outcomes include the following:
- Client demonstrates signs of increased tissue perfusion as evidenced by pink mucous membranes, warm skin, normal blood pressure, normal cardiac output, increased alertness.
- Client demonstrates signs of increased blood volume.

Special Considerations in Planning and Implementation

General

Closely monitor clients with coagulopathies or those receiving anticoagulants for bleeding from insertion sites. Do not use heparin with clients who have heparin-induced thrombocytopenia or allergy to heparin. Consult agency policy manual for recommendations for maintaining patency. Institutional policies vary regarding use of saline or heparin solution.

Pediatric

Follow agency policy.

Geriatric

Frequently assess the skin of elderly clients because it is thinner and more vulnerable to trauma. Vessels may be sclerosed and hard, requiring close monitoring for complications at the site.

End-of-Life Care

Use of aggressive diagnostic and monitoring procedures is limited for dying clients if there has been time for planning and discussion with the client and family. It is generally used only in critical situations, often requiring quick decisions by family members. Provide frequent and sensitive communication with the client and family to help them to cope, as often they are torn about the use of aggressive therapy when death is imminent.

Delegation

Only RNs may perform hemodynamic monitoring procedures. Special training or certification may be required.

Implementation

Action	Rationale
1. Explain procedure to client.	*Reduces anxiety*
2. Perform hand hygiene and organize equipment.	*Reduces microorganism transfer; promotes efficiency*
Performing System Calibration	
3. Place the client in a supine position.	*Facilitates leveling of transducer at appropriate point*
4. Level the transducer for air reference point of the phlebostatic axis (the intersection of the fourth intercostal space and midchest) (Fig. 7.20).	*Levels the transducer*
5. Secure the system to a pole mount or to the client's chest or arm. Mark the phlebostatic axis on client's skin with indelible marker if pole mount is used.	*Ensures that air-filled interface zeroing stopcock is maintained at the level of the phlebostatic axis; reduces erroneous readings (readings will be falsely elevated if stopcock is below the axis and falsely low if stopcock is above the axis)*

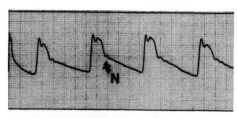

n = dicrotic notch

FIGURE 7.20

Action	Rationale
6. Zero the arterial line stop-cock to establish a circuit between the transducer and the air.	
• Turn stopcock off to the client and open to air. Push the "Zero" button on the hemodynamic monitor.	*Opens it to air*
• Wait for the reading to register zero (and the waveform to reach the zero level).	*Ensures accuracy of the system with the correct reference point*
• Return the stopcock position off to air and open to the client.	*Re-establishes the circuit between the transducer and the client*
7. While observing wave-form, rapidly flush solu-tion through the line to perform the dynamic re-sponse (square wave test).	*Indicates whether system is correctly dampened*
8. Set upper and lower alarm limits based on client's hemodynamic values.	*Activates bedside and central alarm system*

Measuring Arterial Pressure

9. Position extremity in straight position.	*Facilitates accurate reading*
10. Ascertain that arterial waveform is of normal character, noting wave-form height and appear-ance of dicrotic notch (see Fig. 7.20).	*Verifies correct catheter placement*
11. Note and record monitor readings of blood pressure and mean arterial pressure.	*Obtains arterial pressure readings*

Collecting Blood Specimen

12. Perform hand hygiene and apply clean gloves.	*Reduces risk of infection transmission*
13. Assess appearance of site and monitor waveform.	*Verifies that site is without hematoma and that catheter is intact and ready for use*
14. Remove protective cap from port and gently twist and se-cure a 3-mL syringe to port.	*Allows access to blood drawing port*

Action	Rationale
15. Turn stopcock toward the fluid flush line (off to flush tubing, open to client).	*Accesses blood line*
16. Aspirate 3 to 5 mL blood from arterial catheter line and quickly turn stopcock a half-turn toward the client. (Follow agency policy regarding specific discard volumes. Withdraw an additional volume of 5 mL to be discarded if drawing blood for PT/PTT.)	*Removes heparinized blood before actual specimen collection*
17. Quickly discard syringe into appropriate receptacle for blood disposal (if within reach; otherwise, place syringe of blood on paper towel and away from possible exposure to self or others on bedside table until end of procedure).	*Discards unneeded blood without recontamination of stopcock port*
18. Turn stopcock toward the fluid flush line (off to flush tubing, open to client).	*Accesses blood line*
19. Aspirate appropriate volume of blood into syringe (1.5 mL or more depending on required test), and turn stopcock off to client immediately.	*Withdraws blood for sample*
20. While holding syringe between two nondominant fingers, turn stopcock off to client, place gauze at opening of syringe attachment port, then rapidly flush syringe attachment port.	*Flushes blood from stopcock opening*
21. Turn stopcock to open flush infusion line between flush bag and client and perform a rapid flush of the line. Check to make sure line is clear of blood.	*Clears catheter of blood*
22. Apply new protective cap to stopcock attachment port.	*Prevents port contamination*

Action	Rationale
23. Transfer blood to appropriate tube (for routine blood drawing) or place cap over syringe port and place syringe in appropriate receptacle containing ice (for arterial blood gas analysis).	*Prepares specimen for appropriate lab analysis*
24. Discard all supplies, perform hand hygiene, and position client appropriately with siderails raised and call light within reach.	*Prevents infection transmission and promotes client safety*

Dressing Change

Action	Rationale
25. Explain procedure to client.	*Reduces anxiety*
26. Assess peripheral and neurovascular status of area distal to insertion site.	*Identifies possible complications associated with arterial catheter insertion*
27. Perform hand hygiene and gather equipment.	*Reduces microorganism transfer; promotes efficiency*
28. Open packages, keeping supplies sterile.	*Prevents contamination of catheter site*
29. Don clean mask, goggles, or face shield and gloves.	*Avoids exposure to blood under a high-pressure infusion system*
30. Remove tape and previous dressing, taking care to maintain secure placement of catheter.	*Removes soiled dressing; prevents dislodgment of catheter and potential bleeding and hematoma*
31. Assess appearance of site.	*Determines status of catheter*
32. Remove old gloves and apply sterile gloves.	*Prevents cross-contamination*
33. Beginning at catheter insertion site and wiping outward to the surrounding skin, clean insertion site with antiseptic agent.	*Removes microorganisms from site*
34. Apply antimicrobial ointment to site, if ordered, and cover with sterile occlusive dressing.	*Provides antimicrobial protection*
35. Remove gloves, goggles, and mask (or face shield) and discard.	*Reduces risk of infection transmission*
36. Place tape or label over top of dressing.	*Determines next site care (required every 48 to 72 hours)*

Action	Rationale
37. Raise side rails, position client appropriately, and perform hand hygiene.	*Promotes client safety and comfort; prevents spread of microorganisms*

Evaluation

Were desired outcomes achieved? Examples of evaluation include:
● Desired outcome met: Right femoral arterial site clean without redness, hematoma, or drainage.
● Desired outcome met: Right leg and foot warm to touch.
● Desired outcome met: Client verbalized no complaints of pain or numbness in right leg.
● Desired outcome met: Femoral and pedal pulses were 2+ bilaterally.
● Desired outcome met: Client demonstrated normal arterial waveform.
● Desired outcome met: BP maintained at 130/70 mm Hg.

Documentation

The following should be noted on the client's chart:
● Date and time of catheter insertion
● Location of catheter
● Care and maintenance procedures performed
● Equipment used with catheter
● Current blood pressure and mean arterial pressure reading
● Status of peripheral vascular circulation in extremity in which arterial line is inserted
● Neurovascular assessment of extremity
● Appearance of arterial insertion site
● Client tolerance of procedure
● Teaching performed

Sample Documentation
Date: 2/17/05
Time: 2100

Arterial catheter dressing changed at left radial site. No redness, edema, discoloration, drainage, or pain noted at site. Left hand warm, nailbeds pink, capillary refill time 2 seconds, no c/o pain or numbness. BP readings 120/68 mm Hg and as per flow sheet.

Managing Blood Transfusion

Purpose

Provides replacement of blood products to increase client's fluid volume, hemoglobin, and hematocrit for improved circulation and oxygen distribution

Prevents overadministration of blood products or the development of complications associated with a transfusion

Equipment

- Blood transfusion tubing (blood Y set with in-line filter)
- 250- to 500-mL bag/bottle normal saline
- Packed cells or whole blood, as ordered
- Blood warmer or coiled tubing and pan of warm water (optional)
- Order slips for blood
- Flow sheet for vital signs (for frequent checks)
- Nonsterile gloves
- Materials for IV start (see Nursing Procedures 7.4 and 7.5)
- Alcohol or povidone swabs, or approved antiseptic cleansing agent

Assessment

Assessment should focus on the following:
- Baseline vital signs; circulatory and respiratory status
- Skin status (e.g., rash)
- Physician's orders for type, amount, and rate of blood administration
- Size of IV catheter or need for catheter insertion
- Baseline laboratory studies, such as complete blood count, type and cross-match
- History of blood transfusions and reactions (including type of reaction, treatment, and client's response to treatment), if any
- Religious or other personal objections that client has to receiving blood
- Compatibility of client to blood (matching blood sheet numbers to name band)

Nursing Diagnoses

Nursing diagnoses may include:
- Activity intolerance related to weakness (associated with low hemoglobin and hematocrit)
- Deficient fluid volume related to hemorrhage
- Impaired tissue perfusion related to decreased hemoglobin

- Risk for injury related to transfusion reaction
- Deficient knowledge related to procedure and signs and symptoms to report

Outcome Identification and Planning

Desired Outcomes

Sample desired outcomes include the following:
- Blood pressure, pulse, respirations, and temperature are within normal range for client within 48 hours.
- Client ambulates in hallway without complaints of dyspnea.
- Client demonstrates adequate circulation, as evidenced by capillary refill time of 2 to 3 seconds, pink mucous membranes, and warm, dry skin.
- Client remains free of any signs and symptoms of transfusion reactions.
- Client verbalizes reasons for blood transfusion and signs and symptoms to report.

Special Considerations in Planning and Implementation

General

Two RNs should check that the correct blood is being given to the correct client. Client identification procedures should involve a verbal verification between the nurses and the client, when possible. Refer to agency policy. Closely monitor clients with a history of previous transfusions and those with altered levels of consciousness (e.g., confusion or coma) for a transfusion reaction. Confused or comatose clients often cannot communicate discomfort. Infuse a unit of packed red blood cells (PRBCs) or whole blood over no longer than 4 hours (the maximum transfusion time). Begin the blood transfusion within half an hour after obtaining the blood from the blood bank; otherwise, the blood cannot be reissued. If infusing blood rapidly, it should be warmed because infusion of cold blood can lower body temperature.

Pediatric

Carefully assess small children for a transfusion reaction because they often cannot communicate discomfort.

Geriatric

Administer blood transfusions slowly in clients who are fluid-sensitive because they may not tolerate a rapid change in blood volume.

End-of-Life Care

The use of aggressive therapies such as blood transfusions is limited in dying clients if there has been time for planning and discussion with the client and family. When used, it is generally in a critical situation, often requiring quick decisions on the part of family members. Provide frequent and sensitive communication with the client and family to help them to cope, as often they are torn about the use of aggressive therapy when death is imminent.

Home Health

Remain with the client during the entire transfusion period and for 1 hour afterward. Double-check the date, time, and transfusion information on the blood bag and blood bank slip at two separate points in time or ask the client or relative to verify that the transfusion data are identical. Have epinephrine on hand in case an anaphylactic reaction occurs (see agency policy regarding dosage amounts for children and adults).

Transcultural

Some religious groups or denominations hold varying opinions about the use of blood transfusions. Jehovah's Witnesses do not allow blood transfusion, and Christian Scientists and Pentecostals avoid certain aspects of hospital treatment and secular medicine. Communicate clearly with the client and family members if a blood transfusion is needed; opinions may vary among specific denominations and groups as to the use of transfusions.

Delegation

Unlicensed personnel may be helpful in taking frequent vital signs during the transfusion, but they should play NO part in checking client identification or initiating or administering the transfusion. THE NURSE IS RESPONSIBLE FOR ALL ASPECTS OF CARE, INCLUDING MONITORING FOR COMPLICATIONS.

Implementation

Action	Rationale
1. Perform hand hygiene and organize equipment.	*Reduces microorganism transfer; promotes efficiency*
2. Explain procedure to client, particularly the need for frequent vital sign checks.	*Helps decrease anxiety*
3. Prepare blood transfusion tubing (Fig. 7.21):	
• Open tubing package and close drip regulators/roller clamps (which may be a clamp, roller, or screw). Note colors of caps over tubing spikes.	*Prepares for infusion of saline before and after transfusion*

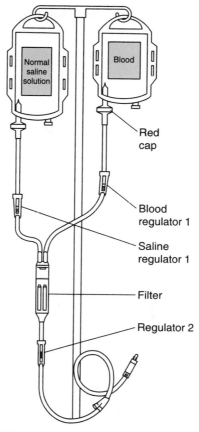

FIGURE 7.21

Action	Rationale
• Remove cap to reveal spike on one side of blood tubing. Remove tab from normal saline bag/bottle and insert tubing spike. Remove cap from end of tubing, open saline regulator 1, prime drip chamber and	*Establishes connection between tubing and saline solution; clears air from tubing*

Action	Rationale
tubing with saline, and close saline regulator.	
• Replace cap on tubing end and place on bed near IV catheter.	*Maintains sterility of system*
4. Insert IV if one is not already present (see Nursing Procedure 7.4); if IV catheter is present, verify that it is of adequate size (catheter should be 20 gauge or larger).	*Decreases hemolysis; allows free flow of blood*
5. Don gloves if not already on and remove dressing enough to expose catheter hub.	*Reduces risk of infection transmission; permits access for connection of blood tubing*
6. Disconnect infusion tubing from hub and connect blood tubing to catheter hub; discard or place needle cap over previous infusion tubing tip.	*Connects blood tubing directly to catheter; preserves previous infusion tubing for future use*
7. Open saline regulator/ roller clamp fully and regulate to a rate that will keep vein open (15 to 30 mL/hr) until blood is available.	*Maintains patency of catheter*
8. Obtain blood and perform safety checks:	
• When blood arrives, check blood and client information, comparing blood package with order slip and checking client name, hospital number, blood type, computerized blood ID number, and expiration date.	*Verifies that the client's name, ABO group, Rh type, and unit number and computer match*
• Check client's name band: name and hospital number (or emergency department number on name band if typing and crossmatching were done in emergency department). If discrepancies are noted, notify the blood bank immediately and postpone	*Ensures transfusion to correct client*

Action	Rationale
transfusion until problems are resolved.	
• Check for correct identification information WITH A SECOND NURSE AND AT CLIENT'S BEDSIDE. Identify client first and do so verbally as well as by checking appropriate written forms of identification. Include the client in the verbal identification process.	*Prevents transfusion of unmatched blood. Failure to identify the blood product or client properly is often linked to severe transfusion reactions. Recent JCAHO guidelines reflect the goal of better client identification procedures, including verbal verification.*
9. Complete blood bank slip with date and time of transfusion initiation and nurses checking information.	*Provides legal record of blood verification*
10. Check and record pulse, respirations, blood pressure, and temperature.	*Provides baseline vital signs before transfusion*
11. Remove cap to reveal spike on other side of blood tubing and insert spike into port on blood bag.	*Accesses blood for administration*
12. Close regulator/roller clamp (#1) on normal saline side of tubing and open blood regulator/roller clamp (#1) on blood side of tubing	*Prevents saline from infusing into blood bag and allows blood tubing to fill with blood*
13. Regulate drip rate to deliver the following:	
• A maximum of 30 mL of blood within the first 15 minutes	*Identifies possible reaction. Most reactions occur within the first 15 minutes of the infusion.*
• One half to one quarter of the volume of blood each hour (62 to 125 mL/hr—depending on client tolerance of volume change and volume of blood to be infused)	*Delivers blood volume in 2 to 4 hours*
• If client has poor tolerance to volume change, check to see if blood bank will divide unit in half so 8 hours may be used to infuse the total unit.	*Allows slower infusion of total unit without violating 4-hour transfusion time limit*

Action	Rationale
14. Check vital signs and temperature again 15 minutes after beginning the transfusion, then every half hour or hourly until transfusion is completed (see agency policy); check at the completion of delivery of each unit of blood.	*Allows prompt detection of transfusion reaction*
15. When blood transfusion is complete, clamp off blood regulator/roller clamp (#1), open saline regulator/roller clamp #1, and begin infusing saline solution. Remove empty blood bag and recap blood tubing spike.	*Clears blood line for infusion of other fluid; maintains sterility for future transfusions*
16. Fill in time of completion on blood bank slip, and place copy of slip with empty bag, or place other copy of slip on chart. (If no further blood is to be given, replace blood transfusion tubing with IV tubing or infusion cap.)	*Complies with agency regulations for confirmation of blood administration*
17. During and after transfusion, monitor client closely for signs of a transfusion reaction (Table 7.4). Check vital signs every 4 hours for 24 hours (or per agency policy).	*Allows for prompt detection and early intervention should a problem arise*
18. Position client appropriately and raise side rails if indicated.	*Promotes client comfort and safety*
19. Discard supplies, remove gloves, and perform hand hygiene.	*Prevents spread of microorganisms*

Evaluation

Were desired outcomes achieved? Examples of evaluation include:
• Desired outcome met: Blood pressure, pulse, respirations, and temperature were within normal range for client within 48 hours.
• Desired outcome met: Client's activity increased to ambulation in hallway without dyspnea.

Table 7.4 Transfusion Reactions

Type of Reaction	Signs and Symptoms	Actions
Allergic reaction—*indicates incompatibility between transfused red cells and host cells*	Rash, chills, fever, nausea, or severe hypotension (shock)	Turn off blood transfusion (*decreases further infusion of incompatible or contaminated blood*). Remove blood tubing and replace with tubing primed with normal saline (*maintains catheter patency*). Infuse normal saline at slow rate (*maintains IV patency*). Notify physician immediately.
Pyrogenic reaction—*indicates sepsis and subsequent renal shutdown*	Nausea, chilling, fever, and headache (usually noted toward end of or after transfusion)	See Allergic reaction.
Circulatory overload—*indicates acute pulmonary edema or heart failure*	Cough, dyspnea, distended neck veins, and crackles in lung bases	Slow blood transfusion rate and notify the physician (*decreases workload of the heart and avoids further overload*). Take vital signs frequently (every 10 to 15 minutes until stable), and perform emergency treatment as needed or ordered (*detects and treats resulting shock or cardiac insufficiency*). Remove and send remaining blood and blood tubing to blood bank with completed blood transfusion forms. Send first voided urine specimen to laboratory (*confirms hemolytic reaction if red blood cells are present*). Monitor I&O, particularly urinary output (*detects renal shutdown secondary to reaction*).

• Desired outcome met: Client exhibited adequate circulation, as evidenced by capillary refill time of 2 to 3 seconds, pink mucous membranes, and warm, dry skin.

Documentation

The following should be noted on the client's chart:
• Date and initiation and completion times for each unit of blood transfused
• Type of blood infused (packed cells or whole blood) and amounts
• Initial and subsequent vital signs
• Presence or absence of transfusion reaction and actions taken
• State of client after transfusion and current IV fluids infusing, if any
• IV catheter size and location; condition of IV site
• Instructions given and client's understanding of instructions

Sample Documentation
Date: 2/17/05
Time: 0400

One unit of packed red blood cells (Unit #R46862, O positive) hung at 0345; BP 120/70 mm Hg; pulse 80 bpm and regular; respirations 20 breaths/min and nonlabored; temperature 98.4°F after first 15 minutes of transfusion. Blood infusing into 18-gauge angiocath in right antecubital space at 100 mL/hr; infused over 3 hr. No signs of transfusion reaction or fluid overload noted. IV site clean, dry, and intact without evidence of redness or inflammation.

● **Nursing Procedure 7.16**

Inserting a Nasogastric/Nasointestinal Tube 🧤

Purpose

Permits nutritional support through gastrointestinal tract
Allows evacuation of gastric contents
Relieves nausea

Equipment

- Nasogastric (NG) tube (14 to 18 French sump tube) or nasointestinal (8 to 12 French, small-bore feeding tube)
- Water-soluble lubricant
- Ice chips or glass of water
- Appropriate-sized syringe:
  NG tube: 30- or 60-mL syringe with catheter tip OR
  Small-bore nasointestinal tube: 20- to 30-mL Luer-lok syringe
- Nonsterile gloves
- pH test strips
- 1-inch tape (two 3-inch strips and one 1-inch strip)
- Washcloth, gauze, cotton balls, cotton-tipped swab
- Petroleum jelly
- Emesis basin
- Tissues

Assessment

Assessment should focus on the following:
- Physician's order for type and use of tube
- Size of previous tube used, if any; history of gastrointestinal problems requiring use of tube
- History of nasal or sinus problems
- Gastrointestinal status, including nausea, vomiting, or diarrhea, bowel sounds, abdominal distention and girth, passage of flatus

Nursing Diagnoses

Nursing diagnoses may include the following:
- Imbalanced nutrition, less than body requirements, related to dysphagia
- Nausea related to absence of bowel peristalsis

Outcome Identification and Planning

Desired Outcomes

Sample desired outcomes include the following:
- Client gains 1 to 2 lb per week.
- Client voices no complaints of nausea or vomiting.

Special Considerations in Planning and Implementation

General

Check agency policies on acceptable methods of verifying tube placement. The best verification is by x-ray, and when in doubt, obtain an order for an x-ray. NEVER INSTILL ANYTHING INTO THE TUBE WITHOUT VERIFYING PLACEMENT. Tape

the tube to the side of the client's face rather than to the nostril
to prevent nasal ulceration.

Pediatric

Be prepared to use protective devices or enlist family members
to prevent the child from pulling on the NG tube. If the NG tube
is plastic, change it every 3 days.

Delegation

Check agency policy. Unlicensed personnel are not usually
skilled in NG tube insertion.

Implementation

Action	Rationale
1. Perform hand hygiene and organize equipment.	*Reduces microorganism transfer; promotes efficiency*
2. Explain procedure to client.	*Reduces anxiety; promotes cooperation and participation*
3. Place client in semi-Fowler's position.	*Facilitates passage of tube into esophagus instead of trachea*
4. Check nasal patency:	
• Ask client to breathe through one naris while the other is occluded. Repeat with other naris.	*Determines patency of nasal passages*
• Have client blow nose with both nares open. Clean mucus and secretions from nares with moist tissues or cotton-tipped swabs.	*Clears nasal passage without pushing microorganisms into inner ear*
5. Measure length of tubing needed by using tube and measure distance from tip of nose to earlobe and then from earlobe to sternal notch. Mark the location on the tubing with a small piece of tape (Fig. 7.22).	*Indicates distance from nasal entrance to pharyngeal area and then to stomach. Tape indicates depth to which tube should be inserted. Ice water makes tube less pliable and facilitates insertion.*
• If necessary, place tube in ice-water bath.	
• If a feeding tube with weighted tip is used (small-bore feeding tube), measure for distance as instructed with package insert. Insert guidewire and prepare the tube as instructed	

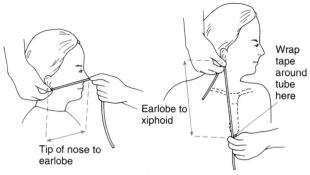

Wrap tape around tube here

Earlobe to xiphoid

Tip of nose to earlobe

FIGURE 7.22

Action	Rationale
on package insert (usually by flushing with 10 to 20 mL of saline irrigation solution).	
6. Don gloves and use water-soluble lubricant or dip feeding tube in water to lubricate tip.	*Reduces risk of infection transmission; promotes smooth insertion of tube*
7. Ask client to tilt head backward; insert tube into clearer naris.	*Facilitates smooth entrance of tube into naris*
8. As tube is advanced, have client hold head and neck straight and open mouth	*Decreases possibility of insertion into trachea and allows visualization of tube in pharynx*
9. When tube is seen and client can feel tube in pharynx, instruct client to swallow (offer ice chips or sips of water, unless contraindicated).	*Facilitates passage of tube into esophagus*
10. Continue to advance tube further into esophagus as client swallows (if client coughs or tube curls in throat, withdraw tube to pharynx and repeat attempts); between attempts, encourage client to take deep breaths.	*Prevents trauma from forcing tube and prevents tube from entering trachea; maintains oxygenation*
11. When tape mark on tube reaches entrance to naris,	*Indicates that tube is in stomach and not curled in mouth*

Action	Rationale
stop tube insertion and check placement by: • Having client open mouth for tube visualization • Aspirating with syringe (Fig. 7.23), noting color of secretion return, and checking pH of drainage (pH between 1 and 5 may indicate gastric secretions; pH of 7 or higher may indicate intestinal placement) or for old tube feeding (if reinsertion)	
12. Secure tube by attaching commercially prepared tube holder or by: • Splitting 2 inches of long tape strip, leaving 1 inch of strip intact • Applying 1-inch base of tape on bridge of nose	*Maintains tube placement with client movement*

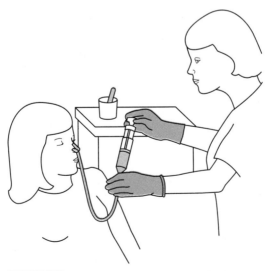

FIGURE 7.23

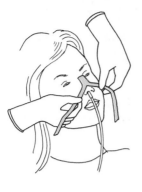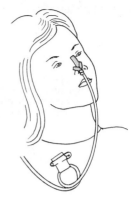

FIGURE 7.24

Action	Rationale
• Wrapping first one and then the other side of split tape around tube (Fig. 7.24).	
13. Tape loop of tube to side of client's face (if feeding tube) or pin to client's gown (if sump tube).	*Decreases pull on client's nose and possible dislodgment*
14. Obtain order for chest x-ray; delay tube feeding or flushing with fluid until physician reads x-ray.	*Confirms placement of tube in stomach or duodenum; prevents aspiration*
15. Store stylet from small-bore feeding tube in a plastic bag at the bedside after correct placement is confirmed by x-ray.	*Allows for reuse of stylet*
16. Begin suction or tube feeding as ordered.	*Initiates therapy*
17. Replace or discard equipment.	*Maintains a neat environment; prevents infection transmission*
18. Reposition client for comfort.	*Facilitates comfort*
19. Perform hand hygiene.	*Removes microorganisms*

Evaluation

Were desired outcomes achieved? Examples of evaluation include:
• Desired outcome met: Client gained 1 to 2 lb per week.
• Desired outcome met: Client had no complaints of nausea or vomiting.

Documentation

The following should be noted on the client's chart:
- Date and time of tube insertion
- Color and amount of drainage return
- pH result
- Size and type of tube
- Client tolerance of procedure
- Confirmation of tube placement by x-ray
- Suction applied (amount) or tube feeding started and rate

Sample Documentation
Date: 2/17/05
Time: 2100

Salem-Sump tube (#18) inserted via left naris, with no obstruction or difficulty. Tolerated insertion with no visible problems or complaints. Gastric aspirate reveals acidic pH of 4 with scant green drainage noted. Radiograph obtained with placement confirmed by Dr. Wey. Connected to suction at 80 mm Hg.

● Nursing Procedures 7.17, 7.18

Maintaining a Nasogastric Tube (7.17)

Discontinuing a Nasogastric Tube (7.18)

Purpose

Maintaining a Nasogastric Tube

Minimizes damage to naris from tube
Maintains proper tube placement
Promotes proper gastric suctioning or tube feeding

Discontinuing a Nasogastric Tube

Terminates nasogastric (NG) therapy based on indications that adequate gastrointestinal function has resumed

Equipment

- Syringe and container with saline (irrigation kit)
- Tape or tube holder
- Washcloth, gauze, cotton balls, cotton-tipped swabs
- Petroleum jelly or ointment
- Towel or linen saver
- 500- or 1,000-mL bottle of saline or ordered irrigant
- Mouth moistener
- Nonsterile gloves

Assessment

Assessment should focus on the following:
- Size and type of tube
- Purpose of tube
- Physician's orders regarding type and frequency of tube irrigation
- Type and rate of tube feeding
- Presence or absence of nausea and vomiting; gastrointestinal functioning
- Status of skin at tube insertion site

Nursing Diagnoses

Nursing diagnoses may include the following:
- Imbalanced nutrition, less than body requirements, related to dysphagia
- Risk for aspiration related to malpositioned tube
- Risk for impaired skin integrity related to pressure on naris

Outcome Identification and Planning

Desired Outcomes

Sample desired outcomes include the following:
- Client will have no episodes of nausea or vomiting.
- Tubing patency is maintained.
- No signs of aspiration are noted.
- Client experiences no skin breakdown at area of tube placement.

Special Considerations in Planning and Implementation

General

Monitor client closely for aspiration, a primary problem with NG tubes. Clients at risk for aspiration are those with decreased levels of consciousness, those with an absent or diminished cough reflex, and those who are noncommunicative and recumbent most of the time. Provide oral and nares care frequently to promote comfort and minimize risk for breakdown. If NG tube is plastic, change every 3 days. Tape the tube to the side of the client's face rather than to the nostril to prevent nasal ulceration.

Pediatric

Use a protective device or enlist a family member to prevent the child from pulling on the NG tube.

Geriatric

Physiologic changes associated with aging result in a decrease in gastrointestinal motility. Be alert for possible intolerance of enteral feeding formulas. Always check for gastric residuals, especially in the elderly, to prevent or decrease regurgitation and aspiration during feeding. Due to fragility of skin, be particularly careful in monitoring for breakdown at the NG insertion site. Be scrupulous in monitoring for diarrhea. Perform frequent oral care to prevent drying and cracking of mucous membranes if the elderly client cannot orally ingest liquids.

End-of-Life Care

Assess whether the client desires to receive feeding and hydration by non-natural means. Review the benefits and disadvantages concerning fluids and nutrients for dying clients for palliative purposes and for the management of symptoms associated with dehydration. Provide scrupulous mouth care. Respect the client's wishes regarding the use of enteral tube feedings. Living wills help to clarify the client's preferences if personal communication is no longer possible.

Home Health

When NG therapy is long term, include in plan of care replacement of tube at specified intervals to avoid complications such as sinusitis, electrolyte imbalances, and esophagitis. Assess clients frequently for complications. Teach home caregivers signs of and ways to avoid aspiration. Advise caregivers to clean the area around the tube daily with warm water and mild soap. Teach family and client how to assess placement, assess drainage, record drainage amounts, ensure suction device is set correctly as needed, and change or clean canister.

Transcultural

Assess cultural view of feeding per nasogastric tubes.

Cost-Cutting Tips

Use a 60-mL syringe, because the plastic outer casing that holds the syringe can be used to hold irrigation fluid, thus eliminating the need for an irrigation kit.

Delegation

Unlicensed personnel may perform NG tube feeding procedures if skilled in the process. Consult agency policy.

Implementation

Action	Rationale

Maintaining a Nasogastric Tube

1. Ask the client if there is any discomfort from the tube and determine whether it needs to be adjusted.

Increases client comfort; allows client to participate in care

2. Inspect tube insertion site for signs of irritation or pressure.

Indicates need to adjust or remove tube from current site

3. Don gloves.

Reduces risk of infection transmission

4. Check tube placement before irrigation or medication administration and every 4 to 8 hours of tube feeding (see Nursing Procedure 7.16).

Reduces risk of aspiration

5. Cleanse nares with moist gauze or cloth and apply ointment or oil to site.

Maintains skin integrity and helps prevent skin breakdown

6. Every 4 hours, perform mouth care: apply lubrication to oral cavity and lips.

Maintains integrity of oral mucous membranes

7. Irrigate tube (if ordered) with 20 to 30 mL of saline every 3 hours.
   - Disconnect tube from suction or tube feeding and attach saline-filled syringe to tube and slowly and gently instill fluid into the tube.

   Allows fluid to clear the tube without rupturing it

   - Aspirate fluid gently, noting appearance; discard fluid. Repeat irrigation and aspiration if necessary.

   Removes irrigant and helps assess for gastric bleeding

   - Reconnect tube to suction or tube feeding.

   Re-establishes therapy

8. Remove and reapply tape if loose or soiled.

Promotes cleanliness and secures tube in place

9. If naris is irritated, remove tube and reinsert in other naris if clear.

Prevents further skin breakdown

Action	Rationale
10. Every 2 hours, check suction for proper pressure (usually 80 to 100 mm Hg = low suction) and frequency (i.e., constant or intermittent).	*Prevents damage to gastric mucosa*
11. Monitor drainage in tubing and container for color, consistency, and odor.	*Indicates presence of bleeding or infection or need for irrigation*
12. Each shift, mark drainage level (if bottle or canister is used) or empty and measure amount of drainage to maintain accuracy of output.	*Removes suction pressure so canister can be emptied; allows for recording of drainage*
• To empty drainage bag (if 75% to 100% full), first turn off suction and wait until suction meter returns to 0. Measure and record drainage in a appropriate graduated container.	
• *If using canister suction* (wall or floor suction), loosen seal and remove cap (disconnect tubing leading to NG tube if disposable lining is used). Empty contents into graduated container and rinse canister (or discard plastic liner and obtain fresh one). Reseal cap and reconnect NG tubing.	
• *If using vacuum suction,* open door to suction machine (Omnibus) and remove bag and cap from bag port. Pour contents into graduated container. Replace cap and place bag into suction machine. Reseal door to suction machine. Reset and initiate appropriate suction pressure.	

Action	Rationale
13. Every 24 hours (or per institutional policy) replace drainage bag (if used) and clean canister.	*Reduces accumulation of microorganisms*
14. Discard supplies and perform hand hygiene.	*Reduces risk of contamination*

Discontinuing a Nasogastric Tube

Action	Rationale
1. Explain procedure to client.	*Decreases anxiety; promotes cooperation*
2. Place client in semi-Fowler's position.	*Opens glottis to aid in tube removal*
3. Place waterproof pad or linen saver over client's chest.	*Prevents soiling of bedclothes*
4. Turn off suction or discontinue feeding, if applicable.	*Terminates suction or feeding*
5. Don gloves.	*Reduces risk of infection transmission*
6. Remove tape securing tube to cheek or attaching tube to gown and remove or loosen tape across bridge of nose.	*Facilitates smooth removal of tube*
7. Place towel under nose and drape over tube.	*Prevents client from seeing appearance of tube during removal*
8. Clamp tube by pinching off or folding over on itself.	*Prevents gastric contents from leaking into lungs during withdrawal*
9. Slowly withdraw tube in one motion until completely removed. Wrap tube in towel and place tube in trash.	
10. Perform nose and mouth care.	*Promotes skin integrity and comfort*
11. Position client with head of bed elevated 45 degrees and call light within reach.	*Facilitates comfort and gastric emptying*
12. Instruct client to call if nausea or discomfort is experienced.	*Facilitates early detection of gastric distention or distress*
13. Monitor bowel sounds every 4 hours and as needed, and note flatulence.	*Indicates adequate bowel activity*
14. Replace or discard equipment.	*Maintains neat environment*

Action	Rationale
15. Reposition client for comfort.	*Promotes comfort*
16. Perform hand hygiene.	*Removes microorganisms*

Evaluation

Were desired outcomes achieved? Examples of evaluation include:
- Desired outcome met: Client had no episodes of nausea or vomiting.
- Desired outcome met: NG tube remained patent and positioned properly.
- Desired outcome met: No signs of aspiration.

Documentation

The following should be noted on the client's chart:
- Type of NG tube and therapy (suction or tube feeding)
- Status of tubing patency and security of placement
- Type and amount of drainage (or of residual if tube feeding)
- Time of NG tube removal
- Status of skin at naris and where secured
- Irrigation solution, frequency and ease of irrigation
- Client tolerance of continued therapy or tube removal
- Client status after removal
- Gastrointestinal functioning during therapy and after NG removal when appropriate

---

Sample Documentation

Date: 2/17/05
Time: 1400

NG to suction intact per Omnibus suction at 80 mm Hg continuous pressure. Thin green drainage noted, with scant amounts this shift. Tube in right naris, with surrounding skin intact. Bowel sounds hypoactive in all 4 quadrants. Bilateral nares cleaned and ointment applied.

Time: 1800

NG tube removed per orders. Mouth care performed with mouthwash. Active bowel sounds noted. Sips of water provided and tolerated without nausea.

Managing a Gastrostomy/ Jejunostomy Tube 🧤

Purpose

Provides a patent access for the delivery of nutrients

Equipment

- Cotton-tipped applicators
- Luer-lok or catheter tip syringe, 30 mL or larger
- Skin sealants or protectant, if indicated
- Normal saline
- Soap and warm water
- Towel and washcloth
- Disposable tape measure
- Tape
- 4 × 4 gauze squares or split gauze dressing
- Disposable gloves (several pairs)
- Stethoscope
- Pin for dating and labeling dressing
- Infusion pump for continuous feedings, if indicated
- pH strips
- 50 to 75 mL water in cup or irrigation receptacle

Assessment

Assessment should focus on the following:
- Abdominal assessment (bowel sounds, abdominal tenderness, pain or tenderness at or around stoma site)
- Skin around and under stoma site
- Signs or symptoms of dehydration, diarrhea, regurgitation, or aspiration
- Respiratory status
- Signs and symptoms associated with bowel obstruction and protracted vomiting
- Confirmed placement of tube
- Intake and output

Nursing Diagnosis

Nursing diagnosis may include the following:
- Risk for impaired skin integrity related to external feeding tube placement
- Risk for aspiration related to placement of enteral tube
- Deficient knowledge related to care of tube

Outcome Identification and Planning

Desired Outcomes

Sample desired outcomes include the following:
● Client displays no evidence of skin breakdown or infection at site.
● Client experiences no regurgitation and shows no signs of aspiration.
● Client and caregiver verbalize information related to care of tube and site.

Special Considerations in Planning and Implementation

General

Do not allow air to enter tube when irrigating or checking for residual, or during medication administration. Irrigate with 30 to 60 mL of water before or after checking for residual, before and after medication administration, and before and after feeding. Use aseptic technique when caring for the insertion site until healed; thereafter, soap and water may be used. If client reports GI distress or is experiencing abdominal distention and an increase in residuals, stop feeding and notify physician. Administer feeding at room temperature (see Nursing Procedure 7.20).

Pediatric

To promote comfort and to lessen the potential for dislodgment, consider using a low-profile tube, also known as a gastrostomy button. Enlist the aid of an additional person to help prevent infants or toddlers from pulling at or pulling out the tube. Consider the developmental stage and age of child when teaching about the tube. Discussion should center on need for placement of tube, allowing child to understand that he or she is eating and receiving nourishment in a very special way. Closely monitor infants and young children who are vulnerable to fluid volume deficit and overload. Assess for diarrhea. Use care when flushing tube, carefully recording the exact amount of water used. If an enteral tube is being used for feeding of children, see Nursing Procedure 7.20.

Geriatric

Always check for gastric residuals in the elderly because of decreased gastric emptying and to prevent or decrease regurgitation and aspiration during feeding. Due to fragility of skin, be particularly careful in monitoring for breakdown and for diarrhea. Provide frequent oral care to prevent drying and cracking of mucous membranes for clients who cannot orally ingest liquids.

End-of-Life Care

Assess for client desires and ability for feeding and hydration by non-natural means. Review benefits and disadvantages concerning fluids and nutrients for dying clients for palliative purposes and for the management of symptoms associated with dehydration. Provide scrupulous mouth care.

Home Health

Teach client and caregiver how to clean insertion site daily with warm water and mild soap. Instruct caregiver or client to remove any buildup of crusts around site with hydrogen peroxide diluted with water (50% H_2O_2:50% H_2O) and cotton-tipped applicators for cleansing around and under the stoma site. Have client or caregiver use a clean washcloth to cleanse the stoma site once healed. Teach caregivers to crush pills thoroughly and to adequately mix with water before administration through tube, particularly if using a large-bore tube. Emphasize the need to prevent air from entering the tube when irrigating before and after medications, feedings, and checks for residual. Instruct caregivers to keep records of daily intake and output.

 Transcultural

Assess cultural view of feeding per gastrostomy/jejunostomy.

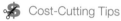 Cost-Cutting Tips

Use a 60-mL syringe when possible because the plastic outer casing that holds the syringe can be used to hold irrigation fluid, thus eliminating the need for an irrigation kit.

Delegation

Maintenance and care of gastrostomy/jejunostomy tubes may be delegated to unlicensed assistive personnel who have been trained, if agency policy allows. However, the patency of the tube should always be checked and verified by licensed personnel.

Implementation

Action	Rationale
1. Perform hand hygiene and organize equipment.	*Reduces microorganism transfer; promotes efficiency*
2. Confirm physician's order for formula frequency, route and rate of any feedings, and residual volume parameters. Assess for allergies to food.	*Ensures accuracy of treatment; prevents allergic responses*
3. Provide privacy and explain procedures to client.	*Alleviates anxiety; helps to build knowledge base, establish rapport, and foster client participation in care*
4. Adjust bed to comfortable working height.	*Prevents back and muscle strain in nurse*

Action	Rationale
5. Place or assist client into appropriate position. If client is receiving continuous feedings, maintain head of bed elevation at 30 to 45 degrees at all times, even when performing site care. Elevate the head of the bed in high Fowler's position during and for at least 30 minutes after feeding. Position head in lateral position if elevation is prohibited.	*Prevents aspiration*
6. Assess abdomen, noting presence of bowel sounds. Assess skin at tube insertion site.	*Verifies gastrointestinal functioning and reduces complications of skin breakdown such as from pressure or weight of tube, drainage, or secretions*
7. Don gloves.	*Reduces microorganism transfer*
8. Remove old dressing over site if in place, discard, and inspect insertion site and surrounding area.	*Allows for early detection of infection*
9. Remove gloves and discard. Perform hand hygiene, and apply a clean pair of gloves.	*Avoids cross-contamination*
10. Measure tube length at regular intervals.	*Verifies tube position. If gastric contractions draw tube toward pylorus, signs and symptoms of bowel obstruction may be evident (e.g., acute protracted vomiting). If tube migration has occurred or is suspected, deflate balloon and notify doctor.*
11. Assess for placement of tube and patency every 4 hours for continuous feeding and every 4 hours and before feedings for intermittent feeding.	*Verifies placement and patency of tube*
12. Check the residual volume (aspirating with a large-bore syringe). Clamp or crimp tube and place tip of syringe into end of appropriate port of tube; release clamp and withdraw GI fluid con-	*Determines if feeding solution being propelled through GI tract*

Action	Rationale
tent. Place a small amount (2 to 5 mL) of residual in small cup and set aside to check pH.	
• If residual volume is 100 mL or less, replace and proceed to next step to flush with water; for residuals over 100 mL, withhold feeding and notify physician for follow-up orders.	*Prevents fluid and electrolyte imbalance*
13. Assess pH of gastric contents every 4 hours. For clients who have jejunostomy tubes, aspirate intestinal contents, observing for appearance and checking for pH.	*Determines acidity. For continuous feedings, pH may be elevated. A client who has not had a gastric inhibitor and has fasted for 4 or more hours usually will have a pH varying from 1 to 4.*
14. Withdraw water from water receptacle and flush tube with 30 mL of water at least every 4 to 6 hours; also perform flushing before and after administering medications.	*Prevents clogging of tube*
15. Reclamp end of ostomy tube.	*Prevents backflow of GI contents through tube*
16. Rotate gastrostomy tube daily by gently twisting between thumb and first finger. Notify physician if unable to rotate tube.	*Alleviates pressure on skin* *Inability to rotate could indicate displaced tube.*
17. Remove gloves, perform hand hygiene, and apply clean pair of gloves.	*Prevents cross-contamination*
18. Cleanse tube insertion site with soap and water, saline, or ordered solution in circular pattern beginning at center and working outward using aseptic technique until site is healed.	*Prevents cross-contamination and helps reduce risk of infection*
19. Leave site open to air unless drainage occurs, or apply clean dressing if indicated and secure with tape. Change dressing as often as necessary or as ordered.	*Prevents reservoir for moisture conducive to the growth of microorganisms; promotes cleanliness and healing*

Action	Rationale
20. Elevate head of bed unless contraindicated, raise side rails, and position client appropriately.	*Prevents regurgitation and aspiration; provides for safety and comfort*
21. Remove gloves, discard equipment, and perform hand hygiene.	*Reduces risk of infection transmission*

Evaluation

Were desired outcomes achieved? Examples of evaluation include:
• Desired outcome met: Site remains free of infection; no signs of irritation or drainage.
• Desired outcome met: Client experiences no regurgitation or and shows no signs of aspiration.
• Desired outcome met: Client and caregiver verbalize information related to care of tube and site.

Documentation

The following should be noted on the client's chart:
• Type of tube and location
• Use of feeding, including type, formula, rate of administration
• Tube patency, including irrigations if any
• Appearance and condition of insertion site
• Bowel sounds
• Pain or tenderness at site or generally in abdominal area
• Any negative or adverse effects and overall response of client
• Residual volume, if any, and orders from physician if indicated
• Withholding of excess residual and discontinuance of any feedings
• pH result
• Intake and output amount

Sample Documentation
Date: 2/17/05
Time: 2100

Stoma site inspected with no drainage noted, residual less than 100 mL, flushed with 30 mL water.

Managing Enteral Tube Feeding

Purpose

Provides nutrition supplementation to clients who cannot ingest
adequate amounts of nutrients orally

Equipment

- Stethoscope
- pH paper (optional)
- Irrigation set with a 60-mL piston-type syringe
- Washcloth and towel
- Disposable gavage feeding set (bag and tubing appropriate for pump)
- Tube feeding product ordered by physician (at room temperature)
- Administration pump
- Nonsterile gloves
- Glass or cup

Assessment

Assessment should focus on the following:
- Nutritional status (skin turgor, urine output, weight, caloric intake, pertinent lab values)
- Gastrointestinal functioning (abdominal distention, bowel sounds)
- Elimination pattern (diarrhea, constipation, date of last bowel movement)
- Response to previous enteral nutritional support
- Medical diagnoses that may affect tolerance to product or administration
- Physician's orders for nutritional product and route of delivery
- Confirmation of tube location
- Residual feeding amounts
- Condition of skin at site of enteral tube insertion

Nursing Diagnoses

Nursing diagnoses may include the following:
- Imbalanced nutrition, less than body requirements, related to inability to ingest nutrients due to biologic factors (status post cerebral vascular accident resulting in altered level of consciousness)
- Risk for aspiration related to impaired swallowing

Outcome Identification and Planning

Desired Outcomes

Sample desired outcomes include the following:
- Formula is infused by prescribed route at appropriate volume and rate.
- Client reports no complaints of nausea and exhibits no signs of aspiration.
- Client gains 1 to 2 lb per week or maintains desired weight.
- Client has decreased edema with albumin level within normal limits.
- Client maintains normal elimination pattern.

Special Considerations in Planning and Implementation

General

If the client has an endotracheal or tracheostomy tube and is receiving enteral feedings, ensure that the tracheostomy cuff is inflated during and 30 minutes after feeding to prevent aspiration. Increase the volume and concentration of formula slowly. Many tube feeding formulas cause diarrhea. If diarrhea persists, report to physician and administer antidiarrheal medications, if ordered. Be careful with gastrostomy tube irrigations. Depending on the surgery, irrigation may be contraindicated. Verify this with the physician. Closely monitor residual feeding amounts to prevent aspiration because some medications (e.g., sedatives, narcotics) and some physiologic conditions (e.g., electrolyte imbalances, gastroparesis, pharmacologic vasoconstriction) can contribute to slowed GI motility. Do not discontinue or change tube feeding in clients experiencing diarrhea until other possible causes are examined. Diarrhea may be associated with infections (*Clostridium difficile, Giardia*), formula contamination, or medications (e.g., magnesium-based antacids, antibiotics, hyperosmolar elixirs). Determining the cause of the diarrhea is important to prevent unnecessary disruption of nutritional support. Administer antidiarrheal medication as ordered. Anticipate the need for regular flushing of small-bore feeding tubes with water to maintain patency; these tubes have an increased incidence of clogging. Always administer a tube feeding at room temperature.

Pediatric

Provide care based on the child's developmental level. Demonstrate the procedure using a doll or stuffed toy. Allow the child to express concerns and understanding through play. Feeding time is normally a time for interaction with an infant or child, so the nurse or family member administering the tube feeding should hold, cuddle, and establish eye contact with the child during feeding (Fig. 7.25). Expect to use intermittent feedings for infants; continu-

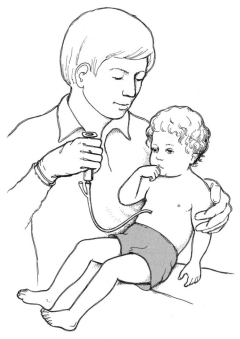

FIGURE 7.25

ous feedings have the potential to cause irritation of mucous membranes and perforation of the stomach. A decrease in the volume of feedings and an increase in the frequency of feedings are needed due to the decreased capacity of the stomach and intestines of an infant/small child. The immature muscle tone of the lower esophageal sphincter causes the small child/infant to be prone to regurgitation after feeding. Use a pediatric volume-control device or pediatric enteral infusion set to control the volume of feeding, in addition to setting the infusion device for infusion of small doses of feeding, then reset for the next volume of feeding.

Geriatric

Physiologic changes associated with aging result in a decrease in GI motility. Monitor for intolerance to enteral formulas, which also may occur in the elderly.

End-of-Life Care

Respect the client's wishes regarding the use of enteral tube feedings. Living wills help to clarify the client's preferences when personal communication is no longer possible.

Home Health

Instruct client or caregiver how to administer feeding via an enteral tube. Ensure understanding and correct technique by return demonstration.

Delegation

Unlicensed personnel may be delegated to perform tube feeding if they are properly trained and agency policy permits. However, the licensed professional is responsible for monitoring client response and residual feeding levels.

Implementation

Action	Rationale
Managing Continuous Feeding	
1. Perform hand hygiene and organize equipment. Confirm orders for formula frequency, route, and rate of feedings:	*Reduces microorganism transfer; promotes efficiency*
• Change disposable gavage feeding sets every 24 hours or per manufacturer's guidelines or agency policy.	*Prevents introduction of pathogens from contaminated equipment*
• Select tubing that is compatible with feeding bag and pump (if used).	*Promotes proper functioning of equipment*
• Determine amount of free water to be infused and pour into cup.	*Minimizes risk of fluid overload*
2. Explain procedure to client; provide for privacy.	*Decreases anxiety and embarrassment*
3. Adjust bed to comfortable working height.	*Prevents back and muscle strain in nurse*
4. Place or assist client into appropriate position. The head of the bed should be elevated in high Fowler's position during and for at least 30 minutes after the feeding.	*Prevents aspiration*
5. Don gloves.	*Reduces microorganism transfer*
6. Assess abdomen, noting the presence of bowel sounds. Assess skin at site enteral tube enters body (naris or	*Verifies GI functioning; prevents skin breakdown*

Action	Rationale
abdomen). Provide site care per physician's orders or agency policy, if appropriate.	
7. Verify tube placement.	*Prevents infusion of formula into pharynx or pulmonary tree*
8. To administer a continuous tube feeding:	
• Prepare formula: Remove formula from refrigerator 30 minutes before hanging (if applicable).	*Prevent muscle cramps from infusion of cold solution*
• Rinse bag and tubing with water.	*Checks for leaks in bag or tubing*
• Close roller clamp on gavage tubing and pour a 4-hour volume of formula in bag.	*Prevents leakage and spoilage of formula hanging without refrigeration*
• Open roller clamp and allow formula to flow to end. Clamp tubing and insert into pump mechanism, if used (Fig. 7.26).	*Replaces air with formula*
9. Attach feeding bag tubing to enteral tube attached to client.	*Establishes closed system for tube feeding*
10. Set pump to deliver appropriate volume and check infusion every 1 to 2 hours.	*Ensures infusion of proper volume per hour*

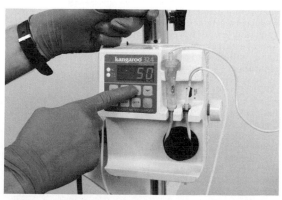

FIGURE 7.26

Action	Rationale

11. Every 4 hours:
  • Stop infusion; slowly aspirate gastric contents, taking care not to pull on tube; and note amount of residual feeding.
    ○ If residual is greater than specified amount per orders (commonly 100 mL), discard aspirated volume from stomach, cease feedings, and notify physician.
    ○ If residual feeding is within acceptable level, return to stomach.
	Determines degree of absorption of feeding; prevents distention of abdomen, possible aspiration, and electrolyte loss

• Monitor bowel sounds in all abdominal quadrants.	*Determines presence of peristalsis*
• Perform mouth care.	*Provides client comfort and prevents accumulation of microorganisms*
12. Irrigate tube every 2 to 3 hours and before and after medication administration with 30 to 60 mL of water, or as per doctor's orders or agency policy.	*Maintains patency of tube*
13. Once each shift, while irrigating enteral tube after completing a dose of formula, rinse bag and gavage tubing with water.	*Clears accumulated feeding from bag and tubing*
14. Remove gloves. Wash hands and properly store equipment.	*Reduces microorganism transfer; enhances cleanliness of environment*

Managing Intermittent Feeding

1. Follow Steps 1 to 7 above.	
2. Check for residual.	
3. Crimp tube and connect syringe to enteral tube and aspirate small amount of contents to fill tube and lower portion of syringe.	*Prevents infusion of air into stomach*
4. Fill syringe with formula and allow to flow slowly	*Assists flow of feeding by gravity; maintains tube patency*

Action	Rationale
into enteral tube. Infuse formula, holding syringe 6 inches above tube insertion site (nose or abdomen). Follow with water.	
5. Do NOT allow syringe to empty until formula and water have completely infused.	*Prevents air from entering stomach*
6. Clamp enteral tube, remove syringe, and remind client to stay in semi-Fowler's or high Fowler's position for at least 30 minutes after the feeding.	*Decreases reflux of feeding and possible aspiration*
7. Check enteral tube placement and residual feeding before each tube feeding.	*Prevents aspiration of formula*
8. Remove gloves. Wash hands and properly store equipment.	*Reduces microorganism transfer; enhances cleanliness of environment*

Evaluation

Were desired outcomes achieved? Examples of evaluation include:
- Desired outcome met: Formula is infused by prescribed route at appropriate volume and rate.
- Desired outcome met: Client reports no complaints of nausea and exhibits no signs of aspiration.
- Desired outcome met: Client gains 1 to 2 lb per week or maintains desired weight.
- Desired outcome met: Client has decreased edema with albumin level within normal limits.
- Desired outcome met: Client maintains normal elimination pattern.

Documentation

The following should be noted on the client's chart:
- Assessment of tube placement and method of confirmation
- Assessment of site of tube entry
- Amount of residual feeding
- Amount and type of product given
- Amount of water given with or between feedings
- Route and method of delivery
- Client position during and after administration of product
- Client tolerance of procedure
- Teaching performed

Sample Documentation

Date: 2/17/05
Time: 0800

Active bowel sounds noted in all four quadrants. Dobhoff feeding tube placed; placement confirmed by x-ray. Head of bed at 45 degrees. Continuous tube feeding initiated with Ensure infusing per pump at 30 mL/hr. 10 mL residual before initiation of feeding.

Time: 1200

No residual feeding aspirated. Tube flushed with 60 mL water. Abdomen nondistended, bowel sounds present in all 4 quadrants. Dobhoff tube remains taped to left naris. Skin on naris intact. Client denies nausea. Ensure infusion increased to 50 mL per order.

8

Elimination

OVERVIEW

- Adequate elimination of body waste is an essential function to sustain life.
- Inadequate bladder and bowel elimination ultimately affects the body's delicate balance of fluids, electrolytes, and acid–base level.
- Various means are available clinically to help assess and maintain adequate elimination status.

- Factors that affect bowel and bladder elimination status include food and fluid intake; age; psychological barriers; medications; activity level; personal hygiene habits; educational level; cultural practices; pathology of the renal, urinary, or gastrointestinal system; surgery; hormonal variations; muscle tone of supporting organs and structures; and concurrent medical problems, such as decreased cardiac output or motor disturbances.
- Alterations in bowel and bladder elimination mandate careful assessment and monitoring of the upper and lower abdomen, as well as of amounts and appearance of body excretions.
- Procedures related to adequate bladder elimination usually require the use of sterile technique to prevent contamination of the highly susceptible urinary tract.
- Because clients on peritoneal dialysis or hemodialysis are using final means of adequate renal excretion, the nurse must perform these procedures with precision.
- Various concentrations of dialysate affect osmolality, rate of fluid removal, electrolyte balance, solute removal, and cardiovascular stability.
- Elimination is very personal to the client; therefore, privacy and professionalism should be maintained when assisting clients with elimination needs.
- Clients with colostomies frequently experience body image and self-concept alterations. Psychological support and teaching are crucial in resolving these problems.
- All procedures involving elimination of body waste require the use of gloves and occasionally other protective barriers.
- When planning a procedure, the nurse should determine whether same-sex or opposite-sex contact with genitalia is culturally offensive to the client.
- Some major nursing diagnostic labels related to elimination are impaired urinary elimination, urinary retention, bowel incontinence, constipation, diarrhea, risk for impaired skin integrity, and urinary incontinence (functional, reflex, urge, stress, or total).
- For procedures that can be delegated to unlicensed assistive personnel, emphasis should be placed on procedural accuracy so correct determinations can be made concerning the client's diagnosis and progress.

Collecting a Midstream Urine Specimen 🖐

Purpose

Obtains urine specimen using aseptic technique for microbiologic analysis

Equipment

- Basin of warm water
- Soap
- Washcloth
- Towel
- Antiseptic swabs or cotton balls
- Sterile specimen collection container
- Specimen container labels
- Bedpan, urinal, bedside commode, or toilet
- Nonsterile gloves
- Pen

Assessment

Assessment should focus on the following:
- Characteristics of the urine
- Symptoms associated with urinary tract infections (e.g., pain or discomfort on voiding, urinary frequency)
- Temperature increase
- Ability of client to follow instructions for obtaining specimen
- Time of day of specimen collection
- Fluid intake and output

Nursing Diagnoses

Nursing diagnoses may include the following:
- Risk for infection related to poor technique in cleaning perineum
- Impaired urinary elimination: frequency related to urinary tract infection

Outcome Identification and Planning

Desired Outcomes

Sample desired outcomes include the following:
- Client shows no signs or symptoms of urinary tract infection.
- Client verbalizes relief of discomfort within 3 days.

Special Considerations in Planning and Implementation

General

Midstream urine collection is frequently performed by the client, so instructions must be clear to obtain reliable laboratory results. Perhaps the most frequent error the client commits is poor cleaning technique. Be certain women understand to cleanse from the front to the back of the perineum, and men from the tip of the penis downward. If possible, a specimen should be obtained on first voiding in the morning.

Pediatric

Parental or staff supervision and assistance should be provided for young children during the procedure to reduce specimen contamination.

Delegation

This procedure may be delegated to unlicensed personnel or to the client or a family member. Emphasize the importance of procedural accuracy.

Implementation

Action	Rationale
1. Perform hand hygiene.	*Reduces microorganism transfer*
2. Explain procedure to client.	*Decreases anxiety*
3. Provide privacy.	*Decreases embarrassment*
4. Put on clean gloves.	*Reduces nurse's exposure to client's body secretions*
5. Wash perineal area with soap and water, rinse, and pat dry.	*Reduces microorganisms in perineal area*
6. Cleanse meatus with antiseptic solution in same manner as for catheterization in males (see Procedure 8.5, steps 15 to 17) and females (see Procedure 8.6, steps 20 and 21).	*Reduces microorganisms at urethral opening*
7. Ask client to begin voiding.	*Flushes organisms from urethral opening*
8. After stream of urine begins to flow, place specimen collection container in place to obtain 30 mL of urine.	*Collects urine at point at which urine is least contaminated*
9. Remove container before client stops voiding.	*Prevents end-stream organisms from dripping into container*

Action	Rationale
10. Allow client to complete voiding using urinal, bedpan, or toilet.	*Decreases retention of urine and additional risk for infection*
11. Dry perineum or wash perineal area again if stain-producing antiseptic was used.	*Removes antiseptic solution; promotes general comfort*
12. Label specimen container with date, time, and client identification information.	*Notes time and date of collection; ensures that specimen and results are associated with correct client*
13. Fill out agency requisition form for specimen.	*Facilitates proper logging and charging in lab*
14. Send specimen to lab immediately.	*Avoids sending old specimen in which urine constituents may have changed*
15. Discard equipment and gloves.	*Reduces spread of infection*
16. Perform hand hygiene.	*Reduces microorganism transfer*

Evaluation

Were desired outcomes achieved? Examples of evaluation include:
- Desired outcome met: Client shows no signs or symptoms of urinary tract infection.
- Desired outcome met: Client verbalizes relief of discomfort.

Documentation

The following should be noted on the client's chart:
- Signs or symptoms of urinary infection
- Amount, color, odor, and consistency of urine obtained
- Specimen collection time
- Total amount voided
- Teaching performed regarding technique for cleaning genitalia

Sample Documentation
Date: 1/1/05
Time: 1100

Clean-catch urine specimen obtained and sent to laboratory: 30 mL of cloudy, yellow urine with slightly foul odor noted. Total amount voided, 120 mL. Client reports slight perineal burning. Instructed client on procedure for cleaning; client verbalized understanding.

Collecting a Timed Urine Specimen 🖐

Purpose

Preserves urine specimens obtained over a designated period of time to ensure proper storage for laboratory analysis

Equipment

- Basin of ice (if required)
- Laboratory-designated sterile specimen collection container
- Graduated container (optional if specimen container is graduated)
- Specimen container labels
- Catheter bag, bedpan, urinal, bedside commode, or toilet
- Nonsterile gloves
- Pen

Assessment

Assessment should focus on the following:
- Test ordered and associated lab protocols
- Characteristics of urine
- Symptoms associated with urinary tract infections (e.g., pain or discomfort upon voiding, urinary frequency)
- Ability of client to follow instructions for obtaining specimen
- Time of day of specimen collection
- Fluid intake and output

Nursing Diagnoses

Nursing diagnoses may include the following:
- Risk for infection related to poor technique in cleaning perineum
- Impaired urinary elimination: frequency related to urinary tract infection

Outcome Identification and Planning

Desired Outcomes

Sample desired outcomes include the following:
- Client shows no signs or symptoms of urinary tract infection.
- Client verbalizes relief of discomfort within 3 days.

Special Considerations in Planning and Implementation

General

Timed urine collection requires careful planning and precision to avoid delayed diagnosis due to delayed or repeated specimen collection secondary to improper timing in collection or storage errors. It is often best to begin a timed specimen collection at the beginning of the day so that it will end in the morning and can be transported directly to the lab.

Delegation

This procedure may be delegated to unlicensed personnel or to the client or a family member. Emphasize the importance of procedural accuracy, particularly proper storage and timing of beginning and completion of urine collection.

Implementation

Action	Rationale
1. Perform hand hygiene.	*Reduces microorganism transfer*
2. Explain procedure to client, emphasizing the importance of saving all urine voided over the designated period.	*Decreases anxiety*
3. Put on gloves.	*Reduces nurse's exposure to client's body secretions*
4. Discard first voided specimen and note the initiation time on specimen collection container.	*Prevents collection of urine held in the bladder for unknown period of time*
5. Ask client to notify nurse each time he or she voids. OR, if specimen is obtained from a catheter, collect urine from the drainage port every 2 to 4 hours.	*Ensures urine is placed in proper storage solution shortly after being voided*
6. With each voiding or each urine collection period, remove the top from the collection container, pour urine specimen from urinal/bedpan or catheter bag into collection container, then tightly recap container.	*Collects urine shortly after voiding; prevents spilling if container turns over*
7. If laboratory procedure requires cooling of specimen, place container in a	*Maintains specimen for analysis, since some elements degrade over time without preservatives or cold*

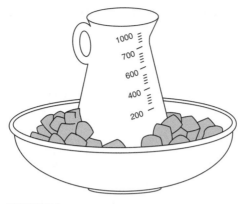

FIGURE 8.1

Action	Rationale
bucket of ice and keep on ice throughout specimen collection period (Fig. 8.1).	
8. After the last specimen is collected, inform client that collection will no longer be needed (if applicable, explain that recording of urine will continue).	*Releases client from continuing rigid specimen collection regimen*
9. Label specimen container with date and time of last voiding and client identification information (if not previously labeled).	*Notes time and date of collection; ensures that specimen and results are associated with the correct client*
10. Fill out agency requisition form for specimen.	*Facilitates proper logging and charging in lab*
11. Send specimen to lab immediately.	*Avoids sending old specimen in which urine constituents may have changed*
12. Discard disposable equipment and gloves.	*Reduces spread of infection*
13. Perform hand hygiene.	*Reduces microorganism transfer*

Evaluation

Were desired outcomes achieved? Examples of evaluation include:

● Desired outcome not met: Client continues to show symptoms of urinary tract infection.

- Desired outcome not met: Client verbalizes discomfort and burning still noted with urination.

Documentation

The following should be noted on the client's chart:
- Signs or symptoms of urinary infection
- Amount, color, odor, and consistency of urine obtained
- Specimen collection times
- Total amount voided
- Teaching performed regarding technique for cleaning genitalia

Sample Documentation
Date: 1/1/05
Time: 1100

24-hour urine specimen collection concluded at 10:30 am. Specimen sent to laboratory: 30 mL of cloudy, yellow urine with slightly foul odor noted. Client reports slight perineal burning.

● Nursing Procedure 8.3

Collecting a Urine Specimen From an Indwelling Catheter 🖐

Purpose

Obtains sterile urine specimens for microbiologic analysis

Equipment

- Sterile 3-mL syringe with 23- or 25-gauge needle
- Nonsterile gloves
- Alcohol swab
- Sterile specimen collection container
- Specimen container labels
- Pen
- Catheter clamp
- Linen saver
- Antiseptic solution

Assessment

Assessment should focus on the following:
- Specimen collection protocols for ordered urine test
- Characteristics of urine
- Symptoms associated with urinary tract infections (e.g., pain or discomfort on voiding, urinary frequency)
- Temperature increase
- Fluid intake and output

Nursing Diagnoses

Nursing diagnoses may include the following:
- Risk of infection related to long-term indwelling catheter
- Acute pain related to urinary tract infection

Outcome Identification and Planning

Desired Outcomes

Sample desired outcomes include the following:
- Client shows no signs of urinary tract infection.
- Client verbalizes lack of perineal discomfort within 3 days.

Special Considerations in Planning and Implementation

General

If a specimen is needed and a new catheter is to be inserted, obtain the specimen during the catheter insertion procedure (see Procedure 8.5 or Procedure 8.6).

Pediatric

Catheterization may be required if a sterile specimen is needed from a pediatric client or a client who cannot follow directions. Obtain assistance to maintain the sterility of the specimen and catheter.

Geriatric

If a specimen is needed from a confused client or a client who cannot follow directions, catheterization may be indicated. Obtain assistance to maintain the sterility of the specimen and catheter.

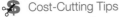 Cost-Cutting Tips

Rubber bands may be used to clamp off the catheter.

Delegation

This procedure can be delegated to nonlicensed personnel with appropriate knowledge and skills. Emphasize the importance of procedural accuracy.

Implementation

Action	Rationale
1. Perform hand hygiene.	*Reduces microorganism transfer*
2. Explain procedure to client.	*Decreases anxiety*
3. Provide privacy.	*Decreases embarrassment*
4. Put on clean gloves. Proceed to next step for closed-system method or open-system method.	*Reduces nurse's exposure to client's body secretions*

Using the Closed-System Method

5. Fold or clamp drainage tubing about 4 inches below junction of drainage tubing and catheter.	*Facilitates trapping of urine in tubing at specimen port*
6. Allow urine to pool in drainage tubing; if urine does not pool in tubing immediately, leave it clamped for urine to collect over a period of time (usually 10 to 30 minutes).	*Allows urine to pool in tubing at specimen port for collection*
7. Cleanse specimen collection port of drainage tubing with alcohol swab or antiseptic solution recommended by agency. (If no collection port is visible, catheter tubing is probably designed with a self-sealing material, so specimen may be obtained from catheter itself by cleansing and piercing catheter tubing close to junction. However, check package label and instructions. If catheter tubing is self-sealing, cleanse catheter tubing close to junction of drainage tubing.)	*Reduces microorganisms at insertion port*
8. Carefully insert sterile needle of syringe into specimen collection port or self-sealing catheter tubing at a 45-degree angle; insert needle slowly, taking care not to puncture the other side of the catheter tubing (Fig. 8.2).	*Prevents accidental puncture of drainage tubing or catheter*

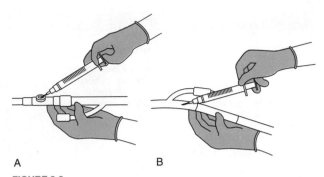

A   B

FIGURE 8.2

Action	Rationale
9. Pull back on plunger of syringe and obtain 3 to 10 mL of urine.	*Draws urine into syringe*
10. Slowly squirt urine into sterile specimen collection container; do not touch inside of specimen container.	*Places urine in container, maintaining sterility of container and specimen*
11. Proceed to step 12.	

Using the Open-System Method

Action	Rationale
5. Place linen saver under tubing at junction of catheter and drainage tubing. Remove cap from specimen bottle, and place bottle on linen saver.	*Prevents soiling of linens; allows easy access to bottle for insertion of specimen*
6. Cleanse junction with antiseptic solution such as Betadine (or antiseptic recommended by agency).	*Reduces microorganisms*
7. Carefully disconnect catheter from drainage tubing at junction. Hold drainage tubing and catheter 1.5 to 2 inches from junction, being careful not to contaminate either end.	*Disconnects catheter to allow for specimen collection; avoids system contamination*
8. Place specimen container under catheter opening	*Allows urine to run into container; avoids contamination*

Action	Rationale
and allow urine to run into container; do not allow catheter tip to touch container.	
9. Place specimen container on bedside table after urine is obtained.	*Prevents contamination of catheter line*
10. Wipe catheter and drainage tubing again with antiseptic solution.	*Reduces microorganism transfer*
11. Firmly reconnect drainage tubing and catheter at junction.	*Reconnects to closed system*
12. Replace top of specimen container.	*Prepares urine specimen for transport*
13. Label container with date and time of collection and client identification information.	*Notes time and date of collection; ensures that specimen and results are associated with the correct client*
14. Fill out agency requisition form for specimen.	*Facilitates proper logging and charging in lab*
15. Send to lab immediately.	*Avoids sending old specimen in which urine constituents may have changed*
16. Discard disposable equipment and gloves.	*Reduces spread of infection*
17. Perform hand hygiene.	*Reduces microorganism transfer*

Evaluation

Were desired outcomes achieved? Examples of evaluation include:
- Desired outcome partially met: Client shows decreased signs of urinary tract infection; urine remains cloudy.
- Desired outcome met: Client verbalizes lack of perineal discomfort.

Documentation

The following should be noted on the client's chart:
- Urine specimen obtained via closed catheter method
- Amount, color, odor, and consistency of urine obtained
- Specimen collection time
- Total amount of urine collected
- Signs or symptoms of urinary infection
- Disposition of specimen to lab

Sample Documentation
Date: 1/1/05
Time: 1100

~~Sterile urine specimen obtained via indwelling catheter~~
~~and sent to laboratory.~~ Specimen is 30 mL of cloudy,
yellow urine, with slightly foul odor noted. Client reports
no perineal burning.

● **Nursing Procedure 8.4**

Applying a Condom Catheter

Purpose

Provides for noninvasive method of urine collection

Equipment

- Nonsterile gloves
- Washcloth
- Towel
- Basin of warm, soapy water
- Condom catheter
- Velcro adhesive strip or elastic adhesive strip
- Urine drainage bag with tubing

Assessment

Assessment should focus on the following:
- Ability of client to void without incontinent episodes
- Appearance of penis (skin intactness, no edema)

Nursing Diagnoses

Nursing diagnoses may include the following:
- Urinary incontinence related to neuromuscular disorder
- Self-care deficit related to confusion and physical debilitation

Outcome Identification and Planning

Desired Outcomes

Sample desired outcomes include the following:
- Client voids without spillage of urine.
- Client experiences no skin breakdown in area of penile shaft.

● Client experiences no constriction of blood flow in area of penile shaft.

Special Considerations in Planning and Implementation

Geriatric

Many geriatric clients have condom catheters applied because of confusion coupled with discomfort of soiled skin and linens. Reorient client as necessary to facilitate cooperation with maintaining catheter.

Pediatric

Infant/pediatric boys may receive a condom catheter to facilitate specimen collection or accuracy of output.

Home Health

Clients and caregivers should be taught the procedure and the importance of reassessing the penis at intervals during the day.

Delegation

This procedure may be delegated to unlicensed assistive personnel. Emphasize the importance of removal during bath and inspection of the penis at intervals. The primary responsibility for inspection, however, lies with the nurse.

Implementation

Action	Rationale
1. Perform hand hygiene.	*Reduces microorganism transfer*
2. Explain procedure to client.	*Decreases anxiety*
3. Provide privacy and drape client to provide access to penis.	*Decreases embarrassment while allowing easy access for procedure*
4. Lower side rails and place client in low Fowler's or supine position.	*Facilitates comfort for client and access to full penis length*
5. Place urinary drainage bag on bed so tubing lies on bed, loops off mattress toward bedframe, and hooks onto bedframe (should not be looped through or onto bed rail).	*Facilitates placement of drainage system so it is easily accessible for connection to condom catheter; prevents entanglement in rails to avoid pulling from penis*
6. Put on clean gloves.	*Reduces nurse's exposure to client's body secretions*
7. Remove drape, then wash and dry penis well.	*Cleans skin, removing debris; facilitates adherence of condom catheter*

Action	Rationale
8. Hold shaft of penis firmly using nondominant hand.	*Positions penis for placement of catheter*
9. Obtain condom catheter with dominant hand and roll onto penis from distal tip up the shaft, leaving 2.5 to 5 cm (1 to 2 in) of open space between distal tip of penis and the end of the catheter to be attached to drainage tubing (Fig. 8.3).	
10. Holding condom catheter in place with nondominant hand, place Velcro or elastic adhesive completely around the top end of the condom catheter that is on the penis. Velcro/elastic adhesive should be placed on the rubber catheter, not the penis itself, and should be snug but not too tight (Fig. 8.4). Ask client if condom is too tight and observe for constriction.	*Positions condom catheter and secures in place with appropriate apparatus; avoids constriction of penile shaft*
11. Connect end of catheter to drainage tubing (Fig. 8.5).	*Directs drainage into bag rather than onto client's skin or bed linens*
12. Arrange drainage tubing so it is loose but not pulling, with drainage bag hanging freely (see Fig. 8.5).	*Avoids accidental pulling off of catheter due to weight of tubing*
13. Position client for comfort.	*Facilitates comfort*
14. Raise side rails.	*Promotes safety*
15. Place call light within reach.	*Allows communication*
16. Discard basin of water and disposable bathing supplies.	*Cleans bedside area*

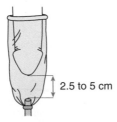

2.5 to 5 cm

FIGURE 8.3

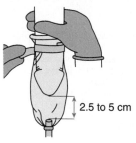

2.5 to 5 cm

FIGURE 8.4

Action	Rationale
17. Discard gloves and wash hands.	*Reduces microorganism transfer*
18. Reassess security of placement, position of catheter on penis, and status of penis and skin every 4 hours.	*Maintains placement and assesses for penile constriction that could cause skin damage or constricted blood flow*
19. Remove condom catheter for half-hour during daily bath or every 24 hours.	*Allows for skin care and full inspection of penis*

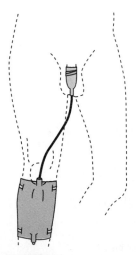

FIGURE 8.5

Evaluation

Were desired outcomes achieved? Examples of evaluation include:
- Desired outcome met: Client voided without spillage of urine.
- Desired outcome not met: Client experienced redness and irritation on penile shaft.
- Desired outcome met: Client experienced no constriction of blood flow in area of penile shaft.

Documentation

The following should be noted on the client's chart:
- Amount, color, odor, and consistency of urine
- Appearance of penis (skin, edema, discharge)
- Client comfort
- Tolerance of procedure
- Teaching done and understanding indicated

Sample Documentation
Date: 1/1/05
Time: 1100

Condom catheter applied with drainage bag. 300 mL clear yellow urine in bag. No edema of penis noted, but slight redness and irritation noted on penile shaft. No discharge noted. No c/o pain. Catheter secured snugly without constriction. Tolerated procedure well. Teaching done regarding care of condom catheter. Client demonstrated correct care.

● Nursing Procedure 8.5

Performing a Male Catheterization 🖑

Purpose

Allows emptying of bladder
Allows sterile urine specimens to be obtained
Allows amount of residual urine in bladder to be determined

Allows for continuous, accurate monitoring of urinary output
Provides avenue for bladder irrigations

Equipment

- Urethral catheterization set (includes sterile gloves, specimen collection container, catheter, two drapes, graduated measurement receptacle, antiseptic solution, cotton balls, forceps, lubricating jelly) *OR* indwelling catheterization set (all the items in the urethral catheterization kit except the graduated measurement receptacle, plus a drainage collection system [tubing and bag that connect to the catheter] and a prefilled saline syringe for balloon inflation)
- Basin of warm, soapy water
- Washcloth
- Large towel
- Nonsterile gloves
- Sheet for draping
- Linen saver
- Tape
- Bedpan, urinal, or second collection container
- Specimen container, if specimen is needed
- Goggles (for client unable to maintain urinary control during procedure)
- Extra lighting

Assessment

Assessment should focus on the following:
- Type of catheterization ordered (e.g., straight, Foley, residual)
- Status of bladder (distention before catheter insertion)
- Abnormalities of genitalia or prostate gland
- History of conditions that may interfere with smooth insertion of catheter (e.g., prostate enlargement, urethral stricture)
- Client allergy to iodine-based antiseptics (e.g., Betadine)

Nursing Diagnoses

Nursing diagnoses may include the following:
- Acute pain related to bladder distention
- Urinary retention related to neuromuscular dysfunction

Outcome Identification and Planning

Desired Outcomes

Sample desired outcomes include the following:
- Client attains and maintains urine output of at least 250 mL per shift during hospital stay.
- Client verbalizes relief of lower abdominal pain within 1 hour of catheter insertion.

Special Considerations in Planning and Implementation

General

Never force a catheter if it does not pass through the urethral canal smoothly. If the catheter still does not pass smoothly after using the suggested troubleshooting methods, discontinue the procedure and notify the physician. Forcing the catheter may result in damage to the urethra and surrounding structures.

Pediatric

The bladder is higher and more anterior in an infant than in an adult. Common catheter sizes are 8 and 10 French. Catheterization is a very threatening and anxiety-provoking experience for children, so they need explanations, support, and understanding.

Geriatric

A common pathologic feature in elderly men is enlargement of the prostate gland, which often makes inserting a catheter difficult.

Home Health

Because indwelling catheterization is used on a long-term basis for the homebound client, the potential for infection is high. Be alert for early signs and symptoms of infection and adhere to a strict schedule for changing catheters. Explore the possibility of an external catheter as an alternative to the indwelling catheter. If the client uses intermittent self-catheterization, store sterilized catheters in sterilized jars.

Cost-Cutting Tips

When replacing a Foley catheter, note the size of the previous catheter to avoid waste from inserting too small a catheter. This occurs frequently with clients on long-term catheterization.

Delegation

In some agencies, catheterization may be delegated to specially trained personnel. Note agency policies concerning delegation of this procedure (e.g., what level of personnel).

Implementation

Action	Rationale
1. Perform hand hygiene.	*Reduces microorganism transfer*
2. Explain procedure to client.	*Decreases anxiety*
3. Determine if client is allergic to iodine-based antiseptics.	*Avoids allergic reactions*
4. Provide privacy.	*Decreases embarrassment*
5. Put on nonsterile gloves.	*Reduces nurse's exposure to client's body secretions*

Action	**Rationale**
6. If catheterization is being done for residual urine, ask client to void in urinal, and measure and record the amount voided; empty urinal.	*Determines amount of urine client is able to void without catheterization*
7. Lower side rails, assist client into a supine position, and place linen saver under client's buttocks.	*Avoids soiling linens*
8. Wash genital area with warm, soapy water, rinse, and pat dry with towel.	*Decreases microorganisms around urethral opening*
9. Discard gloves, bath water, washcloth, and towel; perform hand hygiene.	*Decreases clutter; reduces microorganism transfer*
10. Drape client so only penis is exposed.	*Provides privacy; reduces embarrassment*
11. Set up work field:	
• Open catheter set and remove from outer plastic package.	*Removes kit without opening inner folds*
• Tape outer package to bedside table with top edge turned inside out.	*Provides waste bag*
• Place catheter kit beside client's knees and carefully open outer edges.	*Places items within easy reach*
• Ask client to open legs slightly.	*Relaxes pelvic muscles*
• Remove full drape from kit with fingertips and place across thighs, plastic side down, just below penis; keep other side sterile.	*Provides sterile field*
• If catheter and bag are separate, use sterile technique to open package containing bag and place bag on work field.	*Promotes establishment of sterile closed catheter system*
12. Put on sterile gloves.	*Avoids contaminating other items in kit*
13. Prepare items in kit for use during insertion as follows:	
• Pour iodine solution over cotton balls.	*Prepares cotton balls for cleaning*
• Separate cotton balls with forceps.	*Promotes easy manipulation*

Action	Rationale
• Lubricate 6 to 7 inches of catheter tip and place carefully on tray so tip is secure in tray.	*Prevents local irritation of meatus during catheter insertion; promotes ease of insertion*
• If inserting indwelling catheter, attach prefilled syringe of sterile water to balloon port of catheter.	*Connects to balloon port the syringe needed to inflate balloon*
• Inject 2 to 3 mL of sterile water from prefilled syringe into balloon and observe balloon for leaks as it fills.	*Tests balloon for defects*
• If any leaks are noted, discard and obtain another kit.	*Prevents catheter from dislodging after insertion*
• Deflate balloon, and leave syringe connected.	*Leaves syringe within reach*
• Attach catheter to drainage container tubing (or, if drainage tubing is already attached to the catheter, place tubing and bag securely on sterile field, close to the other equipment).	*Facilitates organization while maintaining sterility*
• Check clamp on collection bag to be sure it is closed. Place catheter and collection tray close to perineum.	*Prevents loss of urine before measurement*
• Open specimen collection container and place on sterile field.	*Places container within easy reach for specimen collection*
14. Remove fenestrated drape from kit and place penis through hole in drape with nondominant hand. KEEP DOMINANT HAND STERILE.	*Expands sterile field*
15. Pull penis up at a 90-degree angle to client's supine body.	*Straightens urethra*
16. With nondominant hand, gently grasp glans (tip) of penis; retract foreskin, if necessary.	*Provides grasp of penis, preventing contamination of sterile field later*
17. With forceps in dominant hand, cleanse meatus and glans with cotton balls, be-	*Cleanses meatus without cross-contaminating or contaminating sterile hand*

Action	Rationale
ginning at urethral opening and moving toward shaft of penis; make one complete circle around penis with each cotton ball, discarding cotton ball after each wipe (Fig. 8.6).	
18. After all cotton balls have been used, discard forceps.	*Prevents contamination of sterile field*
19. With thumb and first finger, pick catheter up about 1.5 to 2 inches from tip.	*Gives nurse good control of catheter tip (which easily bends)*
20. Carefully gather additional tubing in hand.	*Gives nurse good control of full catheter length*
21. Ask client to bear down as if voiding and to take slow, deep breaths; encourage him to continue to breathe deeply until catheter is inserted.	*Opens sphincter; relaxes sphincter muscles of bladder and urethra*
22. Insert tip of catheter slowly through urethral opening 7 to 9 inches (or until urine returns).	*Inserts catheter*
23. Lower penis to about a 45-degree angle after catheter is inserted about halfway and hold open end of catheter over collection container (if it is not connected to a drainage bag).	*Places penis in position for urine to be released into collection container so accurate amount is measured*
24. If resistance is met:	
• Stop for a few seconds.	*Allows sphincters to relax and reduces anxiety*

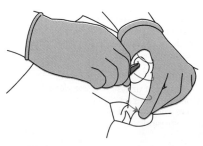

FIGURE 8.6

Action	Rationale
• Encourage client to continue taking slow, deep breaths.	*Promotes relaxation of the client and sphincter muscles*
• Do not force; remove catheter tip and notify doctor if above sequence is unsuccessful.	*Prevents injury to prostate, urethra, and surrounding structures*
25. After catheter has been advanced an appropriate distance, advance another 1 to 1.5 inches.	*Ensures that catheter is advanced far enough not to be dislodged*
26. For straight catheterization:	
• Obtain urine specimen in specimen container, if ordered.	*Obtains sterile specimen*
• Allow urine to drain until it stops or until maximum number of milliliters specified by agency (usually 1,000 to 1,500 mL) has drained into container; use second container, bedpan, or urinal, if necessary.	*Empties bladder; obtains residual urine amount*
27. For an indwelling catheter, inflate balloon with attached syringe and gently pull back on catheter until it stops (catches).	*Secures catheter placement*
28. Secure catheter loosely with tape to lower abdomen on side from which drainage bag will be hanging (preferably away from door); make certain that tubing is not caught on railing locks or obstructed.	*Stabilizes catheter; prevents accidental dislodgment*
29. Clear bed of all equipment.	*Removes waste from bed*
30. Reposition client for comfort, and replace linens for warmth and privacy.	*Promotes general comfort*
31. Raise side rails.	*Prevents falls*
32. Measure amount of urine in collection container or drainage bag and discard urine and disposable supplies.	*Provides assessment data*

Action	Rationale
33. Gather all additional equipment and discard gloves.	*Promotes clean environment*
34. Perform hand hygiene.	*Reduces microorganism transfer*

Evaluation

Were desired outcomes achieved? Examples of evaluation include:
- Desired outcome met: Urine output 250 mL per shift maintained during hospital stay.
- Desired outcome met: Client verbalized relief of lower abdominal pain within 1 hour of catheter insertion.

Documentation

The following should be noted on the client's chart:
- Presence of distention before catheterization
- Assessment of genitalia, if abnormalities noted
- Type of catheterization
- Size of catheter
- Amount, color, and consistency of urine returned upon catheterization
- Amount of urine returned before catheterization (if residual urine catheterization)
- Difficulties encountered, if any, in passing the catheter smoothly
- Reports of unusual discomfort during insertion
- Urine specimen obtained for culture

Sample Documentation
Date: 1/1/05
Time: 1100

Client complained of lower abdominal pain, slight bulge palpable. Catheter (#16 French Foley) inserted without resistance or report of discomfort. Procedure yielded 700 mL straw-colored urine without sediment or foul odor. Tolerated procedure well. Client indicates pain relieved after catheterization.

Performing a Female Catheterization 🖑

Purpose

Allows emptying of bladder
Allows sterile urine specimens to be obtained
Allows amount of residual urine in bladder to be determined
Allows for continuous, accurate monitoring of urinary output
Provides avenue for bladder irrigations

Equipment

- Urethral catheterization set (includes sterile gloves, specimen collection container, catheter, two drapes, graduated measurement receptacle, antiseptic solution, cotton balls, forceps, lubricating jelly) *OR* indwelling catheterization set (all the items in the urethral catheterization kit except the graduated measurement receptacle, plus a drainage collection system [tubing and bag that connect to the catheter] and a prefilled saline syringe for balloon inflation)
- Basin of warm, soapy water
- Washcloth
- Large towel
- Nonsterile gloves
- Sheet for draping
- Linen saver
- Tape
- Bedpan, urinal, or second collection container
- Specimen container, if specimen is needed
- Extra lighting

Assessment

Assessment should focus on the following:
- Type of catheterization ordered (e.g., straight, Foley, residual)
- Status of bladder (distention before catheter insertion)
- Abnormalities of genitalia
- Client allergy to iodine-based antiseptics (e.g., Betadine)

Nursing Diagnoses

Nursing diagnoses may include the following:
- Acute pain related to bladder distention
- Urinary retention related to neuromuscular dysfunction

Outcome Identification and Planning

Desired Outcomes

Sample desired outcomes include the following:
- Client attains and maintains a urine output of at least 250 mL per shift during hospital stay.
- Client verbalizes relief of lower abdominal pain within 1 hour of catheter insertion.

Special Considerations in Planning and Implementation

General

Never force a catheter if it does not pass through the urethra smoothly. If the catheter still does not pass smoothly after using the suggested troubleshooting methods, discontinue the procedure and notify the physician. Forcing the catheter may result in damage to the urethra and surrounding structures.

Pediatric

In the baby girl, the urethra hooks around the symphysis in a C shape. Common catheter size is 8 or 10 French. Catheterization is a very threatening and anxiety-producing experience. Children need explanations, support, and understanding.

Home Health

Because indwelling catheterization is used on a long-term basis for the homebound client, the potential for infection is high. Be alert for early signs and symptoms of infection and adhere to a strict schedule for changing catheters. If the client uses intermittent self-catheterization, store sterilized catheters in sterilized jars.

Cost-Cutting Tips

For female clients, time and money may be saved by using clean gloves to locate the meatus before opening the sterile kit. This minimizes the chance of sterile glove contamination. If replacing a Foley catheter, note the size of the previous catheter to avoid waste from insertion of too small a catheter. This occurs frequently with clients on long-term catheterization.

Delegation

In some agencies, catheterization may be delegated to specially trained personnel. Note agency policies concerning delegation of this procedure (e.g., what level of personnel).

Implementation

Action	Rationale
1. Perform hand hygiene.	*Reduces microorganism transfer*
2. Explain procedure to client, emphasizing need to maintain sterile field.	*Decreases anxiety*
3. Determine if client is allergic to iodine-based antiseptics.	*Avoids allergic reactions*
4. Provide privacy.	*Decreases embarrassment*
5. Put on nonsterile gloves.	*Reduces nurse's exposure to client's body secretions*
6. If catheterization is for residual urine, ask client to void in bedpan, and measure and record the amount voided; empty bedpan.	*Determines amount of urine client is able to void without catheterization*
7. Lower side rails, assist client into supine or side-lying position, and place linen saver under client's buttocks.	*Provides access to urethra; avoids soiling linens*
8. Place light to enhance visualization.	*Promotes clear identification of anatomical parts*
9. Separate labia to expose urethral opening: • If using dorsal recumbent position (Fig. 8.7A), separate labia with thumb and forefinger by gently lifting upward and outward (Fig. 8.7B). • If using side-lying position (Fig. 8.8), pull upward on upper labia minora.	*Allows nurse to identify urethral opening clearly before area is cleansed.*
10. Wash genital area with warm, soapy water, rinse, and pat dry with towel.	*Decreases microorganisms around urethral opening*
11. Discard bath water, washcloth, and towel.	*Decreases clutter; reduces microorganism transfer*
12. If inserting an indwelling catheter in which the drainage apparatus is separate from the catheter (not preconnected): • Check for closed clamp on collection bag.	*Places drainage tubing within immediate and easy reach, decreasing chance of catheter contamination once inserted*

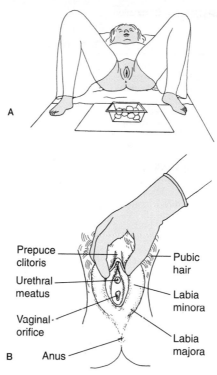

Prepuce clitoris	Pubic hair
Urethral meatus	Labia minora
Vaginal orifice	Labia majora
Anus	

B

FIGURE 8.7

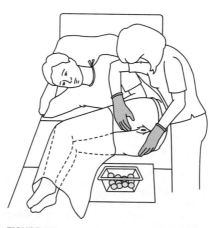

FIGURE 8.8

485

Action	Rationale
• Secure drainage collection bag to bed frame.	
• Pull tubing up between bed and bed rails to top surface of bed.	
• Check to be sure tubing will not get caught when rails are lowered or raised.	
13. Position client in dorsal recumbent or side-lying position with knees flexed (see Figs. 8.7A and 8.7B); in side-lying position, slide client's hips toward edge of bed.	*Exposes labia*
14. Drape client so only perineum is exposed.	*Provides privacy; reduces embarrassment*
15. Remove gloves and wash hands; lift side rails and cover client before leaving bedside.	*Reduces microorganism transfer; prevents client from falling; reduces embarrassment*
16. Set up field:	
• Carefully open catheter set and remove it from plastic outer package.	*Removes kit without opening inner folds*
• Tape outer package to bedside table with top edge turned inside out.	*Provides waste bag*
• Place catheter kit between client's knees and carefully open outer edges (if using side-lying position, place kit about 1 foot from perineal area near thighs).	*Places items within easy reach*
• Remove full drape from kit with fingertips and place, plastic side down, just under buttocks by having client raise hips; keep other side sterile.	*Provides sterile field*
17. Put on sterile gloves.	*Avoids contaminating other items in kit*
18. Prepare items in kit for use during insertion as follows:	
• Pour iodine solution over cotton balls.	*Prepares cotton balls for cleaning*

Action	Rationale
• Separate cotton balls with forceps.	*Promotes easy manipulation*
• Lubricate 3 to 4 inches of catheter tip and place carefully on tray so that tip is secure in tray.	*Prevents local irritation of meatus during catheter insertion; promotes insertion*
• If inserting indwelling catheter, attach prefilled syringe of sterile water to balloon port of catheter by twisting syringe in clockwise direction.	*Connects syringe needed to inflate balloon to balloon port*
• Inject 2 to 3 mL of sterile water from prefilled syringe into balloon, and observe balloon for leaks as it fills.	*Tests balloon for defects*
• If any leaks are noted, discard and obtain another kit.	*Prevents catheter from becoming dislodged after insertion*
• Deflate balloon, and leave syringe connected.	*Leaves syringe within reach*
• If inserting closed indwelling system with drainage tubing already attached to catheter, move tubing and bag close to other equipment on work field, making certain that drainage system is on the sterile field only. Place catheter and collection tray close to perineum.	*Facilitates organization while maintaining sterility*
• Check clamp on collection bag to be sure it is closed.	*Prevents loss of urine before measurement*
• Open specimen collection container and place on sterile field.	*Places container within easy reach for specimen*
19. Remove fenestrated drape from kit and place on perineum such that only labia are exposed (or discard the drape if you prefer).	*Expands sterile field*
20. Separate labia minora with nondominant hand in	*Exposes urethral opening*

Action	Rationale
same manner as in step 9 and hold this position until catheter is inserted (dominant hand is the only hand sterile now; contaminated hand continues to separate labia).	
21. With forceps in dominant hand, cleanse meatus with cotton balls: • Making one downward stroke with each cotton ball, begin at labium on side farther from you and move toward labium closer to you. • Afterward, wipe once down center of meatus. • Wipe once with each cotton ball and discard (Fig. 8.9).	*Cleanses meatus without cross-contaminating or contaminating sterile hand*
22. After all cotton balls have been used, discard forceps.	*Prevents contamination of sterile field*
23. Move cleaning tray to end of sterile field and move collection container and catheter closer to client.	*Facilitates organization; prevents accidental contamination of system*

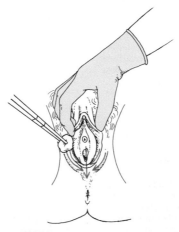

FIGURE 8.9

Action	Rationale
24. With thumb and first finger, pick catheter up about 1.5 to 2 inches from tip.	*Gives nurse good control of catheter tip (which easily bends)*
25. Carefully gather additional tubing in hand.	*Gives nurse good control of full catheter length*
26. Ask client to bear down as if voiding and to take slow, deep breaths; encourage her to continue to breathe deeply until catheter is fully inserted.	*Opens sphincter; relaxes sphincter muscles of bladder and urethra*
27. Insert tip of catheter slowly through urethral opening 3 to 4 inches (or until urine returns), releasing tubing from hand as insertion continues; direct open end of catheter into collection container. If resistance is met, verify position, and if unable to insert past resistance, withdraw catheter and notify physician.	*Inserts catheter*
28. After catheter has been advanced an appropriate distance (3 to 4 inches or until urine returns), advance another 1 to 1.5 inches.	*Ensures that catheter is advanced far enough not to be dislodged*
29. Grasp catheter with thumb and first finger of nondominant hand and hold steady.	*Keeps catheter from being forced out by sphincter muscles; avoids contamination of distal portion of catheter*
30. For straight catheterization: • Obtain urine specimen in specimen container, if ordered, and replace open end of catheter in urine collection container.	*Obtains sterile specimen*
• Allow urine to drain until it stops or until maximum number of milliliters specified by agency (usually 1,000 to 1,500 mL; clamp tube before allowing the remaining urine to flow out) has drained into container; use second	*Empties bladder; obtains residual urine amount; prevents temporary hypovolemic shock state*

Action	Rationale
container, bedpan, or urinal, if necessary. • Remove catheter.	
31. For an indwelling catheter, inflate balloon with attached syringe and gently pull back on catheter until it stops (catches).	*Secures catheter placement*
32. If the indwelling catheter is separate from bag and tubing, remove protective cap from end of tubing and attach drainage tubing to end of catheter.	*Converts system to closed system*
33. Secure catheter loosely with tape to thigh on side from which drainage bag will be hanging (preferably away from door); make certain that tubing is not caught on railing locks or obstructed.	*Stabilizes catheter; prevents accidental dislodgment*
34. Clear bed of all equipment, reposition client for comfort, and replace linens for warmth and privacy; lift side rails.	*Promotes clean environment, comfort, and safety*
35. Measure amount of urine in collection container or drainage bag and discard urine and collection container.	*Provides assessment data*
36. Gather all additional equipment and discard with gloves.	*Promotes clean environment*
37. Perform hand hygiene.	*Reduces microorganism transfer*

Evaluation

Were desired outcomes achieved? Examples of evaluation include:
• Desired outcome not met: Urine output of 150 mL per shift noted; doctor notified.
• Desired outcome not met: Client reports lower abdominal pain 2 hours after catheter insertion.

Documentation

The following should be noted on the client's chart:
• Assessment of lower abdomen before catheterization
• Assessment of genitalia, if abnormalities noted

- Type of catheterization
- Size of catheter
- Amount, color, and consistency of urine returned upon catheterization
- Amount of urine returned before catheterization (if residual urine was collected)
- Difficulties encountered, if any, in passing the catheter smoothly
- Reports of unusual discomfort during insertion
- Specimen obtained for culture

Sample Documentation
Date: 1/1/05
Time: 1100

Voided 100 ccs then straight cath performed for urine residual. Catheter (#16 French Foley) inserted without resistance or report of discomfort. Procedure yielded 200 mL of straw-colored urine without sediment or foul odor.

● **Nursing Procedure 8.7**

Caring for a Urinary Catheter

Purpose

Decreases bacterial contamination of bladder and urinary tract infection
Maintains skin integrity

Equipment

- Urethral catheter care kit (includes nonsterile gloves, drapes, antiseptic solution, cotton balls, forceps)
- Extra lighting (optional)

If a urethral catheter kit is unavailable or not preferred, substitute the following materials:
- Basin of warm, soapy water
- Washcloth or cotton balls
- Large towel
- Nonsterile gloves
- One sheet for draping
- Linen saver

- Roll of tape
- Bacterial ointment (optional)
- Antiseptic solution (optional)

Assessment

Assessment should focus on the following:
- Physician's orders for specific catheter care (antiseptic solutions or ointment)
- Status of bladder (distention indicating decreased catheter patency)
- Abnormalities of genitalia (e.g., swelling, redness, drainage)
- Urine color, odor, and amount
- Client allergy to latex gloves or antiseptics (e.g., Betadine)
- Client's emotional reaction and feelings related to catheter and care

Nursing Diagnoses

Nursing diagnoses may include the following:
- Impaired urinary elimination: decreased output related to catheter encrustation
- Risk for infection related to invasive catheter
- Risk for impaired skin integrity, related to infection and pressure from catheter

Outcome Identification and Planning

Desired Outcomes

Sample desired outcomes include the following:
- Client maintains urine output of at least 250 mL per shift during hospital stay.
- Client demonstrates minimal discomfort and no signs of infection while catheter is maintained.

Special Considerations in Planning and Implementation

General

Soap and water are usually used for catheter care as clients may be allergic to povidone-iodine or other antiseptic solutions. Refer to institution policy for proper protocol and recommended solutions. If the client has local inflammation related to the catheter, assess for latex allergy, and remove the catheter if the client has a positive history and reinsert a latex-free catheter. If the catheter slips out from the urethra, do not reinsert the same catheter.

Pediatric

Use a doll to demonstrate care first. If the child has a history of abuse, involve the child's therapist. Demonstrate and teach catheter care procedure to an adult caregiver if the catheter will remain in place after discharge.

Geriatric

Contractures, arthritis, and other conditions causing stiffness and pain may make it difficult to position the client; special care is needed when moving the client's joints.

Home Health

When indwelling catheterization is used on a long-term basis, there is a high potential for infection. Be alert for early signs and symptoms of infection and adhere to a strict schedule for perineal care and catheter changes.

Delegation

Catheter care and perineal cleansing may be delegated to unlicensed assistive personnel after proper instruction and supervision. The nurse should be notified about the appearance of catheter drainage and any problems with catheter tubing, such as leaks. Ultimately, the responsibility for monitoring the client for signs of infection and catheter complications remains with licensed personnel.

Implementation

Action	Rationale
1. Perform hand hygiene.	*Reduces microorganism transfer*
2. Explain procedure to client, emphasizing the need to clean around the catheter and manipulate tubing.	*Prepares client and decreases anxiety*
3. Determine if client is allergic to antiseptics or soap (inquire or check records).	*Avoids allergic reactions*
4. Prepare warm water and linens (prepare to change bed linens, if indicated).	*Increases efficiency by performing catheter care with hygiene and bed change*
5. Provide privacy.	*Protects client's dignity and decreases embarrassment*
6. Apply nonsterile gloves.	*Reduces nurse's exposure to client's body secretions*
7. Lower side rails and place linen saver under client's buttocks.	*Avoids soiling linens*
8. Position client supine in a dorsal recumbent or lateral position. (For female client, separate legs.)	*Provides easy access to perineal area*
9. Cleanse suprapubic and pubic area with soapy cloth and rinse with water. Rinse washcloth.	

Action	Rationale
10. Examine catheter insertion site for redness, and ask client if burning or discomfort is present.	
11. For a female client, open labia and cleanse entrance to urinary meatus with soapy cloth or cotton ball using a circular motion. Clean from the innermost surface outward. If there is excessive purulent drainage, use non-irritating antiseptic solutions on cotton balls to cleanse the area.	*Cleanses from clean to dirty areas; decreases contamination of clean area and risk of recontamination*
Wash and rinse the inside of the labia, using one cotton ball on each side or a fresh area of the washcloth on each side and using a downward stroke.	*Promotes removal of debris without recontamination from soiled cloth or cotton ball*
For a male client, grasp the shaft of the penis firmly. Being careful not to pull on the catheter, cleanse urinary meatus and glans with cotton balls or soapy washcloth beginning at urethral opening (retract foreskin if necessary). Cleanse in a circular motion, moving from the meatus outward toward the shaft of the penis (Fig. 8.10).	*Cleanses meatus without cross-contaminating*

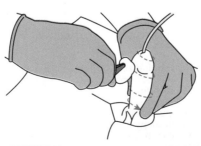

FIGURE 8.10

Action	Rationale
12. Clean around catheter and clean the catheter tube from the insertion site distal to 4 inches (10 cm). Be careful not to pull on the catheter. Note and remove any dried secretions.	*Cleans from clean to dirty area of catheter*
13. Rinse area thoroughly. If irritation is present and if ordered, apply bacteriostatic ointment around catheter site.	*Removes potentially irritating agents; retards growth of bacteria and infection*
14. Dry genital area with a towel.	*Decreases microorganisms around urethral opening*
15. Discard bath water, washcloth, and towel.	*Decreases clutter; reduces microorganisms*
16. Secure catheter loosely with tape to thigh on side from which drainage bag will be hanging (preferably away from door); make certain that tubing is not kinked, twisted, caught on railing locks, or obstructed.	*Stabilizes catheter; prevents accidental dislodgment*
17. Clear bed of all equipment, reposition client for comfort, and replace linens for warmth and privacy; lift side rails.	*Promotes clean environment, comfort, and safety*
18. Gather all additional equipment and discard gloves.	*Promotes clean environment*
19. Perform hand hygiene.	*Reduces microorganism transfer*

Evaluation

Were desired outcomes achieved? Examples of evaluation include:
- Desired outcome met: 300 mL clear urine noted from night shift.
- Desired outcome met: Client reports absence of lower abdominal pain 2 hours after catheter insertion.

Documentation

The following should be noted on the client's chart:
- Assessment of genitalia, if abnormalities noted
- Size of catheter
- Status of catheter (presence of secretions or dried substances)

- Condition of skin surrounding catheter (redness, swelling, excoriation)
- Amount, color, and consistency of urine returned upon catheterization
- Amount of urine returned before catheterization (if residual urine was collected)
- Reports of unusual discomfort during care

Sample Documentation
Date: 1/1/05
Time: 1100

Perineal care and catheter care performed. #16 catheter in place. Catheter insertion site and genitalia intact without redness, irritation, or report of discomfort. Clear yellow urine noted without sediment or foul odor.

● **Nursing Procedure 8.8**

Removing an Indwelling Catheter

Purpose

Terminates urinary catheterization
Permits return of client-controlled voiding

Equipment

- Syringe (appropriate size to remove water from balloon on catheter)
- Graduated container
- Pair of clean gloves
- Basin of warm water
- Soap
- Washcloth
- Towel
- Linen saver

Assessment

Assessment should focus on the following:
- Length of time catheter has been in place and agency policy regarding maximum length of time before catheter removal or change
- Order for catheter removal and parameters for removal (e.g., after specimen obtained, when client is ambulatory)
- Client's knowledge of catheter removal procedure

- Size of catheter and balloon
- Characteristics of urine (e.g., color, clarity, odor, amount)
- Amount of urine output
- Distention, pain, or tenderness of lower abdomen

Nursing Diagnoses

Nursing diagnoses may include the following:
- Acute pain related to urethral irritation from catheter
- Impaired urinary elimination
- Deficient knowledge regarding perineal care

Outcome Identification and Planning

Desired Outcomes

Sample desired outcomes include the following:
- Client verbalizes minimal discomfort during catheter removal.
- Client voids within 6 hours of catheter removal.

Special Considerations in Planning and Implementation

General

If swelling is noted around the catheter entry site, consult physician before removing catheter.

Geriatric and Home Health

If catheter has been in place for an extended period, bladder training may be beneficial before catheter removal to improve sphincter control.

Delegation

Unlicensed assistive personnel can remove catheters. Nurse should observe perineal area and urinary output and assess that client voids within 4 hours of catheter removal.

Implementation

Action	Rationale
1. Explain procedure to client.	*Promotes cooperation and decreases anxiety*
2. Provide privacy.	*Protects client's dignity and decreases embarrassment*
3. Apply nonsterile gloves.	*Reduces nurse's exposure to client's body secretions*
4. Place client in supine or lateral position, and place linen saver under client's buttocks.	*Provides access to catheter and prevents soiling linens*

Action	Rationale
5. Obtain urine specimen if ordered (see Procedure 8.3).	*Permits removal of sterile specimens before loss of access*
6. Insert syringe into balloon port inflation valve.	*Provides access to remove water from the balloon to deflate it*
7. Aspirate total amount of fluid that was used to inflate the balloon. If unsure if balloon is fully deflated, cut the inflation port and allow water to drain.	*Fully deflates balloon to prevent damage to urethra during removal process*
8. Remove tape or catheter holder.	*Allows removal of catheter*
9. Instruct client to relax and take slow deep breaths. Slowly and smoothly pull catheter out onto towel.	*Promotes relaxation of sphincter muscles; prevents trauma to urethral mucosa*
10. Hold catheter up until urine has drained into bag.	*Permits collection of urine and prevents spilling of urine onto client*
11. Measure amount of urine in collection container or drainage bag, noting color and consistency of urine, and discard catheter and drainage bag by wrapping them in a linen saver.	*Provides assessment data; decreases exposure to body waste; properly disposes of contaminated substances*
12. Position client for comfort and discard all disposable equipment with gloves.	*Promotes clean environment*
13. Perform hand hygiene.	*Reduces microorganism transfer*
14. Instruct client to notify nurse of next voiding and to save urine.	*Allows nurse to assess ability to void after catheter removal*

Evaluation

Were desired outcomes achieved? Examples of evaluation include:
- Desired outcome not met: Client complained of intense pain during catheter removal.
- Desired outcome not met: Client has not voided for the past 6 hours since removal of catheter.

Documentation

The following should be noted on the client's chart:
- Assessment of lower abdomen before removal of catheter
- Assessment of genitalia, if abnormalities noted
- Size of catheter

- Amount, color, and consistency of urine draining from catheter
- Any difficulties encountered when removing catheter
- Reports of unusual discomfort during removal
- Status of catheter
- Time and amount of first voiding
- Specimen obtained (catheter tip sent to lab, if applicable)

Sample Documentation
Date: 1/1/05
Time: 1100

Catheter (#16 French Foley) removed as ordered with 150 ml cloudy yellow urine noted. Swelling and redness noted around urinary meatus. Client complains of "bladder fullness" with palpable mass in lower abdomen after 4 hours. Unable to void despite warm water to perineum. Doctor notified. Client sitting in bedside chair. If client unable to void will insert straight catheter to drain bladder, as ordered.

Nursing Procedure 8.9

Irrigating a Bladder/Catheter

Purpose

Decreases urinary tract infection (particularly when antiseptic irrigant used)
Clears debris, tissue, and blood from bladder/catheter
Maintains patent catheter and urinary drainage

Equipment

- Two-way indwelling catheter set *OR* three-way indwelling catheter set
- Solution ordered for irrigation
- Catheter irrigation kit (includes large catheter-tip syringe with protective cap, sterile linen saver, graduated irrigation container)
- Medication additives, as ordered
- Medication labels

- IV tubing
- IV pole
- Two pairs of clean gloves
- Basin of warm water
- Soap
- Washcloth
- Towel
- Linen saver (optional)
- Betadine (or recommended antiseptic solution for cleansing irrigation port)
- Catheter clamp or rubber band

Assessment

Assessment should focus on the following:
- Type of irrigation ordered
- Characteristics of urine before irrigation (e.g., hematuria)
- Amount of urine output
- Distention, pain, or tenderness of the lower abdomen
- Signs of inflammation or infection of bladder and perineal structures
- Status of catheter (if already inserted) before irrigations

Nursing Diagnoses

Nursing diagnoses may include the following:
- Acute pain related to bladder inflammation
- Urinary retention related to bladder outlet obstruction from blood clots

Outcome Identification and Planning

Desired Outcomes

Sample desired outcomes include the following:
- Client verbalizes decrease in lower abdominal discomfort within 24 hours of irrigation.
- Client maintains urine output of at least 250 mL per shift.

Special Considerations in Planning and Implementation

General

When calculating urine output for a client receiving bladder irrigations, subtract the amount of irrigation solution infused within a designated period of time from the total amount of fluid accumulated within the bag.

Pediatric

A child's bladder is small; therefore, irrigation should be performed carefully with small volumes to avoid discomfort.

Delegation

Unlicensed assistive personnel can help with emptying the catheter bag, but irrigation fluid should be hung only by the nurse.

Implementation

Action	Rationale
Irrigating the Bladder	
1. Perform hand hygiene.	*Reduces microorganism transfer*
2. Explain procedure to client.	*Decreases anxiety*
3. Determine if client is allergic to iodine-based antiseptics or additives to be injected into irrigation fluid.	*Avoids allergic reactions*
4. Prepare irrigation fluid:	
• Remove fluid and IV tubing from outer packages.	*Prepares irrigation solution for infusion*
• Close roller clamp on tubing.	*Promotes control of irrigation fluid*
• Insert additives, if ordered, into fluid container additive port.	*Prepares medicated irrigation fluid as ordered*
• Insert spike of tubing into insertion port of fluid bag and place on IV pole.	*Establishes fluid for flow into catheter*
• Pinch fluid chamber until fluid fills chamber halfway.	*Prevents infusion of air into bladder*
• Remove protective cover from end of tubing line, taking care not to contaminate end of tubing or protective cover.	*Prepares tubing for sterile insertion into catheter port*
• Slowly open roller clamp and fill tubing with fluid.	*Removes air from tubing*
• Close roller clamp and replace protective cover.	*Maintains sterility of tubing*
• Place label on bag of fluid stating type of solution, additives, date, and time solution was opened.	*Identifies contents of irrigant*
5. Provide privacy.	*Decreases embarrassment*
6. If three-way catheter has not already been inserted:	
• Put on clean gloves, place linen saver under buttocks, and wash and dry perineal area.	*Reduces microorganisms in local perineal area before catheter insertion*

Action	Rationale
• Discard gloves, bath water, washcloth, and towel, then perform hand hygiene.	*Decreases bedside clutter; reduces microorganism transfer*
• Insert catheter using Procedure 8.5 for men or Procedure 8.6 for women.	*Inserts catheter for irrigation*
7. Put on clean gloves.	*Reduces nurse's exposure to client's body secretions*
8. Cleanse irrigation port of catheter with antiseptic solution recommended by agency.	*Removes microorganisms from port; decreases contamination*
9. Connect tubing of irrigation fluid to irrigation port of three-way catheter (Fig. 8.11).	*Connects tubing to appropriate catheter port for irrigation*
10. Slowly open roller clamp on tubing and adjust drip rate. Follow steps for intermittent irrigation or for continuous irrigation.	*Sets fluid at appropriate infusion rate for type of infusion*
Performing Intermittent Irrigation	
11. Clamp catheter drainage tubing (or kink tubing and bind with rubber band). Open roller clamp so	*Channels fluid flow into bladder or irrigation; infuses irrigation fluid into bladder*

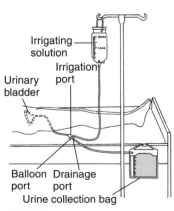

Irrigating solution

Irrigation port

Urinary bladder

Balloon port

Drainage port

Urine collection bag

FIGURE 8.11

Action	Rationale
100 mL of irrigation fluid flows into bladder by gravitational flow; close roller clamp.	
12. Allow fluid to remain for 15 minutes (or amount of time specified by physician's order).	*Allows proper exchange of electrolytes and fluid*
13. Unclamp drainage tubing. Repeat irrigation at frequency ordered. Proceed to step 14.	*Allows fluid to drain from abdomen into drainage bag*

Performing Continuous Irrigation

Action	Rationale
11. Leave drainage tubing open.	
12. Slowly open roller clamp of irrigation fluid tubing.	
13. Adjust irrigation to ordered drip rate (see Procedure 5.5 to review calculation of drip rates).	*Provides continuous flushing of clots and debris from bladder*
14. Remove linen saver.	*Removes soiled linen saver*
15. Discard gloves and wash hands.	*Prevents spread of microorganisms*
16. Record urinary output on intake and output flow sheet.	*Provides accurate record of urine output*

Catheter Irrigation Using a Two-Way Catheter

Action	Rationale
1. Open catheter irrigation kit and remove catheter-tip syringe from sterile container. Remove sterile cap and place syringe back into sterile container. Hold cap between fingers, being careful not to contaminate the open end.	*Ensures continued sterility of syringe tip while allowing use of sterile cap to protect drainage tubing tip*
2. Fill container with saline or ordered irrigant and fill syringe.	*Prepares syringe for irrigation process*
3. Disinfect the drainage tubing/catheter connection using the antimicrobial agent recommended by the institution.	*Decreases microorganisms at connection site*
4. Open sterile linen saver and spread on bed near catheter.	*Provides sterile field*

Action	Rationale
5. Disconnect catheter and drainage tubing. Place cap over drainage tube tip, being careful to keep catheter end sterile. Place capped tubing on linen saver.	*Maintains sterility of drainage tubing for reconnection*
6. Remove syringe from container and insert tip securely into catheter, using sterile technique.	*Reestablishes closed sterile system for irrigation*
7. Slowly infuse irrigant into catheter until full amount of ordered fluid has been infused or client complains of inability to tolerate additional fluid infusion.	*Minimizes discomfort caused by rapid or excessive fluid infusion*
8. Clamp catheter by bending end above syringe tip, and remove the syringe. Disinfect the catheter end with antimicrobial agent. Remove cap from the drainage tubing and insert it into catheter end.	*Prevents leakage of irrigant from catheter; minimizes microorganisms at connection site*
9. Repeat irrigation at frequency ordered.	*Reestablishes closed bladder drainage system*
10. Remove linen saver.	*Removes soiled linen saver*
11. Discard gloves and wash hands.	*Prevents spread of microorganisms*
12. Record urinary output on intake and output flow sheet.	*Provides accurate record of urine output*

Evaluation

Were desired outcomes achieved? Example of evaluation include:
● Desired outcome met: Client verbalized decrease in lower abdominal discomfort from an 8 to a 3 within 24 hours of irrigation.
● Desired outcome met: Client maintained urine output of 350 mL per shift after irrigation.

Documentation

The following should be noted on the client's chart:
● Amount, color, and consistency of fluid obtained
● Type and amount of irrigation solution and any medication additives administered

- Infusion rate
- Abdominal assessment
- Urine output (total fluid volume measured minus irrigation solution instilled)
- Discomfort verbalized by client

Sample Documentation
Date: 1/1/05
Time: 1100

Three-way irrigation catheter inserted and continuous bladder irrigation initiated with 1,000 mL sterile normal saline irrigant. Drip rate 50 mL/hr via infusion regulator. Client reports cramping in lower abdomen as if having spasms, no bladder distention noted. Urine and irrigant clear, without sediment or evidence of blood clots. Irrigant volume 700 mL, drainage 1,100 mL with urine total of 400 mL.

● Nursing Procedure 8.10

Scanning the Bladder

Purpose

Evaluates bladder volume noninvasively to determine need for catheterization to empty bladder
Assists in evaluating general bladder function

Equipment

- Bladder scanning device
- Ultrasound transmission gel
- Gloves
- Washcloth
- Soap

Assessment

Assessment should focus on the following:
- Medical diagnosis (e.g., urinary retention, urinary incontinence, stroke, spinal cord injury, other pertinent diagnosis)
- Physician order for use of bladder scanning

- Bladder palpation for fullness
- Patterns of urine amounts on previous voidings or catheterizations
- Previous residual urine volumes, if applicable
- Time of last bladder emptying

Nursing Diagnoses

Nursing diagnoses may include the following:
- Impaired urinary elimination: incomplete bladder emptying related to urinary incontinence
- Acute pain related to bladder distention from urinary retention

Outcome Identification and Planning

Desired Outcomes

- Client maintains urine output of at least 250 mL per 8 hours.
- Client verbalizes no lower abdominal pain.

Special Considerations in Planning and Implementation

General

Bladder scanning has been associated with fewer urinary tract infections in some research studies. The BVI 3000 is designed for acute care settings, the BVI 5000 for rehabilitation and home settings.

Geriatric

Urinary incontinence is a significant problem for many elderly clients. Bladder scanning is used in many geriatric rehabilitation settings because these clients are prone to urinary tract infections.

Implementation

Action	Rationale
1. Perform hand hygiene and gather equipment: BVI 3000 (Fig. 8.12A) or BVI 5000 (Fig. 8.12B).	*Reduces microorganisms; organizes equipment*
2. Explain procedure to client.	*Reduces anxiety*
3. Apply gloves and assist the client into supine position.	*Positions client for obtaining accurate readings*
4. Expose client's lower abdomen.	*Determines location of bladder*
5. Palpate the symphysis pubis.	*Identifies starting point for scan*
6. Apply gel over bladder area.	*Promotes conduction of scan waves*

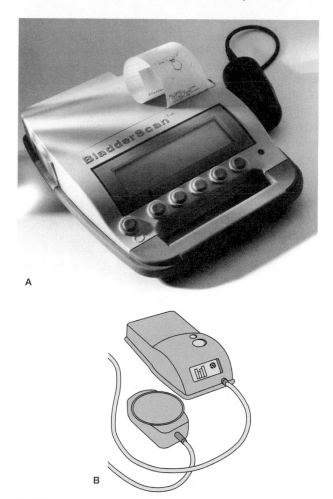

A

B

FIGURE 8.12

Action	Rationale
7. Place the scanhead device on lower abdomen where symphysis pubis is palpated (Fig. 8.13).	

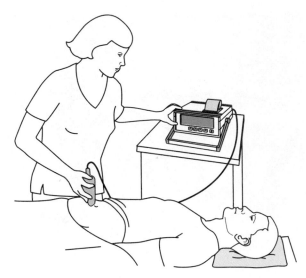

FIGURE 8.13

Action	Rationale
• Hold the scanhead completely still.	
• Do not raise the dome of the scanhead off the client's body.	
8. Press scan button.	*Obtains bladder volume*
9. Check aiming screen.	*Verifies correct position of scanhead*
10. Note the final calculated volume reading on the display screen in 5 seconds (BVI 2500) or 10 seconds (BVI 5000).	*Obtains calculated bladder volume*
11. Press print button (BVI 2500).	*Produces hard (written) copy of results*
12. Turn machine off.	*Discontinues scanning*
13. Wash gel off client.	*Removes gel*
14. Replace cover over abdomen.	*Reclothes client*
15. Clean and store bladder scanning device.	*Prepares scanning equipment for next use*
16. Perform hand hygiene.	*Reduces microorganism transfer*

Evaluation

Were desired outcomes achieved? Examples of evaluation include:
- Desired outcome not met: Client maintains urine output of 150 mL per 8 hours.
- Desired outcome not met: Client continues to complain of lower abdominal pain: doctor notified, straight catheterization ordered.

Documentation

The following should be noted on the client's chart:
- Status of bladder on palpation
- Volume indicated on bladder scan readings
- Complaints of client discomfort
- Disposition of catheterization as intervention for bladder emptying

Sample Documentation
Date: 1/1/05
Time: 1100

Client has not voided since 1200. Bladder distention noted on palpation. Bladder scanning shows volume of 450 mL. Straight catheterization done, with 430 mL clear yellow urine return. No bladder distention noted on palpation.

● Nursing Procedure 8.11

Caring for a Hemodialysis Shunt, Graft, and Fistula ✋

Purpose

Maintains patency of access for dialysis
Detects complications related to infection, occlusion, or cannula separation at a hemodialysis access site

Equipment

- Nonsterile gloves
- Two pairs of sterile gloves

- Antiseptic cleansing agent or antiseptic swabs
- Topical antiseptic, if ordered
- Sterile 4 × 4-inch gauze pads
- Kerlix/Kling wrap
- Cannula clamps

Assessment

Assessment should focus on the following:
- Status of fistula, graft, or cannula site and dressing
- Location of shunt, fistula, or graft
- Vital signs
- Pulses distal to shunt, fistula, or graft
- Color and temperature of extremity in which access is located
- Presence of pain or numbness in extremity in which access is located
- Time of last dressing change

Nursing Diagnoses

Nursing diagnoses may include the following:
- Altered tissue perfusion related to shunt/fistula/graft occlusion or infection
- Risk of peripheral neurovascular dysfunction related to possible shunt/graft/fistula occlusion

Outcome Identification and Planning

Desired Outcomes

Sample desired outcomes include the following:
- A bruit is present on auscultation and a thrill is palpable.
- Client displays no edema, redness, pain, drainage, or bleeding at the hemodialysis access site.

Special Considerations in Planning and Implementation

General

A potential complication related to the presence of the shunt is cannula separation. Hemorrhage can occur if the shunt is not clamped off until a new cannula is inserted; therefore, a pair of cannula clamps should be kept at the client's bedside at all times.

Pediatric and Geriatric

Educate client and caregiver on care of shunt and dressing changes.

Home Health

To enable client to change dressings between nursing visits, secure the dressing with a stockinette dressing that the client can roll down over Kerlix, remove old dressing, and roll up to secure new dressing.

Delegation

This procedure should be performed by the nurse.

Implementation

Action	Rationale
1. Perform hand hygiene.	*Reduces microorganism transfer*
2. Explain procedure to client.	*Decreases anxiety*
3. Open several 4 × 4 packages of gauze, and soak several pads with antiseptic solution, or open antiseptic swabs and position for easy access. Keep one package of gauze dry.	*Facilitates cleaning process; provides gauze to cover shunt*
4. Put on clean gloves.	*Reduces nurse's exposure to client's body secretions*
5. Position client to expose site. Remove old dressing, if present, and check access site.	*Exposes access site*
6. Discard old dressing and gloves.	*Removes contaminated items*
7. Perform hand hygiene and put on sterile gloves.	*Avoids site contamination*
8. Cleanse access area with antiseptic agent recommended by agency. For shunt care, begin at exit areas and work outward, discarding antiseptic swab or folded gauze pad after each wipe.	*Reduces contamination*
9. Lightly place two or three fingertips over access site and assess for presence of thrill (a palpable vibration should be present); assess site for extreme warmth or coolness.	*Tests for adequate blood flow through shunt*
10. Apply topical ointment, if ordered.	*Prevents infection*
11. Place dry sterile gauze pads over access site.	*Reduces site contamination*
12. For shunt, apply Kerlix or Kling wrap over gauze pads and around extremity (wrap firmly enough that dressing is secure but not so tight as	*Prevents accidental dislodgment of cannula; allows for visualization of continuous blood flow*

Action	Rationale
to occlude blood flow) and tape securely; leave small piece of shunt tubing visible.	
13. Discard equipment and gloves, then perform hand hygiene.	*Reduces spread of infection*
14. Place call light within reach.	*Allows communication*
15. Assess status of dressing, access site, and pulses in affected extremity every 2 hours.	*Monitors frequently for complications*
16. During immediate post-operative period, inform client, family, and staff of the following care instructions:	*Prevents loss of access site due to occlusion, infection, or cannula separation*
• If shunt is in arm or leg, keep extremity elevated on pillow until instructed otherwise.	
• Keep extremity as still as possible.	
• Do not apply pressure to or lift heavy objects with extremity. (If shunt is in leg, crutches will be used for a short while when client becomes ambulatory.)	*Prevents rupture and pain*
• Do not allow access area to get wet during showering, bathing, or swimming.	
17. Inform client, family, and staff of the following care instructions:	*Promotes cooperation with care of site; reduces fear; prevents injury*
• Never perform a blood pressure assessment or any procedure that might occlude blood flow on affected extremity.	*Prevents occlusion of blood flow*
• NEVER perform venipuncture or any procedure involving a needlestick. Place a sign over bed prohibiting use of affected extremity for these procedures.	*Prevents injury, clotting, and infection*

Action	Rationale
• Avoid restricting blood flow in affected extremity with tight-fitting clothes, watches, name bands, knee-high stockings, antiembolytic hose, restraints, and so forth.	*Prevents restriction of blood flow and injury to graft/shunt/fistula area*
• Notify nurse immediately if bleeding or cannula disconnection is noted.	*Prevents excessive bleeding*
• Apply cannula clamps if disconnection is noted.	*Prevents hemorrhage*

Evaluation

Were desired outcomes achieved? Examples of evaluation include:
- Desired outcome met: A bruit is present on auscultation, and a thrill is palpable.
- Desired outcome met: Client displays no edema, redness, pain, drainage, or bleeding at the hemodialysis access site.

Documentation

The following should be noted on the client's chart:
- Location of access site
- Status of site and dressing
- Vital signs
- Status of pulses distal to access area
- Color and temperature of extremity in which access is located
- Presence of pain or numbness in extremity in which access is located

---

Sample Documentation
Date: 1/1/05
Time: 1100

Left forearm Goretex graft site care given. Radial pulse normal (3+) in left arm. Left fingers pink with 2-sec capillary refill. Denies pain or numbness of left arm. Thrill palpable at graft site. No swelling or irritation noted at site. Site cleaned with Betadine solution and sterile dressing applied. Site and dressing intact.

Managing Peritoneal Dialysis

Purpose

Instills solutions into peritoneal cavity to remove metabolic end products, toxins, and excess fluid from body when kidney function is totally or partially ineffective

Treats electrolyte and acid–base imbalances

Equipment

- Dialysate fluid bag/bottle(s) ordered
- Medication additives ordered (usually some combination of potassium chloride, heparin, sodium bicarbonate, and possibly antibiotics)
- Syringes for additives
- Medication labels
- Dialysis flow sheet
- Dialysate tubing
- IV pole
- Peroxide or sterile saline
- Antiseptic recommended by agency
- Masks (for each person in room, including client and visitors)
- Clean gown
- Multiple pairs of sterile gloves
- Gauze dressing pads (2×2 inches and 4×4 inches)
- Tape
- Graduated container
- Scale
- Warmer
- Spike
- Clamp

Assessment

Assessment should focus on the following:
- Changes in mental status
- Fluid balance indicators (e.g., vital signs, weight, skin turgor, condition of mucous membranes, presence or absence of edema, intake and output)
- Abdominal status, including abdominal girth
- Cardiopulmonary status
- Status of dressing and catheter site
- Status of skin surrounding site
- Indicators of peritonitis (e.g., sharp abdominal pain, cloudy or pink-tinged dialysate fluid return, increased temperature)
- Laboratory data (e.g., blood gases, potassium, blood urea nitrogen, creatinine, hemoglobin, hematocrit)
- Indicators of electrolyte imbalance

Nursing Diagnoses

Nursing diagnoses may include the following:
- Fluid volume excess related to inability of kidneys to remove excess fluids
- Risk of infection related to peritoneal catheter

Outcome Identification and Planning

Desired Outcomes

Sample desired outcomes include the following:
- After dialysis, the client has a balanced fluid volume.
- Client demonstrates no signs of infection; there is no acute abdominal pain, temperature is within normal range, dialysate return is clear, and there is no redness, edema, or abnormal drainage at catheter insertion site.

Special Considerations in Planning and Implementation

General

Peritonitis is a frequent complication in clients with peritoneal dialysis; therefore, strict aseptic technique must be maintained.

Pediatric

The pediatric client may be anxious, apathetic, or withdrawn. Spend as much time with client as possible and arrange for family members to be present to provide support.

Home Health

Many homebound clients dialyze intermittently at home using a cycler. Many also use continuous ambulatory peritoneal dialysis (CAPD) or continuous cycling peritoneal dialysis (CCPD). Observe return demonstrations until you are certain that the client and family understand the importance of preventing infection.

Cost-Cutting Tips

If not contraindicated by agency's or manufacturer's policy, a blanket warmer may be used to warm dialysate solution, saving time in preparation.

Delegation

Except in agencies where special training or certification is provided (see agency policy), this procedure cannot be delegated to unlicensed personnel. They may, however, assist with obtaining weights, emptying drainage receptacles/graduated containers, and recording output.

Implementation

Action	Rationale
1. Perform hand hygiene.	*Reduces microorganism transfer*
2. Explain procedure to client.	*Decreases anxiety*
3. Weigh client each morning and as ordered for each series of exchanges, and record weight.	*Provides data needed to determine appropriate concentrations of fluids and additives*
4. Place unopened dialysate fluid bag or bottle in warmer if solution is not at least room temperature.	*Enhances solute and fluid clearance; prevents abdominal cramping*
5. Put on mask.	*Reduces spread of airborne microorganisms*
6. Prepare dialysate with medication additives as ordered; prepare each bag according to the five rights of drug administration (client, drug, dosage [concentration], route, time; see Procedure 11.1); place completed medication label on bag.	*Avoids errors that could affect end results of dialysis: concentration affects osmolality, rate of fluid removal, electrolyte balance, solute removal, and cardiovascular stability*
7. Insert dialysate infusion tubing spike into insertion port on dialysate fluid bag or bottle and prime tubing, then place fluid bag or bottle on IV pole. Some tubing spikes are designed like a screw cap with a spike in the center of the cap. Place an antiseptic solution in the cap before spiking the bag.	*Eliminates air, which may contribute to client discomfort*
8. Adjust position of bed so fluid hangs higher than client's abdomen and drainage bag is lower than abdomen (Fig. 8.14).	*Enhances gravitational flow as fluid infuses and drains*
9. Provide privacy.	*Reduces embarrassment*
10. Open and arrange cleaning supplies using inside of packages as sterile field (soak 4 × 4 gauze pads with saline or designated solution, leaving dry pads for covering or other dressing, if ordered).	

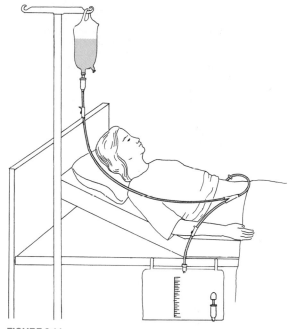

FIGURE 8.14

Action	Rationale
11. Put on clean gown and sterile gloves; instruct each person in room to put on appropriate protective wear (masks for all persons in room, sterile gloves for nurse and assistant handling fluid bags).	*Decreases nurse's exposure to microorganisms and client's exposure to airborne microorganisms; reduces risk of peritonitis*
12. Remove old peritoneal catheter dressing and examine catheter site for catheter dislodgment or signs of infection; if leakage or abnormal drainage is noted, culture site.	*Assesses catheter intactness; facilitates identification of infectious agent*
13. Discard dressing and gloves; perform hand hygiene and put on sterile gloves.	*Reduces microorganism transfer*

Action	Rationale
14. Beginning at catheter insertion site, cleanse site with a circular motion outward, using peroxide or sterile saline on gauze or swab, and allow to dry; apply antiseptic agent recommended by agency or ordered by doctor (discard each gauze or swab after each wipe when cleansing site and applying antiseptic).	*Decreases microorganisms at catheter insertion site; reduces risk of peritonitis*
15. Using sterile technique, apply new dressing and secure with tape.	*Protects site from microorganisms*
16. Discard gloves and perform hand hygiene.	*Reduces microorganisms*
17. Label dressing with date and time of change and your initials.	*Provides data needed to determine when next dressing change is due*
18. Put on sterile gloves.	*Reduces microorganisms*
19. Connect end of dialysate tubing to abdominal catheter.	*Connects tubing to begin dialysate infusion*
20. Clamp tubing from abdominal catheter to drainage bag (outflow tubing).	*Prevents dialysate from running through*
21. Check client's position (abdomen lower than height of fluid, which allows gravity to facilitate flow); check tubing for kinks or bends.	*Removes obstructions that could affect infusion rate*
22. Open dialysate infusion tubing clamp(s) and allow fluid to drain into peritoneal cavity for 10 to 15 minutes. Observe respiratory status and pain status while fluid infuses and while fluid remains in the abdomen (dwell time). Slow or stop infusion as needed to reduce discomfort.	*Infuses dialysate for fluid and electrolyte exchange in peritoneal cavity using volume within client tolerance*
23. Allow fluid to dwell in abdomen for 20 minutes (or amount of time specified by doctor).	*Allows time for exchange of fluids and electrolytes*

Action	Rationale
24. Open clamp leading to drain bag and allow fluid to drain for specified amount of time or until drainage has decreased to a slow drip (if all the fluid does not return, reposition client and recheck tubing leading to drainage bag). • For CAPD, client may fold dialysis bag and secure bag and tubing to abdomen or clothing and allow fluid to dwell while performing daily activities. To drain dialysate, client unfolds and lowers bag and allows fluid to drain from abdominal cavity (same bag is used for infusion and drainage). Measure fluid drainage. A new bag is then hung, and the infusion/dwelling/drainage cycle is repeated continuously.	*Allows end products of dialysis to drain*
25. Record amount of fluid infused and amount drained after each exchange; add balance of fluids infused and drained on appropriate flow sheet (if net output is greater than amount infused by a large margin [200 mL or more] notify doctor).	*Provides accurate record of fluid exchanges for determining fluid balance*
26. Reassess the following client data every 30 to 60 minutes thereafter throughout exchanges: vital signs, output, respiratory status, mental status, abdominal status, appearance of dialysate return, abdominal dressing (should be kept dry), and signs of lethal electrolyte imbalances.	*Alerts nurse to impending complications or need to change fluid and additive concentrations*

Action	Rationale
27. Weigh client at end of ordered number of fluid exchanges.	*Provides data regarding efficiency of exchanges in removing excess fluid*
28. Obtain laboratory data as ordered and as needed (check doctor's orders and agency policy regarding p.r.n. laboratory data).	*Provides data about clearance of metabolic wastes as well as electrolyte status*
29. When the total series of exchanges is completed, empty drainage bag into graduated container, discard bag and tubing, and cap peritoneal catheter.	*Removes fluid waste so other fluid may drain*
30. Discard or restore equipment appropriately.	*Promotes clean environment*
31. Remove and discard gloves and perform hand hygiene.	*Reduces microorganisms*

Evaluation

Were desired outcomes achieved? Examples of evaluation include:
- Desired outcome met: Client demonstrates a balanced fluid volume.
- Desired outcome met: Client demonstrates no signs of infection: no complaints of acute abdominal pain, temperature within normal range, pulse 88, dialysate return clear, no redness, edema, or abnormal drainage at catheter insertion site.

Documentation

The following should be noted on the client's chart:
- Fluid balance indicators (e.g., vital signs, weight, skin turgor, condition of mucous membranes, presence or absence of edema, intake and output) before and after dialysis
- Mental status before and after dialysis
- Cardiopulmonary assessment
- Abdominal assessment, including abdominal girth
- Status of dressing and catheter site
- Status of skin surrounding site
- Indicators of peritonitis (e.g., sharp abdominal pain, cloudy or pink-tinged dialysate fluid return, increased temperature)
- Changes in laboratory data (e.g., blood gases, potassium, blood urea nitrogen, creatinine, hemoglobin, hematocrit)
- Acute indicators of electrolyte imbalance (if present)
- Type and amount of dialysate infused
- Medication additives in dialysate

Sample Documentation
Date: 1/1/05
Time: 1100

First series of dialysis exchanges begun. Weight prior to dialysis 88 kg. Twelve bags of 1.5% dialysate fluid hung to infuse via dialysis cycler. No abdominal distention noted. Dialysis catheter site intact with no signs of infection. Abdominal dressing clean, dry, and intact. Client denies abdominal pain. Dialysate return clear. Postdialysis weight 72 kg. Blood sent to lab for postdialysis evaluation.

● Nursing Procedure 8.13

Caring for Nephrostomy Tubes 🖐

Purpose

Allows urine to drain from the kidney to a drainage bag when the ureters are obstructed by tumors, calculi, strictures, or fistulas

Equipment

- Clean drainage bag and connecting tube
- Disposable gloves
- Alcohol swabs
- Sterile gauze pads
- Sterile saline solution
- Adhesive tape
- Bath basin with soap and water
- Paper bag for disposal of soiled dressing
- Mild detergent and vinegar (for ongoing care)

Assessment

Assessment should focus on the following:
- Continuous flow of urine
- Doctor's order for dressing change
- Client's knowledge of the procedure
- Rise in temperature, purulent discharge at insertion site, malodorous urine, flank pain, integrity of skin around the insertion site

- Appearance of urine
- Client's cognitive status, vision, and manual dexterity
- Caregiver's reliability to care for the tube

Nursing Diagnoses

Nursing diagnoses may include the following:
- Risk for impaired urinary elimination related to urethral diversion
- Risk for infection related to decreased skin integrity around nephrostomy tube

Outcome Identification and Planning

Desired Outcomes

Sample desired outcomes include the following:
- Client maintains adequate urine output.
- Client demonstrates no signs of infection or skin breakdown at the site of nephrostomy tube.

Special Considerations in Planning and Implementation

General

Instruct the client to notify the health care provider immediately if the tube comes out. The tract closes quickly in 2 to 3 hours. Keep the drainage bag lower than the nephrostomy tube to enhance gravitational flow. NEVER irrigate the nephrostomy tube unless ordered.

Pediatric

Enlist the assistance of a parent or assistant when performing this procedure on a small child.

Implementation

Action	Rationale
1. Explain procedure to client.	*Decreases anxiety*
2. Perform hand hygiene.	*Avoids transfer of micro-organisms*
3. Organize equipment within reach.	*Promotes efficiency*
4. Put on disposable gloves.	*Minimizes exposure to client's body secretions*
5. Disconnect the nephrostomy tube from the used tubing and drainage bag. Clean end of the nephrostomy tube with an alcohol swab.	*Reduces microorganism transfer*

Action	Rationale
6. Attach the ends of the nephrostomy tube and the connecting tube securely. Don't touch the ends of the tubes.	*Maintains sterility of system*
7. Check the tubing for kinks.	*Maintains patency of system*
8. Change the dressing daily according to doctor's order. Put soiled dressing in paper bag for disposal.	*Removes medium for micro-organism growth*
9. Gently wash around the nephrostomy tube.	*Decreases microorganisms around the nephrostomy tube*
10. Inspect the skin around the tube. Note color and character of any drainage.	*Redness or white, yellow, or green drainage may indicate infection; drainage that smells like urine may indicate tube displacement; either condition should be reported to the doctor immediately.*
11. Fold several gauze pads in half and place them around the base of the nephrostomy tube. Secure the pads with tape. Cover the nephrostomy tube entry site with a dry sterile 4 × 4 and tape securely.	*Protects the skin and is more comfortable for the client*
12. Bring all the tubing forward, and tape securely to the body.	*Allows the client to turn without obstructing urine flow or dislodging the tube from the kidney*
13. Keep separate output records for each kidney, if both have tubes.	*Promotes more accurate assessment of kidney function*
14. Irrigate the tube gently with 5 mL of sterile warm saline solution, if ordered. Alert doctor immediately if tube is not patent.	*Determines patency*
15. Wash the used bag and connecting tube with a weak detergent daily. Rinse with plain water and hang on clothes hanger to air dry.	*A biodegradable or chlorine product may erode the bag.*
16. Twice weekly, wash the bag and tubing with a solution of one part white vinegar to three parts water.	*Avoids crystalline buildup*
17. Perform hand hygiene after procedure is complete and equipment stored.	*Reduces microorganism transfer*

Evaluation

Were desired outcomes achieved? Examples of evaluation include:
● Desired outcome met: Urine output 10 cc/hour.
● Desired outcome not met: Area surrounding nephrostomy is reddened with initial skin breakdown.

Documentation

The following should be noted on the client's chart:
● Teaching done
● Functional limitations that interfere with performance of procedure
● Client tolerance of procedure
● Condition of insertion site
● Quality and quantity of urinary output
● Plans for future visits
● Discharge planning

Sample Documentation
Date: 1/1/05
Time: 1100

Left flank nephrostomy tube site care given and sterile dressing applied with client assistance. Tolerated procedure well. Client verbalized understanding and demonstrated skill in performance of procedure. Observed continuous flow of clear amber urine. Denies flank pain. Temperature 98.8°F. No redness or drainage noted at insertion site.

● Nursing Procedure 8.14

Removing Fecal Impaction

Purpose

Manually removes hardened stool blocking lower part of colon
Relieves pain and discomfort
Facilitates normal peristalsis
Prevents rectal and anal injury

Equipment

- Three pairs of nonsterile gloves
- Packet of water-soluble lubricant
- Bedpan
- Disposable waterproof bed pad

- Basin of warm water
- Soap
- Washcloth
- Towel
- Room deodorizer

Assessment

Assessment should focus on the following:
- Agency policy and physician's order regarding performance of procedure
- Time of last bowel movement and usual bowel evacuation pattern
- Status of anus and skin surrounding buttocks (e.g., presence of ulcerations, tears, hemorrhoids, excoriation)
- Indicators of impaction (e.g., lower abdominal and rectal pain, seepage of liquid stools, inability to pass stool, general malaise, urge to defecate without being able to do so, nausea and vomiting, shortness of breath)
- Abdominal status
- Vital signs before, during, and after removal
- History of factors that may contraindicate or present complications during impaction removal (e.g., cardiac dysrhythmia or bradycardia, recent rectal or pelvic surgery, spinal cord injury)
- Client's dietary habits (e.g., intake of liquids and fiber), changes in activity pattern, frequency of use of laxatives or enemas
- Client knowledge regarding promotion of normal bowel elimination
- Medications that decrease peristalsis, such as narcotics

Nursing Diagnoses

Nursing diagnoses may include the following:
- Constipation related to immobility, decreased fluid intake, or surgery
- Acute abdominal pain related to bowel distention from impaction or from procedure

Outcome Identification and Planning

Desired Outcomes

Sample desired outcomes include the following:
- Client's rectum is free of impacted stool.
- Client has normal bowel movement within 24 hours.

Special Considerations in Planning and Implementation

General

Consult agency policy and physician's orders regarding the performance of this procedure on any client. Digital removal of impacted stool stretches the anal sphincter, causing vagal stimulation. As a result, electrical impulses may be inhibited at the SA node of the heart, causing a dangerous decrease in heart rate as well as dysrhythmias. Therefore, this procedure is contraindicated in cardiac clients. Certain tube feeding formulas (hypertonic) promote constipation and fecal impaction. Check medication record and nutritional supplement list if impaction occurs.

Pediatric

Use little finger when removing impaction in small children. Young children may view this procedure as punishment; reassure them they have done nothing wrong.

Geriatric

Many elderly clients are especially prone to dysrhythmias and palpitations related to vagal stimulation because of chronic cardiac problems. Observe such clients closely during procedure. Many elderly clients are especially prone to fecal impaction because of decreased metabolic rate, decreased activity levels, inadequate fluid and fiber intake, and tendency to overuse laxatives and enemas as a routine means of promoting bowel evacuation. A thorough history related to these factors should be obtained. Confused elderly clients may not understand the need for the procedure, so assistance may be necessary to carry out this procedure safely.

Delegation

This procedure may be delegated to unlicensed assistive personnel; however, reinforce observation for Valsalva response.

Implementation

Action	Rationale
1. Perform hand hygiene.	*Reduces microorganism transfer*
2. Assemble all equipment near bedside.	*Promotes efficiency and avoids interruptions*
3. Explain procedure to client, explaining that the procedure will cause some discomfort.	*Reduces anxiety*
4. Assess blood pressure and rate and rhythm of pulse.	*Provides baseline data in case of complications*
5. Raise side rail (left) on side facing client.	*Prevents injury due to fall*

Action	Rationale
6. Put on gloves, placing one glove on nondominant hand and two gloves on dominant hand.	*Decreases nurse's exposure to client's body secretions in case hardened fecal mass tears glove*
7. Position client in the left lateral position with knees flexed.	*Facilitates access to rectum*
8. Tuck disposable bed pad beneath left buttock and place bedpan close at hand.	*Prevents soiling of linens; facilitates disposal of fecal mass*
9. Provide privacy; drape client with bed linen so only buttocks are exposed.	*Reduces embarrassment*
10. Generously lubricate first two gloved fingers of dominant hand.	*Prevents injury to anus and rectum upon entry*
11. Gently spread buttocks with nondominant hand.	*Exposes anal opening*
12. Instruct client to take slow, deep breaths through mouth.	*Relaxes sphincter muscles, facilitating entry*
13. Insert index finger into rectum (directed toward umbilicus) until fecal mass is palpable (Fig. 8.15).	*Prevents rectal trauma*
14. Gently break up hardened stool using index or middle finger and remove one piece at a time until all stool is removed; place stool in bedpan as it is removed.	*Manually removes impacted stool*
15. Observe client for untoward reactions or unusual discomfort during stool re-	*Monitors for complications from vagal stimulation*

Impacted stool

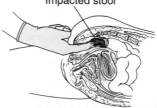

FIGURE 8.15

Action	Rationale
moval; obtain pulse and blood pressure if unusual reaction is suspected.	
16. Remove finger, wipe excess lubricant from perineal area, and release buttocks.	*Promotes comfort*
17. Empty bedpan and discard gloves.	*Promotes clean environment*
18. Perform hand hygiene and put on a new pair of gloves.	*Reduces microorganism transfer*
19. Wash, rinse, and dry buttocks.	*Removes residual stool*
20. Reposition client for comfort and raise side rail.	*Promotes comfort and safety*
21. Leave bedpan within easy reach.	*Impaction removal may have stimulated defecation reflex.*
22. Discard bathwater and gloves.	*Promotes clean environment*
23. Spray room deodorizer at bedside.	*Eliminates odor*
24. Perform hand hygiene.	*Reduces microorganism transfer*

Evaluation

Were desired outcomes achieved? Examples of evaluation include:
- Desired outcome met: Client passed medium soft stool and experienced minimal discomfort during procedure.
- Desired outcome not met: Rectum has hard stool beyond finger reach and the client still complains of mild rectal pressure 2 hours after procedure.

Documentation

The following should be noted on the client's chart:
- Procedure completion with date and time and color, consistency, and amount of stool removed
- Condition of anus and surrounding area before and after procedure
- Vital signs before and after impaction removal
- Abdominal assessment before and after removal
- Description of and interventions for any adverse reactions experienced during the procedure
- Presence of discomfort after procedure
- Client teaching regarding prevention of fecal impaction

Sample Documentation
Date: 1/1/05
Time: 1100

Large amount of hard, dark-brown impacted stool removed
manually, with no signs of adverse effects; passed medium soft
brown stool after impaction removed. Pulse 75 and regular
before removal and 68 and regular afterward. Bowel sounds
auscultated in four quadrants after removal. Abdomen soft
and nondistended. Discussed with client factors preventing
constipation and impaction. Factors verbalized by client.
Client continues to have mild rectal pressure 2 hr after
procedure. Perineal care done; no anal irritation noted.

● Nursing Procedure 8.15

Administering an Enema

Purpose

Relieves abdominal distention, constipation, and discomfort
Stimulates peristalsis
Resumes normal bowel evacuation
Cleanses and evacuates colon

Equipment

- Two pairs of nonsterile gloves
- IV pole and enema setup (administration bag or bucket with rectal tubing, Castile soap, protective plastic linen saver, packet of water-soluble lubricant)
- Solution for enema, as prescribed by physician (for adults, 750 to 1,000 mL; for children, up to 350 mL; for infants, up to 250 mL)
- Bath thermometer
- Bedpan or bedside commode
- Disposable waterproof bed pad
- Basin of warm water
- Soap
- Washcloth
- Towel
- Room deodorizer

Assessment

Assessment should focus on the following:
- Physician's order for type of enema
- Agency policy and physician's order regarding performance of procedure
- Time of last bowel movement and usual bowel evacuation pattern
- Indicators of constipation (e.g., lower abdominal pain; hard, small stools)
- History of factors that may contraindicate enema or present complications during enema administration (e.g., cardiac dysrhythmia or bradycardia, recent rectal or pelvic surgery, spinal cord injury)
- Client's dietary habits (e.g., intake of liquids and fiber), changes in activity pattern, frequency of use of laxatives or enemas
- Abdominal status: presence of bowel sounds
- Client's mental status and any fears associated with procedure
- Status of anus and skin surrounding buttocks (e.g., presence of ulcerations, tears, hemorrhoids, excoriation)
- Vital signs before, during, and after enema
- Client knowledge regarding promotion of normal bowel evacuation
- Client medications that decrease peristalsis, such as narcotics

Nursing Diagnoses

Nursing diagnoses may include the following:
- Constipation related to immobility; decreased food, fiber, or fluid intake; or surgery
- Acute abdominal pain related to bowel distention from constipation or from procedure

Outcome Identification and Planning

Desired Outcomes

Sample desired outcomes include the following:
- Client evacuates moderate to large amount of stool.
- Client verbalizes pain relief within 1 hour.

Special Considerations in Planning and Implementation

Pediatric

Young children may view the procedure as punishment; reassure them they have done nothing wrong. Minimal elevation of fluid above the anus (4 to 18 inches) is needed to achieve adequate influx of solution.

Geriatric

Many elderly clients are especially prone to dysrhythmias and palpitations related to vagal stimulation because of chronic cardiac problems. Observe such clients closely during procedure. Many elderly clients are especially prone to constipation and impaction because of decreased metabolic rate; decreased activity levels; inadequate fluid, food, or fiber intake; and tendency to overuse laxatives and enemas as a routine means of promoting bowel evacuation. A thorough history related to these factors should be obtained. Confused elderly clients may not understand the need for the procedure; assistance may be necessary to carry out the procedure safely.

 Cost-Cutting Tips

If bath thermometer is not available to test solution temperature, use the inner aspect of your forearm.

Delegation

This procedure may be delegated to unlicensed assistive personnel. Emphasize the importance of monitoring client comfort and monitoring closely for Valsalva response.

Implementation

Action	Rationale
1. Perform hand hygiene.	*Reduces microorganism transfer*
2. Explain procedure to client, explaining that the procedure may cause some mild discomfort.	*Reduces anxiety*
3. Explain to client that the enema solution will need to be retained for specified time period.	*Contributes to procedure success*
4. Prepare solution, making certain that temperature of solution is lukewarm (about 100°F to 110°F) by placing solution in warm water bath.	*Reduces abdominal cramping during procedure*
5. Prime tubing with fluid and close tubing clamp; place container on bedside IV pole.	*Prevents distention of colon and abdominal discomfort from air*
6. Lower pole so enema solution hangs no more than 18 to 24 inches above buttocks for adults (Fig. 8.16); for infants and children, solution should hang no more than 4 to 18 inches above anus.	*Slows rate of fluid infusion and prevents cramping*

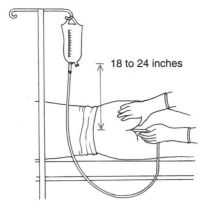

18 to 24 inches

FIGURE 8.16

Action	Rationale
7. Put on gloves.	*Decreases nurse's exposure to client's body secretions*
8. Raise side rail (left) on side facing client.	*Prevents injury due to fall*
9. Position client in side-lying position with knees flexed.	*Allows good exposure of anal opening*
10. Provide privacy by draping client with bed linen or towel so that only buttocks are exposed.	*Reduces embarrassment*
11. Tuck disposable bed pad beneath left buttock.	*Prevents soiling of linens*
12. Lubricate 2 to 4 inches of the rectal tube.	*Reduces anorectal trauma*
13. Place bedpan on bed within easy reach.	*Facilitates disposal of enema solution*
14. Gently spread buttocks with nondominant hand.	*Exposes anal opening*
15. Instruct client to take slow, deep breaths through mouth.	*Relaxes sphincter muscles, facilitating entry*
16. With dominant hand, insert rectal tube into rectum (directed toward umbilicus) about 3 to 4 inches and hold in place with dominant hand (1 to 1.5 inches for infants; 2 to 3 inches for a child).	*Prevents rectal trauma; places tube in far enough to cleanse colon*

Action	Rationale
17. Release tubing clamp.	*Allows solution to flow*
18. Allow solution to flow into colon slowly, observing client closely.	*Avoids cramping*
19. If cramping, extreme anxiety, or complaint of inability to retain solution occurs: • Lower solution container. • Clamp or pinch tubing off for a few minutes. • Resume instillation of solution.	*Decreases or stops solution flow, allowing client to readjust and gain composure*
20. Administer all of solution or as much as client can tolerate; be sure to clamp tubing just before all of the solution clears tubing.	*Delivers enough solution for proper effect; prevents infusion of air*
21. Slowly remove rectal tubing while gently holding buttocks together.	*Prevents accidental evacuation of solution*
22. Remind client to hold solution for amount of time appropriate for type of enema.	*Ensures optimal effect*
23. Reposition client for comfort.	*Facilitates comfort*
24. Place call light and bedpan or bedside commode within easy reach.	*Provides means of contacting nurse; provides receptacle for enema solution*
25. Discard or restore equipment appropriately.	*Promotes clean environment*
26. Remove gloves and perform hand hygiene.	*Reduces microorganism transfer*
27. Check client every 5 to 10 minutes to assess if client is still able to retain enema.	*Reassesses client's condition and retention of enema*
28. Assist client on bedpan or toilet after retention time has expired or when client can no longer retain enema.	*Facilitates evacuation of solution*
29. Apply gloves and perform perineal care with soap and water. Spray room deodorizer after evacuation.	*Removes residual stool soilage; eliminates odor*
30. Perform hand hygiene.	*Reduces microorganism transfer*

Evaluation

Were desired outcomes achieved? Examples of evaluation include:
- Desired outcome met: After enema the rectum was free of hard stool, client expelled gas, and abdomen is now soft.
- Desired outcome met: Client states abdominal pain relieved after enema.

Documentation

The following should be noted on the client's chart:
- Type and amount of solution used
- Procedure completion with date and time and color, consistency, and amount of stool expelled
- Condition of anus and surrounding area before and after procedure
- Vital signs before and after enema
- Description of and interventions for any adverse reactions experienced during the procedure
- Abdominal assessment before and after enema
- Presence of discomfort after enema
- Client teaching regarding prevention of constipation

Sample Documentation
Date: 1/1/05
Time: 1100

Soap suds enema (750 mL) given. Anus intact without irritation. Large amount of dark brown stool returned after enema. No sign of adverse effects. Bowel sounds auscultated in four quadrants before and after procedure. Abdomen soft and nondistended. Vital signs stable before and after enema. Client verbalized measures for promoting normal bowel evacuation.

● **Nursing Procedure 8.16**

Applying a Colostomy Pouch 🧤

Purpose

Maintains integrity of stoma and peristomal skin (skin surrounding stoma)

Prevents lesions, ulcerations, excoriation, and other skin break
   down caused by fecal contaminants
Prevents infection
Promotes general comfort and positive self-image/self-concept
Provides clean ostomy pouch for fecal evacuation
Reduces odor from overuse of old pouch

Equipment

- Three pairs of nonsterile gloves (one pair for client, if needed)
- Graduated container
- Two disposable waterproof bed pads
- Basin of warm water
- Mild soap (without oils, perfumes, or creams)
- Washcloth and towel
- Room deodorizer
- New pouch appliance
- Scissors
- Pen or pencil
- Mirror
- Peristomal skin paste and wafer
- Ostomy pouch deodorizer

Assessment

Assessment should focus on the following:
- Appearance of stoma and peristomal skin
- Presence of bowel sounds
- Characteristics of fecal waste
- Type of appliance needed for type of colostomy, nature of drainage, and client preference
- Teaching needs, ability, and preference of client for self-care

Nursing Diagnoses

Nursing diagnoses may include the following:
- Risk for impaired skin integrity related to fecal diversion
- Deficient knowledge related to lack of information regarding stoma care

Outcome Identification and Planning

Desired Outcomes

Sample desired outcomes include the following:
- Client demonstrates no redness, edema, swelling, tears, breaks, ulceration, or fistulas at stoma area.
- Client performs procedure with 100% accuracy.

Special Considerations in Planning and Implementation

General

Ostomy care alters a person's self-concept significantly.
Perform care unhurriedly, and discuss care in a positive

manner with the client. A wide variety of ostomy appliances are available to meet clients' personal preferences and needs. Minor variations in techniques of application may be needed to ensure adequate skin protection and pouch security. Some ostomy appliances are permanent and should be discarded only every few months. Consult appliance manuals for complete information regarding application and recommended usage time for the pouch. Once client (or family member) shows readiness to learn how to perform ostomy care, supervise client's performance of the procedure until it is accomplished accurately and comfortably.

Delegation

This procedure may be delegated to unlicensed assistive personnel only for an established ostomy. Emphasize importance of observations of stoma for irritation or other problems.

Implementation

Action	Rationale
1. Perform hand hygiene.	*Reduces microorganism transfer*
2. Explain general procedure to client and then explain each step as it is performed, allowing client to ask questions or perform any part of the procedure.	*Reduces anxiety; reinforces detailed instructions client will need to perform self-care*
3. Provide privacy.	*Reduces embarrassment*
4. Put on gloves and offer client gloves.	*Avoids nurse's exposure to client's body secretions*
5. Place disposable waterproof pads around stoma pouch close to stoma, remove old pouch, and discard contents; measure with graduated container; discard gloves.	*Removes old pouch for new pouch application; maintains clean environment*
6. Perform hand hygiene and put on fresh gloves.	*Reduces microorganism transfer*
7. Assess stoma and peristomal skin. Position mirror to permit client to view procedure.	*Provides assessment data; allows client to observe and learn procedure*
8. Perform stoma care (see Procedure 8.18).	*Removes stool soilage and promotes secure pouch application*
9. Place gauze pad over stoma opening to prevent spillage while preparing wafer and pouch.	*Protects skin and linens during procedure*

Action	Rationale
10. Measure stoma with measuring guide (Fig. 8.17). Use measuring guide to trace opening on back of wafer (a flat, platelike piece, without pouch attached, that fits on skin around stoma).	*Provides for accurate fit of pouch*
11. Leaving intact adhesive covering of skin-barrier wafer, cut out circle, allowing an extra ⅛ inch for placement over stoma.	*Cuts barrier to appropriate size for stoma; allows pouch to be placed over stoma without adhering to it*
12. Open bottom of pouch and apply a small amount of pouch deodorizer, if client prefers; reclose pouch securely.	*Reduces odor and embarrassment; avoids leakage of feces*
13. Remove gauze and apply stomal paste around stoma or apply stomal paste to edges of opening in wafer.	*Prevents skin irritation of uncovered peristomal skin*

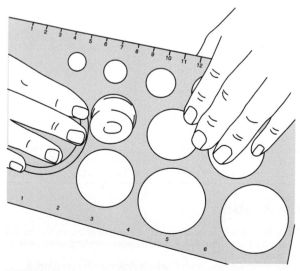

FIGURE 8.17

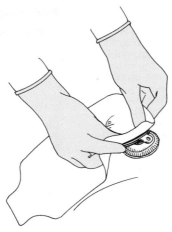

FIGURE 8.18

Action	Rationale
14. Remove adhesive covering of skin-barrier wafer, and place wafer on skin with hole centered over stoma; hold in place for about 30 seconds.	*Adheres barrier wafer to skin; warmth of skin and fingers enhances adhesiveness once wafer makes contact with skin*
15. Center pouch over stoma and place on skin-barrier wafer. If applying a two-piece appliance, snap pouch on the flange of the skin-barrier wafer (Fig. 8.18).	*Secures pouch for collection of feces*
16. Remove gloves and restore or discard all equipment appropriately.	*Promotes clean environment*
17. Spray room deodorizer, if needed.	*Eliminates unpleasant odor*
18. Perform hand hygiene.	*Reduces microorganism transfer*

Evaluation

Were desired outcomes achieved? Examples of evaluation include:
- Desired outcome met: Client displays healing stoma and intact peristomal skin.
- Desired outcome met: Client independently performed pouch change.

Documentation

The following should be noted on the client's chart:
- Color, consistency, and amount of feces in pouch
- Condition of stoma and peristomal skin
- Size of stoma and color and amount of drainage
- Abdominal assessment
- Emotional status of client
- Verbal and nonverbal indicators of altered self-concept during procedure
- Verbal and nonverbal indicators of readiness to perform self-care
- Teaching and client participation in performance of procedure
- Additional teaching needs of client
- Type of appliance client prefers

Sample Documentation
Date: 1/1/05
Time: 1100

New colostomy pouch applied by client with 100% accuracy. Discarded large amount of semiformed brown stool. Stoma 2 cm, pink; surrounding area and abdomen without excoriation or abnormal discharge. Client verbalized anxiety about how wife will accept assisting with his care and stated preference for pouch appliance with flange rings. Discussed self-image concerns.

● Nursing Procedure 8.17

Evacuating and Cleaning a Colostomy Pouch 👋

Purpose

Removes fecal material from ostomy pouch
Cleans pouch for reuse
Maintains integrity of stoma and peristomal skin
Promotes general comfort
Promotes positive self-concept

Equipment

- Three pairs of nonsterile gloves (one pair for client, if necessary)
- Bedpan and/or graduated container
- Two disposable waterproof bed pads
- Room deodorizer
- Two washcloths
- Mirror
- Ostomy pouch deodorizer
- Toilet paper
- Paper towels
- Room deodorizer
- Rubber band

Assessment

Assessment should focus on the following:
- Appearance of stoma (should be pink and moist) and peristomal skin (should be intact with no erythema)
- Characteristics of fecal waste
- Abdominal status
- Type of ostomy appliance (reusable or disposable)
- Teaching needs, ability, and preference of client for self-care

Nursing Diagnoses

Nursing diagnoses may include the following:
- Risk for impaired skin integrity related to fecal diversion
- Deficient knowledge related to lack of information regarding evacuation and cleaning of pouch
- Disturbed body image related to fecal diversion

Outcome Identification and Planning

Desired Outcomes

Sample desired outcomes include the following:
- Client demonstrates no redness, edema, swelling, tears, breaks, ulceration, or fistulas in stoma area.
- Client performs procedure with 100% accuracy within 2 weeks.
- Client verbalizes feelings about fecal diversion.

Special Considerations in Planning and Implementation

General

Ostomy care alters a person's self-concept significantly. Perform care unhurriedly, and discuss care in a positive manner with the client. Once client (or family member) shows readiness to learn how to perform ostomy care, supervise client's performance of the procedure until it is accomplished accurately and comfortably.

 Cost-Cutting Tips

If pouch clamp is not available, use sturdy rubber bands.

Delegation

This procedure may be delegated to unlicensed assistive person-nel only for an established ostomy. Emphasize importance of observations of stoma for irritation or other problems.

Implementation

Action	Rationale
1. Perform hand hygiene.	*Reduces microorganism transfer*
2. Explain general procedure to client and then explain each step as it is per-formed, allowing client to ask questions or perform any part of the procedure.	*Reduces anxiety; reinforces de-tailed instructions client will need to perform self-care*
3. Provide privacy.	*Reduces embarrassment*
4. Position mirror to permit client to view procedure.	*Allows client to observe and learn procedure*
5. Put on gloves.	*Avoids nurse's exposure to client's body secretions*
6. Place disposable water-proof pad on abdomen around and below pouch.	*Prevents seepage of feces onto skin*
7. If using toilet, seat client on toilet or in a chair fac-ing toilet, with pouch over toilet; if using bedpan, place pouch over bedpan.	*Positions client so feces drain into receptacle*
8. Remove clamp on bottom of pouch and place within easy reach. (Fold bottom of pouch up to form a cuff before emptying.)	*Promotes efficiency; cuff keeps bottom of pouch clean, which helps to prevent odor and helps keep hands clean during procedure*
9. Slowly unfold end of pouch and allow feces to drain into bedpan or toilet (Fig. 8.19).	*Removes feces from pouch*
10. Press sides of lower end of pouch together (Fig. 8.20).	*Expels additional feces from pouch*
11. Open lower end of pouch and wipe out with toilet paper.	*Removes excess feces from lower end of pouch*
12. Flush toilet or, if using bedpan, resecure end of pouch with rubber band and then empty bedpan.	*Reduces client embarrassment and room odor*
13. Wash clamp while in bath-room and dry with paper towel.	*Cleans exterior clamp*

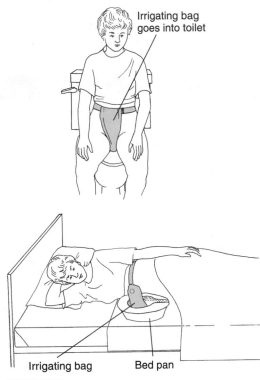

Irrigating bag goes into toilet

Irrigating bag   Bed pan

FIGURE 8.19

Action	Rationale
14. Remove gloves, perform hand hygiene, and reglove.	*Reduces microorganism transfer*
15. Apply pouch deodorizer to lower end of pouch.	*Reduces unpleasant odor*
16. Reclamp pouch with cleaned clamp.	*Prevents leakage of feces*
17. Wipe outside of pouch with clean, wet washcloth; be sure to wipe around clamp at bottom of pouch.	*Completes cleaning of pouch*
18. Remove gloves and restore or discard all equipment appropriately.	*Promotes clean environment*

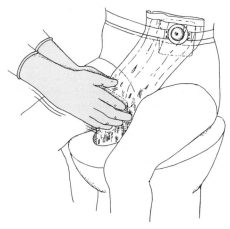

FIGURE 8.20

Action	Rationale
19. Spray room deodorizer, if needed.	*Eliminates unpleasant odor*
20. Perform hand hygiene.	*Reduces microorganism transfer*

Evaluation

Were desired outcomes achieved? Examples of evaluation include:
- Desired outcome met: Client is able to perform procedure independently.
- Desired outcome met: Stoma and surrounding area intact without pain, irritation, or excoriation.
- Desired outcome met: Clients verbalizes positive coping strategies.

Documentation

The following should be noted on the client's chart:
- Color, consistency, and amount of feces in pouch
- Condition of stoma
- Abdominal assessment
- Emotional status of client
- Verbal and nonverbal indicators of altered self-concept during procedure
- Verbal and nonverbal indicators of readiness to perform self-care
- Teaching and client participation in performance of procedure
- Additional teaching needs of client

Sample Documentation
Date: 1/1/05
Time: 1100

Ostomy pouch cleaning and evacuation performed by client with 100% accuracy. Client comfortable with procedure. Discarded large amount of semiformed brown stool. Stoma moist and pink; surrounding area and abdominal area intact without signs of irritation or infection. Client indicates plans to show newly learned procedure to spouse.

● **Nursing Procedure 8.18**

Caring for a Colostomy Stoma

Purpose

Maintains integrity of stoma and peristomal skin
(skin surrounding stoma)
Prevents lesions, ulcerations, excoriation, and other skin break-
down caused by fecal contaminants
Prevents infection
Promotes general comfort
Promotes positive self-concept

Equipment

- Two pairs of nonsterile gloves (add pair for client, if desired)
- Graduated container
- Disposable waterproof bed pad
- Basin of warm, soapy water (soap should be mild without oils, perfumes, or creams)
- Washcloth and towel
- 4 × 4 gauze
- Room deodorizer
- New pouch appliance
- Mirror

Assessment

Assessment should focus on the following:

- Appearance of stoma (should be pink and moist) and peristomal skin (should be intact)
- Dimensions of stoma to ensure correct bag size
- Characteristics of fecal waste
- Abdominal status
- Teaching needs, ability, and preference of client for self-care

Nursing Diagnoses

Nursing diagnoses may include the following:
- Risk for impaired skin integrity related to fecal diversion
- Disturbed body image related to fecal diversion
- Deficient knowledge related to lack of information regarding stoma care

Outcome Identification and Planning

Desired Outcomes

Sample desired outcomes include the following:
- Client demonstrates no redness, edema, swelling, tears, breaks, ulceration, or fistulas at stoma area.
- Client performs procedure with 100% accuracy.
- Client expresses positive feelings about self.

Special Considerations in Planning and Implementation

General

Ostomy care alters a person's self-concept significantly; be sure to perform care unhurriedly, and discuss care in a positive manner with the client. Once client (or family member) shows readiness to begin learning how to perform ostomy care, supervise client's performance of procedure until it is accomplished accurately and comfortably.

Pediatric

Minimal pressure should be used when providing stoma care to children to prevent prolapse of the small stoma.

Delegation

This procedure may be delegated to unlicensed assistive personnel only for an established ostomy. Emphasize the importance of observing the stoma for irritation or other problems and evaluate client's acceptance of the stoma.

Home Health

Homebound clients may dry the skin after cleaning the stoma by using a hair dryer on a low setting.

Implementation

Action	Rationale
1. Perform hand hygiene, organize equipment, and prepare new stoma pouch.	*Reduces microorganism transfer; promotes efficiency*
2. Explain general procedure to client and then explain each step as it is performed, allowing client to ask questions or perform any part of the procedure.	*Reduces anxiety; reinforces detailed instructions client will need to perform self-care*
3. Provide privacy.	*Reduces embarrassment*
4. Position mirror to reveal stoma area to client.	*Permits client to observe and learn procedure*
5. Put on gloves.	*Avoids nurse's exposure to client's body secretions*
6. Place disposable waterproof pad on abdomen around and below stoma opening.	*Prevents seepage of feces onto skin*
7. Carefully remove pouch appliance (bag and skin barrier) and place in plastic waste bag (save tail closure for reuse): remove pouch by gently lifting corner with fingers of dominant hand while pressing skin downward with fingers of nondominant hand; remove small sections at a time until entire barrier wafer is removed. Place 4 × 4 gauze over stoma opening.	*Avoids tearing skin; prevents leakage while changing pouch*
8. Empty pouch; measure waste in graduated container before discarding and record amount of fecal contents (see Procedure 8.17).	*Maintains accurate records*
9. Remove gloves, perform hand hygiene, and re-glove.	*Reduces contamination*
10. Gently clean entire stoma and peristomal skin with gauze or washcloth soaked in warm, soapy water (if some of the fecal matter is difficult to remove, leave wet gauze or cloth on area for a few minutes before gently removing fecal matter); rinse and pat dry.	*Removes fecal matter from skin and stoma opening*

Action	Rationale
11. Dry skin thoroughly and apply new pouch device (see Procedure 8.16).	*Provides skin protection from fecal contaminants*
12. Remove gloves and restore or discard all equipment appropriately.	*Promotes clean environment*
13. Spray room deodorizer, if needed.	*Eliminates unpleasant odor*
14. Perform hand hygiene.	*Reduces microorganism transfer*

Evaluation

Were desired outcomes achieved? Examples of evaluation include:
- Desired outcome met: Stoma healing with no redness, edema, swelling, tears, breaks, ulceration, or fistulas at stoma area.
- Desired outcome not met: Client remains uncomfortable discussing body image changes.
- Desired outcome not met: Client performs procedure with 70% accuracy.

Documentation

The following should be noted on the client's chart:
- Procedure completion with date and time and color, consistency, and amount of stool in pouch
- Condition of stoma and peristomal skin
- Abdominal assessment
- Emotional status of client
- Verbal and nonverbal indicators of altered self-concept during procedure
- Verbal and nonverbal indicators of readiness to perform self-care
- Teaching and client participation in performance of procedure
- Additional teaching needs of client

Sample Documentation
Date: 1/1/05
Time: 1100

Stoma care reluctantly observed by client with poor return demonstration. Discarded large amount of semiformed brown stool. Stoma pink and moist; peristomal and abdominal skin intact without erythema, excoriation, or abnormal discharge. New pouch applied. Client states, "I hate the look of it." Discussed client coping related to body image changes.

Irrigating a Colostomy

Purpose

Facilitates emptying of colon

Equipment

- IV pole or wall hook
- Irrigation bag and tubing
- Irrigation cone
- Water-soluble lubricant
- Toilet (or toilet chair)
- Warm saline or tap water
- Bath thermometer
- Two towels and two washcloths
- Two disposable water-proof bed pads
- Mild soap (without oils, perfumes, or creams)
- Room deodorizer
- Bath basin or sink
- Fresh pouch
- 2 pairs nonsterile gloves

Assessment

Assessment should focus on the following:
- Doctor's order for frequency of irrigation and type and amount of solution
- Type of colostomy and nature of drainage
- Client's ability and preference to perform colostomy care
- Client teaching needs

Nursing Diagnoses

Nursing diagnoses may include the following:
- Constipation related to immobility, decreased fluid intake, or surgery
- Acute abdominal pain related to constipation
- Disturbed body image related to fecal diversion

Outcome Identification and Planning

Desired Outcomes

Sample desired outcomes include the following:
- Client will have a bowel movement after colostomy irrigation.
- Client indicates pain is relieved after irrigation.
- Client will express positive feelings about self.

Special Considerations in Planning and Implementation

General

The procedure can be performed in the bathroom or at the bedside. If no stool returns and irrigant is retained, reposition client and apply drainable pouch, if needed. You may have client ambulate, if permissible. Notify doctor if there is no return or if abdominal distention is noted. Distention of the colon with irrigation fluid can cause a vasovagal reaction (bradycardia, hypotension, and possible loss of consciousness). Therefore, the initial irrigation should be performed with the client in bed.

Pediatric

Routine irrigations are seldom done for the purpose of bowel regulation. Caution should be exercised because of the small size of the stoma.

Home Health

If the homebound client plans to irrigate colostomy while sitting on the toilet, teach client the proper procedure and have the client demonstrate it to you. Correct client's technique, if necessary.

Delegation

This procedure may be delegated to unlicensed assistive personnel only for an established ostomy. Emphasize importance of observations of stoma for irritation or other problems. Check agency policy.

Implementation

Action	Rationale
1. Perform hand hygiene and organize equipment.	*Reduces microorganism transfer; promotes efficiency*
2. Explain procedure to client.	*Reduces anxiety*
3. Obtain extra lighting, if needed.	*Ensures proper amount of light to perform procedure*
4. Provide for warmth and privacy.	*Promotes comfort and reduces embarrassment*
5. Prepare irrigating solution and tubing as follows:	
• Obtain irrigation bag and solution (usually tepid water); use 250 to 500 mL for initial irrigation, 500 to 1,000 mL for subsequent irrigations (minimal amounts are recommended).	*Allows bowel to adjust to fluid pressure*
• Check temperature of solution (should feel warm to touch but not hot). Place in warm water bath if necessary to increase solution temperature.	*Prevents injury from hot solution or cramping from cold solution*

Action	Rationale
• Close tubing clamp. • Fill bag with tap water or ordered solution at appropriate temperature. • Open clamp and expel air from tubing. • Close off clamp. 6. Put on gloves. 7. Place client comfortably in any of the following positions (place disposable waterproof pad under client if performing procedure in bed): • On toilet • Sitting on chair facing toilet • In side-lying position, turned toward side of stomal opening, with head of bed elevated 30 to 45 degrees • In supine position	*Allows for control of fluid flow* *Prepares irrigation solution* *Prevents air from infusing into bowel* *Allows for control of fluid flow* *Prevents nurse's contact with client's body secretions* *Provides for effective irrigation*
8. Gently remove pouch from stomal area.	*Avoids skin irritation or injury*
9. Assess site for redness, swelling, tenderness, and excoriation.	*Determines need for other skin-care measures*
10. Gently wash stoma area with warm, soapy water.	*Removes secretions*
11. Rinse with clear water and dry thoroughly.	*Removes soap and prevents irritation of stoma and surrounding skin area*
12. Apply irrigation sleeve and belt. The round opening of the irrigation sleeve fits over the stoma and the belt fits around the client's waist.	*Holds irrigation bag in place to prevent spillage*
13. Position irrigation bag (with tubing attached) 18 inches above stoma (approximately shoulder level). Lubricate the cone tip of the tubing with water-soluble gel.	*Avoids undue pressure on mucosal tissues from rushing of fluid; prevents irritation of stoma tissue*
14. Place lower end of sleeve into toilet or large bedpan and unclamp.	*Provides receptacle for drainage and begins flow of irrigant*
15. Expose stoma through upper opening of sleeve.	*Provides access to stoma for insertion of irrigation tubing*

Action	Rationale
16. Gently ease lubricated cone into stoma opening (Fig. 8.21). Hold tip securely in place to prevent backflow.	*Prevents escape of bowel contents onto skin*
17. Release irrigation tubing clamp and allow solution to infuse over 10 to 15 minutes (Fig. 8.22).	*Slow infusion prevents cramping from overdistention.*
18. Encourage client to take slow, deep breaths as solution is infusing.	*Relaxes client and decreases cramping of bowel*
19. If client complains of cramping, stop infusion for several minutes; then resume infusion slowly.	*Allows bowel time to adjust to fluid*
20. Clamp tubing and remove after all the solution has emptied out of bag.	*Completes irrigation*
21. Observe for return of fecal material and solution, and assess drainage.	*Indicates effectiveness of irrigation*
22. Remove bottom of sleeve from drainage receptacle and flush toilet or empty and clean bedpan.	*Restores room cleanliness*
23. Dry bottom of sleeve and clamp.	*Prevents soiling and collects further drainage*
24. Remove irrigation sleeve and belt.	*Concludes irrigation procedure*

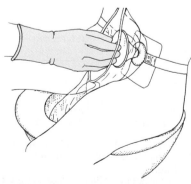

FIGURE 8.21

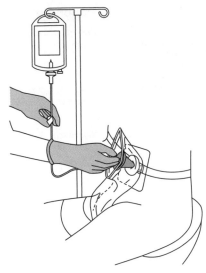

FIGURE 8.22

Action	Rationale
25. Discard or restore equipment.	*Promotes clean, organized environment*
26. Discard old gloves and put on new pair.	*Reduces contamination*
27. Wash, rinse, and dry stoma area.	*Cleanses peristomal area*
28. Apply new dressing or ostomy pouch, if needed. Spray room deodorizer.	*Restores ostomy dressing pouch; removes offensive odors*
29. Remove gloves and perform hand hygiene.	*Reduces microorganism transfer*

Evaluation

Were desired outcomes achieved? Examples of evaluation include:

● Desired outcome met: Client states abdominal pain relieved after irrigation.
● Desired outcome partially met: Client performed procedure accurately but had only small amount of hard formed stool after procedure.
● Desired outcome not met: Client indicates doubt about ability to deal with having a stoma.

Documentation

The following should be noted on the client's chart:
- Condition of stoma site
- Type and amount of irrigant infused
- Date and time and color, consistency, and amount of stool evacuated
- Client tolerance for procedure
- Client teaching accomplished or needed

Sample Documentation
Date: 1/1/05
Time: 1100

Colostomy irrigation done with 600 mL tap water infused. Client tolerated procedure without cramping or pain and states abdominal "fullness" relieved. Client demonstrated correct technique, but only a small amount of hard stool was evacuated. Stoma site clean and moist without irritation.

● Nursing Procedure 8.20

Testing Stool for Occult Blood With Hemoccult Slide 🖐

Purpose

Obtains stool specimen to detect occult blood related to gastrointestinal bleeding and anemia
Serves as a screening test for colorectal cancer

Equipment

- Stool specimen
- Hemoccult specimen collection card
- Chemical reagent (developer)
- Tongue blade
- Nonsterile gloves
- Stop watch or watch with second hand
- Specimen container labels
- Pen

Assessment

Assessment should focus on the following:
● Specific orders regarding specimen collection
● Characteristics of stool
● Manifestations of gastrointestinal bleeding or anemia
● History of gastrointestinal bleeding or anemia
● Dietary intake of foods or drugs that could alter test reliability
● Intake of medications that cause occult bleeding (aspirin, anticoagulants, NSAIDs, or steroids)

Nursing Diagnoses

Nursing diagnoses may include the following:
● Deficient knowledge related to the procedure or need for this test

Outcome Identification and Planning

Desired Outcomes

Sample desired outcomes include the following:
● Client will verbalize the purpose and procedure of this test.
● Client will collect the specimen accurately.

Special Considerations in Planning and Implementation

General

Many clients are placed on special diagnostic diets 2 to 3 days before Hemoccult testing. Emphasize to client the importance of adhering to diet restrictions. Some vitamins and minerals (such as vitamin C and iron) can cause erratic test results. Consult a pharmacy reference for a complete listing of such preparations and the amounts necessary to alter results.

Implementation

Action	Rationale
1. Perform hand hygiene.	*Reduces microorganism transfer*
2. Explain procedure to client.	*Decreases anxiety*
3. Provide privacy.	*Decreases embarrassment*
4. Put on clean gloves.	*Reduces nurse's exposure to client's body secretions*
5. Obtain stool specimen with tongue blade, and after opening the front flap, smear thin specimen onto guaiac test paper:	*Prepares specimen for test*

Action	Rationale
• Smear specimen, taken from inner surface of stool, onto slot A on front of card. • Smear a second specimen from another part of stool onto slot B on front of card • Close front flap of card.	
6. Turn card over and open back flap; apply two drops of reagent (color of reagent bottle label must match color stripe on the card) to slot over both A and B specimens and the control stripe. Wait 60 seconds and ensure control turns blue.	*Activates chemical components necessary for results*
7. Read results (consult product instructions for visual comparison): • If either slot has bluish discoloration, test is positive. • If there is no bluish discoloration, test is negative.	*Determines if results are positive or negative*
8. Restore or discard equipment appropriately (test card may be discarded).	*Promotes clean environment*
9. Remove gloves and perform hand hygiene.	*Reduces microorganism transfer*

Evaluation

Were desired outcomes achieved? Examples of evaluation include:
• Desired outcome not met: Client applied fecal smears to back side of card.
• Desired outcome not met: Additional teaching required.

Documentation

The following should be noted on the client's chart:
• Amount, color, odor, and consistency of stool obtained
• Specimen collection time
• Signs and symptoms consistent with gastrointestinal bleeding

Sample Documentation
Date: 1/1/05
Time: 1100

Large amount of soft, formed, dark brown stool. Client reports no discomfort during defecation. No signs or symptoms of gastrointestinal bleeding. Attempted first stool testing for occult blood with Hemoccult slide. Client did not apply smear correctly; re-education completed.

Activity
and Mobility

OVERVIEW

- The ability to remain physically active and mobile is essential in maintaining health and well-being. Immobility may pose psychological as well as physiologic hazards. Nurses should be alert for the following physical complications of immobility:
  - Hypostatic pneumonia
  - Pulmonary embolism
  - Thrombophlebitis
  - Orthostatic hypotension
  - Pressure ulcers or pressure areas
  - Decreased peristalsis with constipation and fecal impaction
  - Urinary stasis with renal calculi formation
  - Contractures and muscle atrophy
  - Altered fluid and electrolyte status
- Proper positioning and correct support surfaces are important factors in managing tissue loads.
- Psychological hazards of immobility may range from feelings of powerlessness to mild anxiety to psychosis.
- Major nursing diagnostic labels related to activity and mobility include impaired physical mobility, risk for injury, activity intolerance, risk for peripheral neurovascular dysfunction, and risk for disuse syndrome.

- Unlicensed assistive personnel should receive training on how to move or transfer clients and monitor for signs of complications, but routine monitoring remains the responsibility of the nurse.
- Some techniques should be delegated only to assistive personnel who have been specifically trained or certified in physical rehabilitation maneuvers.

● **Nursing Procedure 9.1**

Positioning the Body 🖐

Purpose

Maintains body alignment
Maintains skin integrity (facilitates pressure distribution, prevents friction and shear on tissue)
Prevents injury to and deformities of the musculoskeletal system
Promotes comfort
Promotes optimal lung expansion
Positions client for a variety of clinical procedures

Equipment

- Support devices required by client (e.g., draw sheet, trochanter roll, footboard, heel protectors, sandbags, hand rolls, foam wedges)
- Pillow for head, plus extra pillows for proper alignment and support
- Gloves if contact with body fluids is likely

Assessment

Assessment should focus on the following:
- Client's age and medical diagnosis
- Client's physical ability to maintain position
- Integumentary and musculoskeletal assessment
- Risk for pressure ulcers
- Length of time client has maintained present body positioning
- Doctor's orders for specific restrictions in positioning client or for special position required for procedure

Nursing Diagnoses

Nursing diagnoses may include the following:
- Risk for impaired skin integrity related to mechanical factors (pressure) and physical immobilization
- Impaired physical mobility related to decreased muscle strength

Outcome Identification and Planning

Desired Outcomes

Sample desired outcomes include the following:
- Client's skin is warm, dry, intact, and without discoloration over pressure points.
- Client can perform active right limb range of motion without pain.

Special Considerations in Planning and Implementation

General

To avoid injury when positioning clients, it is important that the client and caregiver have good body alignment and that appropriate body mechanics are used (see Nursing Procedure 1.1). Secure assistance as needed for the safe repositioning of the client. NEVER BECOME SO IMPATIENT THAT YOU TAKE RISKS. Foot drop, pressure ulcers, shoulder subluxation, and internal and external rotation of large joint areas are complications that can be prevented if the client is positioned and supported correctly. Use pillows, trochanter rolls, footboards, and other supportive equipment to maintain body alignment. Prevent joint and ligament pulling. Make sure the head, feet, and hands do not droop and that large joint areas do not rotate internally or externally. Avoid putting excess pressure on any body area. Immobile clients with existing pressure ulcers who are at risk for new ulcers should not be positioned directly on their trochanters. Clients at high risk for skin breakdown may need to be repositioned more frequently than every 2 hours.

Geriatric

Bedridden elderly clients are particularly susceptible to impaired skin integrity if they are not repositioned frequently because they have less subcutaneous fat and skin that is less elastic, thinner, drier, and thus more fragile than that of a younger person.

Home Health

In the home, pillows, sofa cushions, or rolled linens may be used for positioning. A recliner may be used to maintain a Fowler's or semi-Fowler's position. Family caregivers should be taught appropriate body mechanics and proper repositioning techniques. Have them show competency by return demonstration.

End-of-Life Care

Care should be given to prevent complications of immobility that would compromise quality of life. If pain is a consideration, analgesia should be given.

Cost-Cutting Tips

High-topped canvas shoes may be used to maintain neutral ankle position to prevent foot drop.

Implementation

Action	Rationale
1. Obtain assistance, as needed.	*Prevents back and muscle strain in nurse and injury to client*
2. Perform hand hygiene.	*Reduces microorganism transfer*
3. Explain procedure to client, emphasizing the importance of repositioning at least every 2 hours and maintaining the proper position.	*Decreases anxiety; increases compliance; prevents complications of immobility*
4. Provide privacy.	*Decreases embarrassment*
5. Adjust bed to comfortable working height.	*Prevents back and muscle strain in nurse*
6. Place or assist client into appropriate position. Avoid dragging client on sheet or bed. Various positions are illustrated in Figure 9.1 and described in Table 9.1.	*Avoids shearing of skin tissue*
7. Use the following guidelines to reposition client:	
• Secure all equipment, lines, and drains attached to client.	*Prevents accidental dislodgment and injury*
• Close off drains, if necessary (remember to reopen them after positioning client).	*Prevents reflux of drainage*
• Designate an assistant to handle extremities bound by immobilizers (e.g., casts, splints) or equipment that must be moved with client (e.g., traction apparatus).	*Maintains stability of body part; prevents injury and pain*
• Maintain head elevation for clients prone to dyspnea when flat; allow brief rest periods, as needed, during procedure.	*Facilitates breathing and reduces anxiety; prevents overexertion*
• When moving client to side of bed, move major portions of the body sequentially from	*Maintains body alignment; facilitates comfort*

A. Fowler's

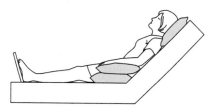

B. Supine

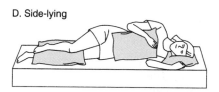

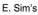

C. Prone

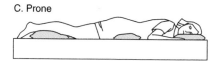

D. Side-lying

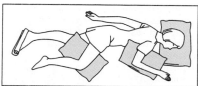

E. Sim's

FIGURE 9.1

F. Lithotomy

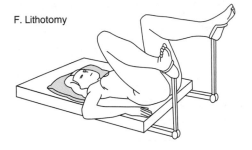

G. Dorsal Recumbent

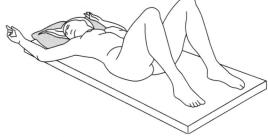

FIGURE 9.1 (continued)

Action	Rationale
top to bottom or vice versa (e.g., head and shoulders first, trunk and hips second, legs last). This method is contraindicated in clients with spinal instability (see Nursing Procedure 9.2).	
• Use pillows, trochanter rolls, and special positioning supports as needed to maintain body alignment and normal position of extremities and to avoid placing undue pressure on vulnerable skin surfaces.	*Maintains correct alignment; prevents injury; promotes comfort; balances weight to manage tissue load*

● Table 9.1 Body Positioning

Position	Purpose	Description
Fowler's (low to high)	Improves breathing capacity Prevents aspiration Promotes comfort	Head of bed up 30 to 90 degrees Client in a semisitting position Knees slightly flexed
Supine	Prevents bending at crucial areas (e.g., groin or spine) after diagnostic procedures	Client flat on back in bed Body straight and in alignment Feet protected with footboard to support 90-degree flexion
Prone	Serves as positioning alternative in turning procedure for immobilized clients	Client flat on abdomen with knees slightly flexed Head turned to side Arms flexed at sides, hands near head Feet over end of mattress or protected with footboard to support normal flexion
Side-lying (lateral)	Serves as position for some procedures and alternative position for turning procedures	Client lying on side with upper leg flexed at hip and knee Top arm flexed Lower arm flexed and shoulder positioned to avoid pulling and excessive weight of body or shoulder
Sims	Serves as position for some procedures and alternative position for turning procedure	Client halfway between side-lying and prone positions with bottom knee slightly flexed Knee and hip of top leg flexed (about 90 degrees) Lower arm behind back Upper arm flexed, hand near head
Lithotomy	Places client in position for vaginal or anorectal exams	Client on back with legs flexed 90 degrees at hips and knees Feet up in stirrups
Dorsal recumbent	Places client in position for vaginal exams and insertion of catheters	Client on back with legs flexed at hips and knees Feet flat on mattress
Modified Trendelenburg's	Places client in "shock" position to increase blood flow to heart and cerebral tissue	Client flat on back with legs straight and elevated at hips Head and shoulders slightly raised

Note: Pillows and other support equipment are placed to support alignment and normal flexion points anc to prevent pressure on any body area.

Action	Rationale
• Be certain that client's face is not pressed into bed or pillow while turning and that body position does not prevent full expansion of diaphragm.	*Maintains adequate respirations*
• Use appropriate body mechanics (see Nursing Procedure 1.1).	*Prevents injury*
8. Assess client's alignment, comfort, and character of respirations; recheck client periodically.	*Determines if position adjustment is needed*
9. Once client is positioned, lift side rails, lock wheels, and place bed in low position. If traction apparatus is being used, be certain that weights are not dragging on floor or touching bed or wall and that line of pull is unchanged.	*Prevents falls; prevents injury or disruption of therapy*
10. Place call light within reach.	*Facilitates communication*
11. Move overbed table close to bed and place frequently used items on table.	*Places items used frequently within easy reach*
12. Perform hand hygiene.	*Decreases microorganism transfer*

Evaluation

Were desired outcomes achieved? Examples of evaluation include:
• Desired outcome met: Client's skin is warm, dry, intact, and without discoloration over pressure points.
• Desired outcome met: Client can perform active right limb range of motion without pain.

Documentation

The following should be noted on the client's chart:
• Client's position
• Any equipment, lines, or drains attached to client
• Client reports of pain, dyspnea, discomfort
• Exertion or dyspnea observed during repositioning
• Abnormal findings on integumentary assessment
• Status of equipment needed for stabilization of body parts (e.g., traction, casts, immobilizers)
• Special positioning supports used
• Teaching regarding importance of maintaining position

Sample Documentation
Date: 2/17/05
Time: 2100

Repositioned into right side-lying position. Slight shortness of breath reported during repositioning. No complaint of pain. Given a brief rest period and no further shortness of breath reported. Skin intact without redness or discoloration over bony prominences.

● Nursing Procedure 9.2

Positioning the Body via Logrolling 🖐

Purpose

Prevents injury to unstable spine by maintaining correct alignment without tension on spinal column, thus maintaining present level of neurologic functioning

Maintains body alignment

Maintains skin integrity (facilitates pressure distribution, prevents friction and shear on tissue)

Prevents injury to and deformities of the musculoskeletal system

Promotes comfort

Promotes optimal lung expansion

Equipment

- Support devices required by client (e.g., drawsheet, trochanter roll, footboard, heel protectors, sandbags, hand rolls, foam wedges)
- Several pillows needed for proper alignment and support
- Gloves if contact with body fluids is likely

Assessment

Assessment should focus on the following:
- Physician's orders for activity (logrolling)
- Neurologic status
- Urinary bladder and bowel function (continence)
- Reports of pain or discomfort

Nursing Diagnoses

Nursing diagnoses may include the following:
- Impaired physical mobility related to musculoskeletal/neuromuscular impairment
- Risk for impaired skin integrity related to physical immobilization
- Risk for disuse syndrome related to prescribed immobilization
- Risk for injury related to physical alterations of the spine

Outcome Identification and Planning

Desired Outcomes

Sample desired outcomes include the following:
- The client's neurologic status is maintained.
- No signs or symptoms of complications of immobility are present (e.g., pressure ulcers or pressure areas, contractures, decreased peristalsis, constipation and fecal impaction, orthostatic hypotension, pulmonary embolism, thrombophlebitis).

Special Considerations in Planning and Implementation

General

Following spinal surgery or trauma, clients who are immobile should be repositioned by logrolling until activity restrictions are clarified with the physician. To maintain cervical spinal alignment, place a pillow under the client's head with the client in the side-lying position. Clients with known or suspected cervical spine injury should wear a cervical collar. Ask the physician if a pillow under the head is allowed in the supine position; this may be contraindicated for some clients.

Pediatric

Demonstrate the procedure using a doll, and instruct the child to perform simple techniques on the doll. Depending on developmental age, the use of orthotics (braces) may required.

Geriatric

Elderly clients are particularly prone to skin breakdown when they are bedridden and not repositioned frequently because they have less subcutaneous fat and their skin is less elastic, thinner, drier, and more fragile than that of a younger person. They also have an increased incidence of other complications related to immobility, such as pneumonia, thrombophlebitis, and constipation.

End-of-Life Care

Care should be given to prevent complications of immobility that would compromise quality of life. If pain is a consideration, analgesia should be given.

Home Health

In the home, pillows, sofa cushions, or rolled linens may be used for positioning. Family caregivers should be taught appropriate body mechanics and repositioning techniques using logrolling. Have them show competency by return demonstration.

Delegation

Ascertain that assistive personnel have been trained in the logrolling technique. Reinforce the importance of monitoring the cardiopulmonary status of clients likely to experience breathing difficulty, chest pain, or general discomfort.

 Cost-Cutting Tips

High-topped canvas shoes may be used to maintain neutral ankle position to prevent foot drop.

Implementation

Action	Rationale
1. Obtain assistance.	*Prevents back and muscle strain in nurse and injury to client*
2. Perform hand hygiene.	*Reduces microorganism transfer*
3. Explain procedure to client, emphasizing importance of maintaining a rigid position with the spine straight and arms folded across the chest while being turned.	*Decreases anxiety; increases compliance; facilitates turning without twisting spine*
4. Provide privacy.	*Decreases embarrassment*
5. Adjust bed to comfortable working height.	*Prevents back and muscle strain in nurse*
6. Use the following guidelines in repositioning client:	
• Secure all equipment, lines, and drains attached to client.	*Prevents accidental dislodgment and injury*
• Close off drains, if necessary (remember to reopen them after positioning client).	*Prevents reflux of drainage*
• The nurse and one assistant stand on the side of the bed opposite the side the client will face following the turn. Another assistant stands on the side of the bed that the client will turn toward.	*Prevents back and muscle strain in nurse and injury to client*

Action	Rationale
• Place pillows between client's legs from thighs to feet. Place pillow in position to support head, preventing lateral flexion. (Have additional pillows available for support following the turn.)	*Maintains body alignment*
• Using appropriate body mechanics (see Nursing Procedure 1.1), move client to side of the bed toward the nurse and assistant.	*Prevents injury; prevents body from being too close to the rail after repositioning*
• Instruct client to fold arms across chest to maintain body in a straight, rigid position.	*Maintains correct alignment; prevents injury*
• The nurse and assistant grasp the drawsheet, turning the client toward the assistant on the opposite side of the bed. The assistant on the other side of the bed grasps the drawsheet, stabilizing the client (Fig. 9.2), while the nurse and other assistant place pillows or other support devices behind the client to maintain the spine in straight alignment. Client is then eased back against support structures.	*Balances weight to avoid shearing of skin tissue; promotes comfort*
• Use pillows, trochanter rolls, and special positioning supports as needed to maintain body alignment in a manner that keeps the spine in a neutral (straight) position, keeps extremities in a normal position, and avoids placing undue	*Maintains correct alignment; prevents injury and promotes comfort; balances weight to manage tissue load*

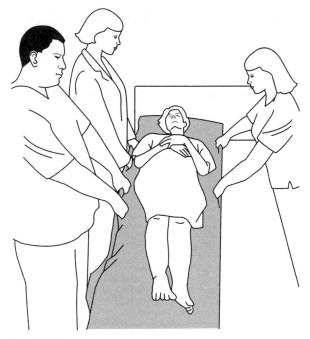

FIGURE 9.2

Action	Rationale
pressure on vulnerable skin surfaces.	
• Be certain that client's face is not pressed into bed or pillow while turning and that body position does not prevent full expansion of diaphragm.	*Maintains adequate respirations*
7. Assess client's alignment, neurovascular status, comfort, and character of respirations. Reassess client periodically.	*Determines if position adjustment is needed*
8. Once client is positioned, lift side rails, lock wheels, and place bed in low position.	*Prevents falls*

Action	Rationale
9. Place call light within reach.	*Facilitates communication while preventing twisting of spine*
10. Move overbed table close to bed and place frequently used items on table.	*Places items used frequently within easy reach*
11. Perform hand hygiene.	*Decreases microorganism transfer*

Evaluation

Were desired outcomes achieved? Examples of evaluation include:
• Desired outcome met: Client's neurologic status is maintained.
• Desired outcome met: No signs or symptoms of complications of immobility are present.

Documentation

The following should be noted on the client's chart:
• Client's position
• Any equipment, lines, or drains attached to client
• Client reports of pain, dyspnea, discomfort
• Exertion or dyspnea observed during repositioning
• Abnormal findings regarding integumentary or neurovascular assessment
• Status of equipment needed for stabilization of body parts (e.g., pillows, foam wedges, orthotics)
• Special positioning supports used
• Teaching regarding importance of maintaining position

Sample Documentation
Date: 2/17/05
Time: 2100

Repositioned via logrolling into right side-lying position. Pillows under head, left arm, and between legs to maintain correct spinal alignment. Denies numbness, tingling, or burning to extremities. Sensation and movement of extremities intact. Urinary bladder and bowel continence intact. Denies dyspnea or pain. Skin intact without redness, bruising, or discoloration over bony prominences. Client states need to keep back straight without twisting to prevent injury to spinal cord.

Performing Range-of-Motion Exercises 👋

Purpose

Maintains present level of functioning and mobility of joints and muscles

Prevents contractures and shortening of musculoskeletal structures

Facilitates circulation and prevents vascular complications of immobility

Facilitates comfort

Equipment

No equipment needed except gloves if contact with body fluids is likely

Assessment

Assessment should focus on the following:
- Medical diagnosis
- Doctor's orders for specific restrictions
- Present range of motion of each area
- Physical and mental ability of client to perform the activity, including normal age-related changes
- History of factors that contraindicate or limit the type or amount of exercise

Nursing Diagnoses

Nursing diagnoses may include the following:
- Impaired physical mobility related to decreased muscle strength and joint stiffness
- Risk for impaired skin integrity related to physical immobilization
- Risk for disuse syndrome related to prescribed immobilization

Outcome Identification and Planning

Desired Outcomes

Sample desired outcomes include the following:
- Client's present range of motion is maintained.
- Range of motion of left elbow increases from 30- to 40-degree flexion.

- No signs or symptoms of complications of immobility are present (e.g., pressure ulcers or pressure areas, contractures, decreased peristalsis, constipation and fecal impaction, orthostatic hypotension, pulmonary embolism, thrombophlebitis).

Special Considerations in Planning and Implementation

General

A client able to perform all or part of a range-of-motion exercise program should be allowed to do so and should be properly instructed. Observe the client performing activities of daily living to determine the limitations of movement and the need, if any, for passive range-of-motion exercise to various joints. When performing a range-of-motion exercise, a joint should be moved only to the point of resistance, pain, or spasm, whichever comes first. Consult doctor's orders before performing a range-of-motion exercise on a client with acute cardiac, vascular, or pulmonary problems or on a client with skin grafts, musculoskeletal trauma, or acute flare-ups of arthritis.

Pediatric

Demonstrate the procedure using a doll, and instruct the child to perform simple techniques on the doll.

Geriatric

For elderly clients with various chronic conditions, use extra caution when performing range-of-motion exercises. Clients with chronic cardiopulmonary conditions should be observed closely during range-of-motion activity for respiratory difficulty, chest pain, and general discomfort. Decreased muscle mass, degenerative changes of joints, and degenerative connective tissue changes result in limited range of motion.

End-of-Life Care

Care should be given to prevent complications of immobility that would compromise quality of life. If pain is a consideration, analgesia should be given.

Home Health

Teach family members how to perform range-of-motion techniques between nurse visits. Have them show competency by return demonstration.

Delegation

Ascertain that assistive personnel have been trained in range-of-motion exercises. Reinforce the importance of monitoring the cardiopulmonary status of clients likely to experience breathing difficulty, chest pain, or general discomfort.

Implementation

Action	Rationale
1. Perform hand hygiene.	*Reduces microorganism transfer*
2. Explain procedure to client.	*Decreases anxiety*
3. Provide privacy.	*Decreases embarrassment*
4. Adjust bed to comfortable working height.	*Prevents back and muscle strain in nurse*
5. Move client to side of bed closest to you.	*Facilitates use of proper body mechanics*
6. Beginning at top and moving downward on one side of body at a time, perform passive (or instruct client through active) range-of-motion exercises of joints in each of the following areas, as applicable for client: • Head and neck (Fig. 9.3A, B) • Spine (Fig. 9.3C) • Shoulder (Fig. 9.3D-F) • Elbow (Fig. 9.3G) • Forearm and hand (Fig. 9.3H) • Wrist (Fig. 9.3I) • Fingers (Fig. 9.3J, K) • Hips (Fig. 9.3L-N) • Knees (Fig. 9.3O, P) • Toes (Fig. 9.3Q, R) • Ankles (Fig. 9.3S, T)	*Exercises all articular areas (joints) and associated muscle groups*
7. For passive range of motion, support the body area being exercised by holding it in the rounded palms of	*Prevents pulling and careless handling of extremity, which could result in pain or injury*

HEAD-NECK

A   Flexion   Extension

FIGURE 9.3

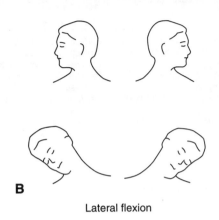

B

Lateral flexion

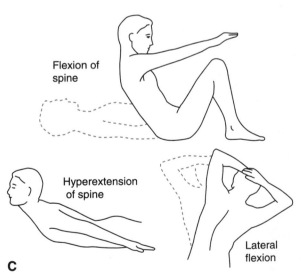

Flexion of spine

Hyperextension of spine

Lateral flexion

C

FIGURE 9.3 (continued)

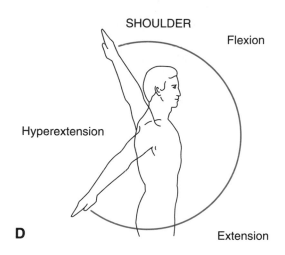

SHOULDER

Flexion

Hyperextension

D

Extension

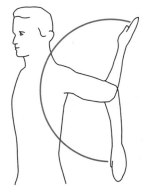

External rotation

E   Internal rotation

FIGURE 9.3 (continued)

SHOULDER *(continued)*

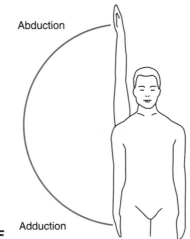

F

ELBOW

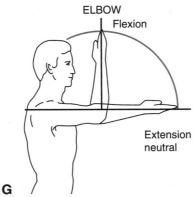

G

FIGURE 9.3 (continued)

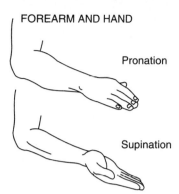

FOREARM AND HAND

Pronation

Supination

H

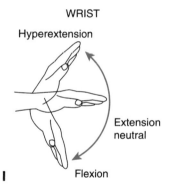

WRIST

Hyperextension

Extension neutral

Flexion

I

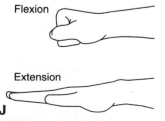

FINGERS

Flexion

Extension

J

FIGURE 9.3 (continued)

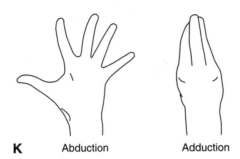

K   Abduction   Adduction

HIPS

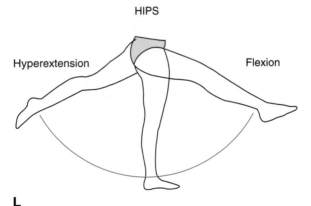

Hyperextension   Flexion

L

FIGURE 9.3 (continued)

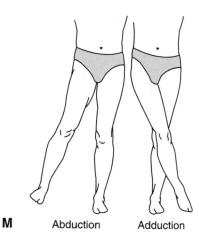

M   Abduction   Adduction

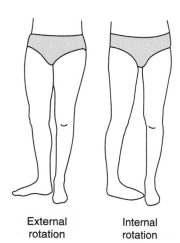

N   External   Internal
        rotation   rotation

FIGURE 9.3 (continued)

KNEE

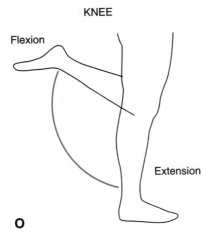

Flexion

Extension

O

KNEE *(continued)*

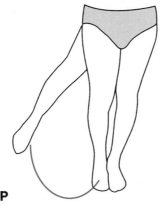

P

FIGURE 9.3 (continued)

TOES

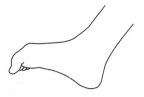

Flexion

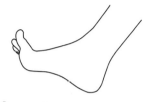

Q   Extension

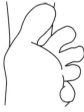   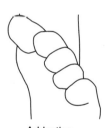

R   Abduction   Adduction

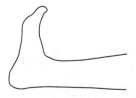   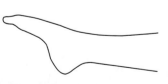

Dorsiflexion   Plantar flexion

S

FIGURE 9.3 (continued)

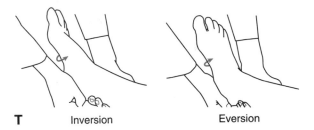

T   Inversion   Eversion

FIGURE 9.3 (continued)

Action	Rationale
your hands as maneuvers are performed (Fig. 9.4): • Arms at elbow and wrist • Legs at knee and ankle • Head at occipital area and chin	
8. Slowly move each area through full range of positions 3 to 10 times or as tolerated by client (Table 9.2 defines each motion).	*Provides adequate exercise of extremity*
9. Observe client for signs of exertion or discomfort while performing range-of-motion exercises.	*Alerts nurse for cues to terminate activity*
10. Return client to middle of bed, replace covers, and position client for comfort and in proper body alignment.	*Promotes comfort; maintains correct alignment*
11. Assess vital signs.	*Provides follow-up data regarding effects of activity on client*

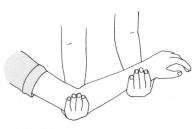

FIGURE 9.4

● Table 9.2 Descriptions of Range-of-Motion Maneuvers

Maneuver	Description	Applicable Areas
Flexion	Bending joint at point or normal anatomic fold	All areas
Extension	Straightening joint into as straight a line as possible	All areas
Hyperextension	Straightening joint into extension, then moving past that point	Neck, fingers, wrists, toes, spine
Abduction	Moving extremity away from midline of body	Arms, legs, fingers, toes
Adduction	Moving extremity toward midline of body	Arms, legs, fingers, toes
Internal rotation	Rotating extremity toward midline of body	Hips, ankles, shoulders
External rotation	Rotating extremity away from midline of body	Hips, ankles, shoulders
Supination	Turning palm upward	Hands
Pronation	Turning palm downward	Hands
Circumduction	Rotating extremity in a complete circle	Shoulders, hips

Action	Rationale
12. Lift side rails, lock wheels, and place bed in low position.	*Prevents falls*
13. Place call light within reach.	*Facilitates communication*
14. Perform hand hygiene.	*Reduces microorganism transfer*

Evaluation

Were desired outcomes achieved? Examples of evaluation include:
● Desired outcome met: Client's present range of motion was maintained.
● Desired outcome met: Range of motion of left elbow increased from 30- to 40-degree flexion.
● Desired outcome met: No signs or symptoms of complications of immobility are present.

Documentation

The following should be noted on the client's chart:
● Areas on which range-of-motion exercises are performed
● Areas of limited range of motion and the degree of limitation

- Areas of passive versus active range of motion
- Reports of pain or discomfort
- Observations of physiologic intolerance to activity

Sample Documentation
Date: 2/17/05
Time: 2100

*Active range-of-motion exercises performed on all
extremities, neck, and spine. Full range of motion of all
joints. No reports of pain or discomfort during exercises.
No signs of activity intolerance.*

● **Nursing Procedure 9.4**

Supporting Axillary Crutch Walking

Purpose

Facilitates mobility and activity for client
Increases self-esteem by decreasing dependence
Decreases physical stress on weight-bearing joints and skeletal
    injuries

Equipment

- Appropriate-size axillary crutches
- Safety belt (gait belt)
- Shoes
- Robe
- Eyeglasses or contacts, if worn

Assessment

Assessment should focus on the following:
- Medical diagnosis
- Doctor's orders for activity restrictions
- Type of crutch and gait movement indicated
- Neuromuscular status (e.g., muscle tone, strength, and range
  of motion of arms, legs, and trunk; gait pattern; body align-
  ment when walking; ability to maintain balance)
- Focal point of injury and reason for crutches
- Measurement parameters of crutches

- Ability of client to comprehend instructions regarding use of crutches
- Additional learning needs of client
- Nature of walking area (e.g., clutter, scatter rugs, traction, adequate rest area)
- General environment for safety hazards that could cause falls

Nursing Diagnoses

Nursing diagnoses may include the following:
- Risk for injury related to altered mobility
- Risk for peripheral neurovascular dysfunction related to mechanical compression (axillary crutches)
- Deficient knowledge regarding crutch-walking principles and techniques related to lack of exposure

Outcome Identification and Planning

Desired Outcomes

Sample desired outcomes include the following:
- Client does not fall while using crutches.
- Client demonstrates correct techniques for crutch-walking maneuvers.

Special Considerations in Planning and Implementation

General

Using crutches on slippery, cluttered surfaces and on stairs can be hazardous. Clients should use the railing of the staircase or walk close to the wall. Clients with visual deficits should wear visual aids. Alterations in balance and strength may prevent some clients from being able to use crutches safely. Walkers provide increased support and stability.

Pediatric

Children are especially prone to injuries from falls because of underdeveloped bones. Use safety belts when assisting these clients with crutch walking.

Geriatric

Older clients are especially prone to injuries from falls because of brittle bones. Use safety belts when assisting these clients with crutch walking. Allow extra time because of decreased muscle strength, decreased coordination, and functional changes in vision.

Home Health

Assess the home environment for hazards and adequate space. Help client rearrange furniture and other items to eliminate hazards while client is on crutches.

Delegation

Crutch walking should be delegated only to assistive personnel who have been trained in physical rehabilitation assistive techniques. Stress the importance of monitoring for fatigue and discomfort.

Implementation

Action	Rationale
1. Perform hand hygiene.	*Reduces microorganism transfer*
2. Explain procedure to client, emphasizing that it will take time to learn the techniques. Stress safety and the importance of moving slowly. Demonstrate the techniques while you explain.	*Decreases anxiety and frustration; increases compliance; prevents injury*
3. Assist client into comfortable shoes with nonskid, hard soles and low heels.	*Prevents falls*
4. Assist client into robe or loose, comfortable clothes.	*Facilitates comfort*
5. Measure client for correct axillary crutch fit:	*Prevents damage to brachial and radial nerves*
• If client is unstable while standing, have client lie flat in bed with proper shoes on (Fig. 9.5).	*Prevents falls*
• Align crutch tips approximately 6 inches to the side of and 6 inches to the front of each foot.	*Promotes stability and balance*
• Make sure the client's wrists are adjacent to the handgrips with the elbows extended.	*Avoids injury to nerves in the wrist*

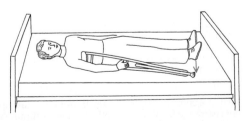

FIGURE 9.5

Action	Rationale
• Make sure the client's elbows are at approximately 30 degrees of flexion when hands are on handgrips; the top of the crutches should be 2 inches below the armpits.	*Avoids damage to brachial plexus, which can result in paralysis of extremity*
• Measure the distance between 2 inches below armpit and 6 inches to the front of and to the side of the foot.	*Determines appropriate length of axillary crutch*
6. Lower bed, lower rails, and lock wheels.	*Prevents falls*
7. Slowly help client into sitting position; assess for dizziness, faintness, or decreased orientation.	*Prevents injury from sudden change in blood pressure when sitting up*
8. Apply safety belt.	*Prevents falls*
9. Instruct client to put all of his or her weight on the handgrips. Client should avoid supporting his or her weight on the top of the crutch (Fig. 9.6).	*Avoids damage to brachial plexus, which can result in paralysis of extremity*
10. Assist client with maneuvers appropriate for type of gait and with other general crutch-walking techniques (see steps 11 and 12). Initially, always have someone stay with the client, but allow greater independence as he or she becomes more proficient and demonstrates ability to walk with crutches in all areas safely. Encourage client to use rails and walk close to wall when climbing stairs.	*Provides assistance and ensures client safety*
11. Demonstrate correct technique for type of gait to be used before client gets out of bed. Have client do a return demonstration. Reinforce instructions and make corrections as client performs crutch walking.	*Permits client to become familiar with maneuvers before attempting them*

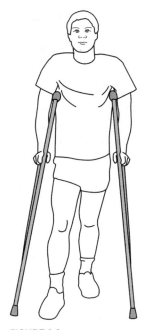

FIGURE 9.6

Action	Rationale
12. Begin demonstrating gait technique from tripod position with crutches 6 inches to side and 6 inches to front of each foot to promote stability and balance (Fig. 9.7).	
a. *Four-point gait:* Advance right crutch, then left foot, then left crutch, then right foot (Fig. 9.8).	*Places weight on legs while crutches provide stability; there are always three points*
b. *Three-point gait:* Advance both crutches and affected extremity at same time, then advance unaffected extremity (Fig. 9.9).	*Places weight on unaffected leg and crutches, with light weight on affected leg*
c. *Two-point gait:* Advance right crutch and left	*Places partial weight on both legs*

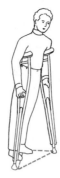

FIGURE 9.7

Action	Rationale
foot together, then left foot and right crutch together (Fig. 9.10). d. *Swing-to or swing-through gait:* Advance both crutches at same time and swing body forward to crutches or past them (Fig. 9.11).	*Provides additional stability for clients with bilateral leg disability*

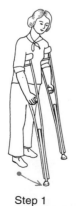 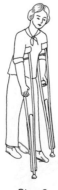 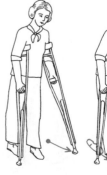 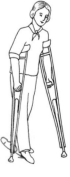

Step 1   Step 2   Step 3   Step 4

FIGURE 9.8

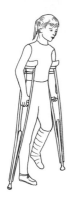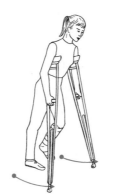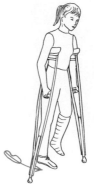

| Step 1 | Step 2 | Step 3 |

FIGURE 9.9

Action	Rationale
13. Demonstrate correct techniques for sitting, standing, and stair walking with crutches (Display 9.1).	
14. Instruct client to ascend stairs by leading with un-affected leg; crutches and affected leg follow together	*Promotes stability and balance*

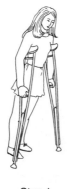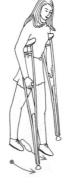

| Step 1 | Step 2 |

FIGURE 9.10

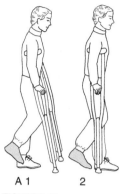 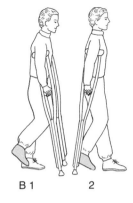

FIGURE 9.11

● Display 9.1 Techniques for General Crutch-Walking Maneuvers

Moving From Sitting to Standing

Place both crutches in hand on affected side (holding crutches together and even).

Push down on stable support base (locked bed, arm, or seat of chair) with free hand, put weight on stronger leg, and lift body.

Stand with a straight back, bearing weight on stronger leg and crutches.

Walking Up Stairs (see Fig. 9.12)

Place both crutches on same level as feet.

Advance unaffected leg to next step while bearing down on crutch handles.

Pull affected leg and crutches up to step while bearing weight on stronger leg.

Moving From Standing to Sitting

Inch backward until backs of lower legs touch bed or center of chair.

Hold crutches together in hand on unaffected side.

Begin easing down onto chair or bed with back straight, using crutches and stronger leg as support.

When close enough, gently hold on to arm of chair and complete the move.

Walking Down Stairs (see Fig. 9.13)

Place both crutches on same level as feet.

Shift weight to stronger leg.

Lower affected leg and crutches to next step while bearing down on crutch handles.

Advance unaffected leg last.

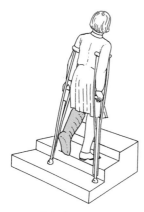

FIGURE 9.12

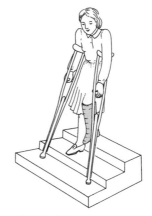

FIGURE 9.13

Action	Rationale
(Fig. 9.12). Descending the stairs is opposite: crutches and affected leg lead and the unaffected leg follows (Fig. 9.13). Remember: "Up with the good, down with the bad."	
15. Observe return demonstrations and help client practice until he or she becomes proficient in crutch walking. Provide praise and encouragement. Encourage rest between activity periods, assisting client, as needed, to a comfortable position.	*Ensures procedure has been learned; provides feedback*
16. Perform hand hygiene and properly store equipment.	*Reduces microorganism transfer; maintains order*

Evaluation

Were desired outcomes achieved? Examples of evaluation include:
- Desired outcome met: Client did not fall while using crutches.
- Desired outcome met: Client demonstrated correct techniques for crutch-walking maneuvers.

Documentation

The following should be noted on the client's chart:
- Gait pattern used
- Crutch height
- Steadiness of gait and amount of assistance needed
- Distance walked by client
- Client tolerance of procedure and comfort level
- Client instruction and return demonstration; additional learning needs of client

---

Sample Documentation
Date: 2/17/05
Time: 2100

Client completed first week of crutch walking. Demonstrates proper use of crutches by supporting weight on handgrips. Efficient with use of four-point gait pattern. Gait steady with good body alignment while on crutches. Walking entire hall length three times per day without fatigue or reports of discomfort. Has not begun stair walking.

● Nursing Procedure 9.5

Caring for a Cast 🖐

Purpose

Prevents neurovascular impairment of areas encircled by cast
Maintains cast for immobilization of injured area
Prevents infection

Equipment

- Washcloth
- Towel
- Soap
- Basin of warm water
- Linen savers for bed
- Pen
- Roll of 1- or 2-inch adhesive tape
- Pillows wrapped in linen saver or plastic bag
- Bed linens with draw sheet
- Gloves

Assessment

Assessment should focus on the following:
- Medical diagnosis
- Doctor's orders for special care of treatment area
- Client's report of pain or discomfort
- Integumentary status
- Neurovascular indicators of status of extremities, particularly of areas distal to cast: color, temperature, capillary refill, sensation, pulse quality, ability to move toes or fingers
- Indicators of infection (e.g., foul odor from cast, pain, fever, edema, extreme warmth over a particular area of cast)
- Indicators of complications of immobility: pressure ulcers or pressure areas, reduced joint movement, decreased peristalsis, constipation, fecal impaction, signs of pulmonary embolism (e.g., chest pain, dyspnea, wheezing, increased heart rate), signs of thrombophlebitis (e.g., redness, heat, swelling, or pain in local area)

Nursing Diagnoses

Nursing diagnoses may include the following:
- Risk for peripheral neurovascular dysfunction related to fracture, mechanical compression (cast), and immobilization
- Deficient knowledge regarding general cast care related to lack of exposure

Outcome Identification and Planning

Desired Outcomes

Sample desired outcomes include the following:
- Signs of neurovascular deficits are detected early.
- Complications resulting from neurovascular deficits are prevented.
- Client verbalizes actions necessary for cast maintenance by time of discharge.

Special Consideration in Planning and Implementation

General

Compartment syndrome may be manifested by severe pain unrelieved by analgesics that is out of proportion to the injury, or a sudden decrease in capillary refill and loss of pulse during first 24 to 48 hours after the cast is in place. Watch for these signs and symptoms. Drying time for synthetic casts is extremely quick (15 minutes) compared to plaster casts (up to 48 hours).

Pediatric

Provide care based on developmental level. Demonstrate the casting procedure using a doll or stuffed toy. Allow child to express concerns and understanding through play (e.g., have child teach doll not to stick things under the cast or get the cast wet).

Geriatric

Watch client closely during initial gait retraining; additional weight of cast could cause lack of balance and result in stress and fracture of fragile bones.

Home Health

Instruct the homebound client to prevent cast from getting wet in order to maintain the integrity of the cast. If the cast does get wet, the client can dry it using a hair dryer on the LOW setting. To prevent skin breakdown, instruct client not to use lotions, oils, or powder under the cast and not to stick objects under the cast.

Delegation

Instruct assistive personnel on transfer or moving of clients with casts. ROUTINE MONITORING OF THE CLIENT'S NEURO-VASCULAR STATUS REMAINS THE RESPONSIBILITY OF LICENSED PERSONNEL.

Implementation

Action	Rationale
1. Perform hand hygiene.	*Reduces microorganism transfer*
2. Place draw sheet and linen savers on bed before client returns from casting area (place these items on bed with each linen change).	*Promotes ease of positioning client; prevents pain when moving client*
3. Explain procedure to client, emphasizing importance of keeping extremity elevated and not handling wet cast. Explain why frequent assessment is important. Instruct client not to insert anything between cast and extremity. Reassure client that the casting material will feel warm as it dries but will cool when drying is complete.	*Decreases anxiety; increases compliance; prevents injury and infection*

Action	Rationale
4. Provide privacy.	*Decreases embarrassment*
5. Put on gloves.	*Avoids contact with body fluids*
6. Handle casted extremity or body area with palms of hands for first 24 to 48 hours or until cast is fully dry (Fig. 9.14).	*Avoids dents, which could result in edema and pressure areas*
7. If cast is slow to dry, place small fan directly facing cast (about 24 inches away). DO NOT PLACE LINEN OVER CAST UNTIL CAST IS DRY.	*Enhances speed of drying; allows air to circulate and assist in drying cast*
8. If cast is on extremity, elevate extremity on pillows (cover pillow with linen savers or plastic bags) so normal curvatures created with casting are maintained.	*Prevents edema; enhances venous return; prevents soiling pillows; prevents creation of flattened areas on cast as it dries; prevents pressure areas*
9. Wash excess antimicrobial agents (e.g., povidone) from skin. Rinse and pat dry.	*Allows for clear skin and vascular assessment*
10. Perform skin and neuro-vascular assessments every 30 minutes to 1 hour for first 24 hours, every 2 hours for next 24 hours, then every 4 hours thereafter. If cast is on extremity, compare to opposite extremity.	*Detects signs of abnormal neuro-vascular function, such as vascular or nerve compression; suggests possible nature of neurovascular deficit*
• If a short-leg cast has been applied, ensure there is sufficient room over the head of the fibula (distal and lateral to patella) to pre-	*Prevents nerve damage that would result in footdrop*

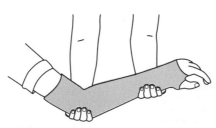

FIGURE 9.14

Action	Rationale
vent peroneal nerve impingement.	
11. If breakthrough bleeding is noted on cast, circle area and write date and time on cast. If there is a moderate to large amount of bleeding, notify doctor; otherwise, follow orders as written for bleeding.	*Provides baseline data for amount of bleeding; facilitates early intervention and prevention of complications*
12. Assess for signs of infection (e.g., purulent drainage, foul odor, fever).	*Detects infectious process at early stage*
13. Reposition client every 2 hours. If client has body or spica cast, secure three assistants to help turn client.	*Prevents client discomfort; makes turning quick, efficient, and safe*
14. Provide back and skin care frequently.	*Prevents skin breakdown*
15. If flaking of cast around edges is noted, remove flakes and apply tape over cast edges: • Cut tape so that one edge is flat and the other is rounded (Fig. 9.15). • Place rounded side of tape on outside of cast and fold flat side of tape over edge of cast. • Continue taping edge of cast, overlapping each "petal" of tape in this manner until the edges of the cast have been covered with tape (Fig. 9.16).	*Prevents accumulation of particles inside cast, which can cause skin breakdown*

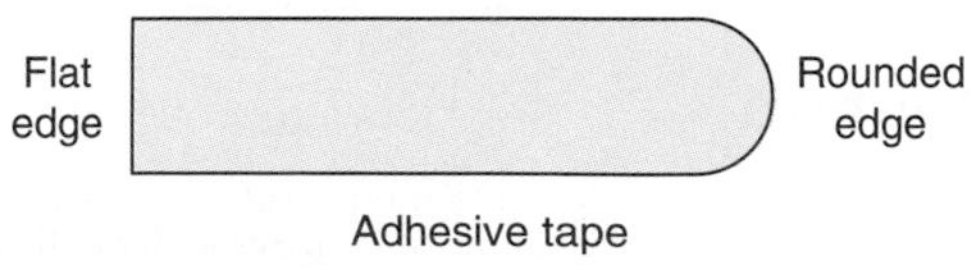

Flat edge   Rounded edge

Adhesive tape

FIGURE 9.15

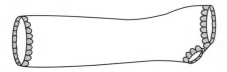

FIGURE 9.16

Action	Rationale
16. Place client with leg or body cast on fracture pan for elimination. For clients with good bowel and bladder control, temporarily line edge of cast close to perineal area with plastic; if client has little or no elimination control (e.g., some pediatric and elderly clients), maintain plastic lining on cast edges and change once a shift.	*Provides for elimination needs; prevents soiling of cast*
17. Perform range-of-motion exercises on all joint areas every 4 hours (except where contraindicated).	
18. Instruct client to cough and deep breathe and reposition client (within guidelines of orders) every 2 hours.	*Prevents pneumonia, decubitus ulcers, and other complications of immobility*
19. Instruct client to keep cast and skin under cast dry. Avoid putting lotion or powder under cast.	*Preserves integrity of cast; prevents skin breakdown*
20. Lift side rails, lock wheels, and place bed in low position.	*Prevents falls*
21. Place call light within reach.	*Facilitates communication*
22. Restore or discard equipment properly.	*Removes waste and clutter*
23. Remove gloves and perform hand hygiene.	*Reduces microorganism transfer*

Evaluation

Were desired outcomes achieved? Examples of evaluation include:
* Desired outcome met: No signs of neurovascular deficits detected.

- Desired outcome met: No complications resulting from neurovascular deficits evidenced.
- Desired outcome met: Client verbalized actions necessary for cast maintenance by time of discharge.

Documentation

The following should be noted on the client's chart:
- Data from neurovascular assessment
- Abnormal data indicating inflammation or infection
- Indicators of complications of immobility
- Frequency of body alignment and repositioning and positions into which client is placed
- Frequency and nature of skin care given
- Frequency of coughing and deep-breathing exercises performed
- Frequency and nature of range-of-motion exercises performed
- Teaching completed and additional teaching needs of client

Sample Documentation
Date: 2/17/05
Time: 2100

Fourth hour since cast application. Left leg full-length cast remains cold and wet. Toes of both left and right feet are pink, warm, and dry. Able to wiggle toes and identify which toe is being touched. Denies numbness, tingling, burning, or pain. Coughing and deep breathing done every hour. Repositioned every 2 hours left side to back to right side alternately. Active range-of-motion exercises performed to all extremities except left leg every 2 hours. Left toes and upper thigh washed with soap and water and dried.

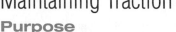

● **Nursing Procedure 9.6**

Maintaining Traction

Purpose

Maintains traction apparatus with appropriate counterbalance
Prevents infection at site of insertion of traction pins

Equipment

- Alcohol wipes
- Antimicrobial agent for cleaning pins (skeletal traction)
- One sterile gauze pad (2 × 2 or 4 × 3) for each traction pin
- Sterile gloves
- Sterile dressings, if needed
- Equipment for supporting body positioning (e.g., trochanter roll, pillows, sandbag, footboard)
- Traction setup

Assessment

Assessment should focus on the following:
- Medical diagnosis
- Doctor's orders for traction weight, line of pull maintained, and pin care
- Type of skin traction or skeletal traction
- Status of weights, ropes, and pulleys
- Reports of pain or discomfort
- Integumentary status
- Neurovascular indicators distal to injury, as well as opposite limb (e.g., skin color and temperature, capillary refill, sensation, presence of pulse, ability to move toes or fingers)
- Indicators of complications of immobility: pressure ulcers or pressure areas, contractures, decreased peristalsis, constipation, fecal impaction, signs of pulmonary embolism (e.g., chest pain, dyspnea, wheezing, increased heart rate), signs of thrombophlebitis (e.g., redness, heat, swelling, or pain in local area)

Nursing Diagnoses

Nursing diagnoses may include the following:
- Risk for infection related to invasive procedure (skeletal traction)
- Risk for constipation related to insufficient physical activity and ingestion of opiates
- Risk for injury related to altered mobility
- Risk for impaired skin integrity related to physical immobilization
- Risk for peripheral neurovascular dysfunction related to fracture and immobilization

Outcome Identification and Planning

Desired Outcomes

Sample desired outcomes include the following:
- No redness, swelling, pain, discharge, or odor occur at pin site.
- Fracture will heal appropriately in a timely manner without complications.

Special Considerations in Planning and Implementation

General

If weights do not swing freely, traction can be counterproductive. Assess status of weights, line of pull, traction ropes, and knots every 1 to 2 hours and after moving client. The line of pull established by the physician should be maintained to prevent disruption of the healing process. Avoid constriction over the head of the fibula (just below the knee) to prevent peroneal nerve damage, which could result in foot drop. Clients in traction should have a trapeze to facilitate repositioning and maintenance of upper extremity strength.

Pediatric

Arrange for quiet play activities of appropriate developmental level to occupy child during confinement. Include child in moving procedure (e.g., by letting child count aloud to time movement). Allow child to express concerns and understanding through play with a puppet or stuffed toy.

Geriatric

Elderly clients are particularly prone to skin breakdown when they are bedridden and not repositioned frequently because they have less subcutaneous fat and their skin is less elastic, thinner, drier, and more fragile than that of a younger person. They also have an increased incidence of other complications related to immobility, such as pneumonia, thrombophlebitis, and constipation.

Delegation

Instruct assistive personnel on moving and assisting with bathing of clients with specific types of traction. ROUTINE MONITORING OF NEUROVASCULAR AND SKIN STATUS REMAINS THE RESPONSIBILITY OF LICENSED PERSONNEL.

Home Health

When the homebound client is mobile, with intermittent traction on an extremity, install traction setup as appropriate (over the door) with a measured source of weight (e.g., flour bag with sand, rocks, bricks).

Implementation

Action	Rationale
1. Perform hand hygiene.	*Reduces microorganism transfer*
2. Explain procedure to client, emphasizing importance of maintaining counter-balance and position.	*Decreases anxiety; increases compliance*
3. Provide privacy.	*Decreases embarrassment*

Action	Rationale
4. Assess traction setup (Fig. 9.17) to ensure accurate counterbalance and function of traction by checking the following: • Line of pull intact as determined by physician • Appropriate amount of weight applied (as ordered) • Weights hanging freely, not touching bed, wall, or floor • Ropes moving freely through pulleys • All knots tight in ropes and away from pulleys • Pulleys and ropes free of entanglements with linens	*Maintains proper therapy; prevents interruption of therapy*
5. Check client's position (head should be near head of bed and properly aligned).	*Maintains proper counterbalance*
6. Assess skin for signs of pressure areas or friction under skin traction belts per institution's protocol (at least every 24 hours).	*Detects early signs of skin breakdown*

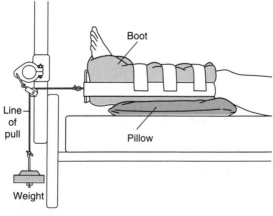

FIGURE 9.17

Action	Rationale
7. Assess neurovascular status of extremity distal to traction. Compare to same area on opposite limb.	*Detects neurovascular complications; provides baseline data*
8. Assess site at and around pin for redness, edema, discharge, or odor.	*Determines presence of infection*
9. Perform hand hygiene.	*Reduces microorganism transfer*
10. Put on gloves.	*Prevents exposure to body fluids*
11. Wash, rinse, and dry skin thoroughly. If permissible, remove skin traction periodically to wash under skin (check doctor's order and agency policy for frequency; weights are removed from skeletal traction only in an emergency).	*Promotes circulation to skin*
12. Discard gloves. Perform hand hygiene.	*Removes microorganisms*
13. Perform pin site care following agency protocol or physician's orders.	*Prevents infection*
14. Change bed linens from the top of the bed to the bottom. (Have client assist as able by pulling up on trapeze while pushing with lower extremity to raise buttocks off bed for linen change and use of bedpan.)	*Prevents interruption of therapy by maintaining correct line of pull; promotes independence; maintains muscle tone*
15. Perform range-of-motion exercises every 4 hours, except areas where contraindicated.	*Prevents pneumonia, pressure ulcers, complications of immobility; maintains articular (joint) mobility and muscle tone*
16. Instruct client to cough and deep breathe, and reposition client (within guidelines for orders) every 2 hours; use trochanter rolls and footboard to prevent internal and external hip rotation and footdrop as needed.	*Facilitates respiratory function; prevents complications related to improper positioning*
17. Lift side rails, lock wheels, and place bed in low position.	*Prevents falls*
18. Place call light within reach.	*Facilitates communication*
19. Perform hand hygiene.	*Reduces microorganism transfer*

Evaluation

Were desired outcomes achieved? Examples of evaluation include:
● Desired outcome partially met: Slight redness at pin site. No swelling, pain, discharge, or odor at pin site.
● Desired outcome met: Fracture healing appropriately in a timely manner without complications.

Documentation

The following should be noted on the client's chart:
● Type of traction, line of pull, and amount of weight used
● Status of ropes and pulleys
● Body alignment of client
● Repositioning (frequency and last position)
● Pin care given
● Skin care given
● Neurovascular assessment
● Coughing and deep-breathing exercises performed
● Range-of-motion exercises performed
● Client teaching completed and additional teaching needs of client

---

Sample Documentation
Date: 2/17/05
Time: 2100

Maintains 20 lb of skeletal traction to right femur in supine position with straight alignment. Pin site care performed with H_2O_2 and normal saline. Sterile 2 × 2 applied to each pin. Skin in perineal area and over bony prominences clean, warm, pink, and dry. Toes of both left and right feet are pink, warm, and dry. Able to identify which toe is being touched bilaterally. Dorsiflexion and plantar flexion intact bilaterally. Range-of-motion exercises of upper and lower extremities (within limitations of right lower extremity traction) performed by client every 4 hr. Coughing and deep breathing every 2 hr; breath sounds clear bilaterally. Large amount of semi-hard, formed, brown stool passed. Oral fluids continue to be encouraged.

Applying Antiembolism Hose

Purpose

Promotes venous blood return to heart by maintaining pressure on capillaries and veins

Prevents development of thrombophlebitis secondary to venous stasis

Equipment

- Antiembolism hose
- Washcloth
- Towel
- Soap
- Basin of warm water
- Tape measure (if not included in package)
- Optional personal items (e.g., talcum powder)
- Gloves, if contact with body fluids is likely

Assessment

Assessment should focus on the following:
- Medical diagnosis
- Physician's order for antiembolism hose
- Reports of pain or discomfort of lower extremities
- Skin status of legs and feet
- Neurovascular indicators of lower extremities (skin color and temperature, capillary refill, sensation, pulse presence and quality)
- Indicators of venous disorders of lower extremities (redness, heat, swelling, or pain in local area)

Nursing Diagnoses

Nursing diagnoses may include the following:
- Risk for peripheral neurovascular dysfunction related to prolonged immobility
- Deficient knowledge regarding application of antiembolism hose related to lack of exposure

Outcome Identification and Planning

Desired Outcomes

Sample desired outcomes include the following:
- Client states two ways to reduce risk of developing venous thrombosis.
- Client remains free of signs of venous thrombosis throughout confinement.

Special Considerations in Planning and Implementation

General

Clients with known or suspected peripheral vascular disorders should not wear antiembolism hose because tissue ischemia or thrombus dislodgment may occur. Poor maintenance of hose could result in circulatory restriction; hose must be applied correctly and remain free of wrinkles, rolls, or kinks.

Geriatric

Elderly clients are particularly prone to circulatory disorders of the lower extremities because of age-related physiologic changes in their vascular tissue. In addition, chronic cardiac and peripheral vascular dysfunction may reduce arterial perfusion or venous return.

End-of-Life Care

Care should be given to prevent complications of immobility that would compromise quality of life. If pain is a consideration, analgesia should be given.

Delegation

After proper training, assistive personnel may apply antiembolism hose. They should be instructed to report pain, skin abnormalities, or discoloration of extremities.

Implementation

Action	Rationale
1. Perform hand hygiene.	*Reduces microorganism transfer*
2. Explain procedure to client, emphasizing the importance of keeping the antiembolism hose on extremity for specified amount of time and wearing hose properly.	*Decreases anxiety; increases compliance*
3. Provide privacy.	*Decreases embarrassment*
4. Measure for correct size of hose (large, medium, small) according to manufacturer's directions.	*Promotes proper functioning of hose; prevents reduced circulation to legs*
5. Wash, rinse, and dry legs; apply light talcum powder, if desired.	*Promotes comfort; promotes clean, dry skin*
6. Turn hose (except foot portion) inside out.	*Promotes proper application of hose*
7. Place foot of hose over toes and foot, ensuring that heel of hose is in appropriate	*Promotes proper functioning of hose; prevents tourniquet effect*

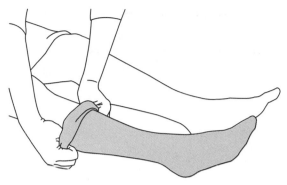

FIGURE 9.18

Action	Rationale
position. Using both hands, slide hose up leg, ensuring that kinks and wrinkles are removed (smooth and straighten hose as it is pulled up; Fig. 9.18). Avoid letting top of hose roll down.	
8. Apply hose to opposite leg in same manner.	*Promotes therapeutic effect*
9. Remove hose twice a day for 20 minutes or per agency policy (ideally during morning and evening care).	*Allows for skin aeration and assessment*
10. Perform hand hygiene.	*Reduces microorganism transfer*

Evaluation

Were desired outcomes achieved? Examples of evaluation include:
- Desired outcome met: Client stated two ways to reduce risk of developing venous thrombosis.
- Desired outcome met: Client showed no signs of venous thrombosis during confinement.

Documentation

The following should be noted on the client's chart:
- Size and length of hose applied

- Lower extremity skin color, temperature, sensation, capillary refill
- Status of pulses in lower extremities
- Presence of pain or discomfort in lower extremities
- Time and duration of hose removal
- Client teaching completed and additional teaching needs of client

---

Sample Documentation
Date: 2/17/05
Time: 2100

Thigh-high antiembolism hose off x1 hour during bath and linen change. New thigh-high hose applied—size, large/long. Skin of both lower extremities warm. No tears or abrasions noted; no complaint of pain in lower extremities. Toes pink, with 2-second capillary refill. Bilateral pedal pulses 2+. Client stated purpose of hose correctly and related care measures, including the importance of avoiding wrinkles or folds in hose.

● **Nursing Procedure 9.8**

Applying a Pneumatic Compression Device

Purpose

Promotes venous blood return to heart by maintaining intermittent pressure on capillaries and veins
Prevents development of thrombophlebitis secondary to venous stasis

Equipment

- Pneumatic compression equipment with comfort stockings or hose
- Washcloth
- Towel
- Soap
- Basin of warm water

Assessment

Assessment should focus on the following:
● Medical diagnosis
● Physician's order for the pneumatic compression device (also called sequential compression device; SCD)
● Reports of pain or discomfort of lower extremities
● Skin status of legs and feet
● Neurovascular indicators of lower extremities (skin color and temperature, capillary refill, sensation, pulse presence and quality)
● Indicators of venous disorders of lower extremities (redness, heat, swelling, or pain in local area)

Nursing Diagnoses

Nursing diagnoses may include the following:
● Risk for peripheral neurovascular dysfunction related to prolonged immobility

Outcome Identification and Planning

Desired Outcomes

Sample desired outcomes include the following:
● Client states two ways to reduce risk of developing venous thrombosis.
● Client remains free of signs of venous thrombosis throughout confinement.

Special Considerations in Planning and Implementation

General

Generally, a pneumatic compression device is applied during surgery or immediately after surgery or after an injury and worn continuously except for hygiene and skin assessment. If application is delayed (72 hours), testing to rule out the presence of thrombi should be done before application. Pneumatic compression equipment should not be placed under skin traction apparatus (e.g., Buck's traction boot).

Geriatric

Elderly clients are particularly prone to circulatory disorders of lower extremities because of age-related physiologic changes that occur in their vascular tissue. In addition, chronic cardiac and peripheral vascular dysfunction may reduce venous return.

Delegation

After proper training, assistive personnel may apply a pneumatic compression device. They should be instructed to report pain, skin abnormalities, or discoloration of extremities.

Implementation

Action	Rationale
1. Perform hand hygiene.	*Reduces microorganism transfer*
2. Review manufacturer's guidelines and directions.	*Alerts caregiver to instructions associated with use of specific product*
3. Explain procedure to client, emphasizing the importance of keeping vinyl sleeves on extremities for specified amount of time.	*Decreases anxiety; increases compliance*
4. Provide privacy.	*Decreases embarrassment*
5. Obtain appropriate-size vinyl sleeves and comfort stockings/hose.	*Promotes proper functioning of device; prevents reduced circulation to legs*
6. Wash, rinse, and dry legs; apply light talcum powder, if desired.	*Promotes comfort; promotes clean, dry skin*
7. Slide vinyl surgical sleeve over each calf or apply Velcro-secured vinyl compression hose under thigh and leg, with knee-opening site under the popliteal area (Fig. 9.19).	*Places source of intermittent compression over the veins of the extremities*

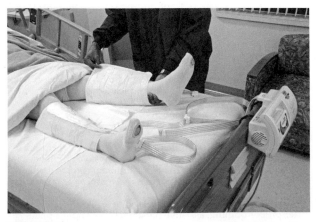

FIGURE 9.19

Action	Rationale
8. Connect the vinyl hose by overlapping the edges and securing the Velcro connectors.	*Establishes air pump source; prepares unit for function*
9. Turn the power on. Follow manufacturer's guidelines regarding setting of inflation pressure as needed.	*Promotes proper functioning of device*
10. Monitor several inflation/ deflation compression cycles.	*Permits early detection of excessive compression*
11. Cover client with bed linen.	*Provides privacy and warmth*
12. Observe extremities every 2 to 3 hours to assess neurovascular status and hose placement.	*Prevents complications*
13. Remove the pneumatic compression sleeves only to provide hygiene and to assess skin integrity, then reapply immediately.	*Allows for skin aeration and assessment*
14. Perform hand hygiene and restore equipment.	*Reduces microorganism transfer; maintains organized environment*

Evaluation

Were desired outcomes achieved? Examples of evaluation include:
- Desired outcome met: Client stated two ways to reduce risk of developing venous thrombosis.
- Desired outcome met: Client showed no signs of venous thrombosis during confinement.

Documentation

The following should be noted on the client's chart:
- Size, length, and location of pneumatic compression sleeve applied
- Lower extremity skin color, temperature, sensation, capillary refill
- Status of pulses in lower extremities
- Presence of pain or discomfort in lower extremities
- Time and duration of device removal
- Client teaching completed and additional teaching needs of client

Sample Documentation
Date: 2/17/05
Time: 2100

Thigh-high SCD hose off x30 minutes during bath and linen change, then reapplied. Skin of both lower extremities warm. No tears or abrasions noted; no complaint of pain in lower extremities. Toes pink, with 2-second capillary refill. Bilateral pedal pulses 2+. Client stated purpose of SCD correctly and related care measures.

● **Nursing Procedure 9.9**

Using a Continuous Passive Motion (CPM) Device

Purpose

Increases range of motion
Decreases effects of immobility
Stimulates healing of articular cartilage
Reduces adhesions and swelling

Equipment

- CPM device
- Softgoods kit (single-client use)
- Tape measure
- Goniometer

Assessment

Assessment should focus on the following:
- Physician's orders for degrees of flexion and extension
- Neurovascular status of extremity before start of CPM (presence of pulses and capillary refill in affected extremity, skin color and temperature, sensation, and movement of extremity)
- Reports of pain or discomfort

Nursing Diagnoses

Nursing diagnoses may include the following:
- Impaired physical mobility related to musculoskeletal impairment, pain, and prescribed movement restrictions
- Risk of peripheral neurovascular dysfunction related to orthopedic surgery and immobilization
- Disturbed sleep pattern related to therapeutic interruption

Outcome Identification and Planning

Desired Outcomes

Sample desired outcomes include the following:
- Client tolerates progressive increase in flexion and extension with CPM device.
- Client demonstrates increasing mobility of affected extremity.

Special Considerations in Planning and Implementation

Geriatric

Elderly clients are particularly prone to skin breakdown and other complications of immobility.

Pediatric

Explain the CPM device clearly, showing how the device works with a doll or stuffed animal. Arrange for quiet play activities that are developmentally appropriate.

Delegation

Instruct assistive personnel in techniques of moving clients with CPM machines in bed.

Implementation

Action	Rationale
1. Perform hand hygiene.	*Reduces microorganism transfer*
2. Organize equipment, and apply softgoods to CPM device (Fig. 9.20).	*Promotes efficiency; prevents friction to extremity during motion*
3. Check doctor's order for degrees of flexion and extension. Speed of device will be determined by client comfort. Begin with a midpoint setting; may change on a daily or per-shift basis as the client progresses.	

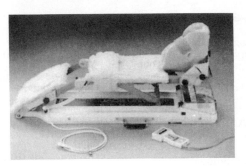

FIGURE 9.20

Action	Rationale
4. Explain procedure to client, emphasizing the importance of maintaining setting and position.	*Decreases anxiety; facilitates cooperation*
5. Using the tape measure, determine the distance between the gluteal crease and the popliteal space.	*Determines the distance to adjust the Thigh Length Adjustment knobs on the CPM device*
6. Measure the length of client's leg from the knee to 0.25 inches beyond the bottom of the foot.	*Determines the distance to adjust the position of the footplate*
7. Position the client in the middle of the bed with the extremity in a slightly abducted position.	*Promotes proper body alignment; prevents CPM device from exerting pressure on opposite extremity*
8. Elevate client's leg and place in padded CPM device.	*Prepares client for therapy*
9. Use the proper anatomic placement of the device by placing the client's knee at the hinged joint of the machine.	*Prevents injuries*
10. Adjust the footplate to maintain the client's foot in a neutral position. Make certain that the leg is neither internally nor externally rotated.	*Prevents injuries*

Action	Rationale
11. Apply the soft restraining straps under CPM device and around extremity loosely enough to fit several fingers between leg and restraint strap.	*Maintains the extremity in position; prevents injury due to compression from strap*
12. Turn unit on at main power switch. Set controls to level prescribed by physician.	*Prepares machine for function*
13. Instruct the client in the use of the GO/STOP button.	*Decreases anxiety*
14. Set CPM device in the ON stage and press the GO button (Fig. 9.21).	*Initiates intervention*
15. Determine angle of flexion when device has reached its greatest height using the goniometer. If unit is not anatomic, there might be a slight difference between the reading on the device and the actual angle of the client's knee.	*Determines maximum point of pull without causing pain*

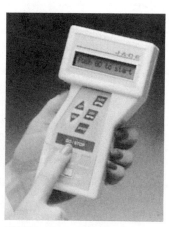

FIGURE 9.21

Evaluation

Were desired outcomes achieved? Examples of evaluation include:
- Desired outcome met: Client tolerated progressive increase in flexion and extension with CPM device with minimal pain verbalized.
- Desired outcome met: Client demonstrated increasing mobility of affected extremity.

Documentation

The following should be noted on the client's chart:
- Onset of therapy
- Tolerance of procedure
- Degree of extension and flexion and speed of machine
- Amount of time client used device
- Neurovascular status of extremity
- Therapeutic aids, immobilizer, and so forth

Sample Documentation
Date: 2/17/05
Time: 1100

CPM device applied to left leg at 0 degrees of extension and 35 degrees of flexion; started at slow speed for 2 hours. Verified by goniometer. Client instructed in use of go/stop button. Both feet warm, nailbeds pink, 3-second capillary refill. No complaint of numbness in left extremity. Denies need for pain medication. Padding to all soft tissue near CPM device. Call bell within reach.

Time: 1400

CPM device removed from left leg. Left lower extremity warm and dry to touch. Distal pulses present; client denies numbness or tingling. Dorsiflexion and plantar flexion intact; no edema noted. Immobilizer applied.

Providing Residual Limb Care Following Amputation

Purpose

Reduces edema
Promotes stump shrinkage and healing in a manner conducive
for prosthetic fitting and application
Prevents contractures

Equipment

- Compression dressings
  - Double-length elastic bandages of appropriate size
    (usually 4-inch wrap for an amputation below the knee
    or 6-inch wrap for an amputation above the knee in
    an adult)
  - Stump shrinker socks (compression dressing) *or*
- Rigid residual limb dressing (casting material usually
  applied at time of surgery; see Procedure 9.5)

Assessment

Assessment should focus on the following:
- Incision (appearance, size, healing status)
- Skin integrity (redness, abrasion, or irritation)
- Range of motion of all limbs
- Phantom limb sensation/pain
- Ability of client to comprehend instructions regarding care
  of residual limb
- Additional learning needs of client
- Psychosocial impact of loss of limb; coping skills

Nursing Diagnoses

Nursing diagnoses may include the following:
- Acute pain related to physical injury (surgery)
- Impaired physical mobility related to musculoskeletal
  impairment
- Disturbed body image related to surgery (below-the-knee
  amputation)
- Deficient knowledge regarding stump care related to lack of
  exposure
- Risk for injury related to altered mobility

Outcome Identification and Planning

Desired Outcomes

Sample desired outcomes include the following:
● The client will demonstrate proper residual limb care.
● The client's residual limb will heal in a timely manner without contracture formation.
● The residual limb will shrink in such a manner as to allow fitting and application of a prosthesis.

Special Considerations in Planning and Implementation

Geriatric

Elderly clients are particularly prone to skin breakdown because they have less subcutaneous fat and their skin is less elastic, thinner, drier, and more fragile than that of a younger person. They also often have decreased range of motion. The caregiver must be vigilant in caring for and positioning the residual limb to prevent skin breakdown and contractures.

Pediatric

Since they heal so rapidly, children often have an immediate postoperative prosthesis (IPOP) applied. This decreases pain and facilitates early ambulation. Demonstrate the appropriate shrinkage device/procedure using a doll or stuffed toy with an "amputation." Allow child to express concerns and understanding through play.

Delegation

Instruct assistive personnel on positioning techniques to prevent formation of contractures. ROUTINE MONITORING OF NEUROVASCULAR, INCISION, AND SKIN STATUS REMAINS THE RESPONSIBILITY OF LICENSED PERSONNEL.

Home Health

Approximately 3 weeks after surgery (clarify timing with physician), client should be instructed to massage residual limb with a rough terry-type cloth to prevent adhesions and desensitize the skin in preparation for prosthesis fitting. If needed, family caregivers should be taught to care for residual limb and techniques to prevent contractures. Have them show competency by return demonstration.

Implementation

Action	Rationale
1. Perform hand hygiene.	*Reduces microorganism transfer*
2. Organize equipment.	*Promotes efficiency*

Action	Rationale
3. Reassure client that phantom limb sensation is normal and usually diminishes over time.	*Reduces anxiety*
4. If client had a lower limb amputation, avoid elevating residual limb unless directed to do so by physician's order (if elevated at all, usually only during the first 24 hours).	*Prevents formation of flexion contractures*
• Avoid positioning client in Fowler's or semi-Fowler's position for extended lengths of time.	*Prevents contractures of hips*
• After the first 24 hours, position client in prone position for 20 minutes at least twice a day.	*Promotes hip/knee extension; prevents flexion contractures*
5. Instruct client on need to maintain extension of the joints in the residual limb.	*Prevents flexion contractures; facilitates function of residual limb*
6. Maintain application of device to shrink stump.	*Reduces edema; promotes shrinkage of residual limb*
• Inspect incision each shift until healed.	*Allows early intervention if complications occur*
• Wash healed incision/ residual limb daily with mild soap and water.	*Reduces microorganisms; promotes good hygiene*
7. Instruct client on correct method to apply shrinkage dressings.	*Promotes appropriate healing*
• Apply elastic bandages in a figure-of-eight configuration with increased constriction at distal end of residual limb and less constriction at proximal end of dressing, taking care not to interrupt perfusion of the distal end of the residual limb. Example: Below the knee, Figure 9.22A Example: Above the knee, Figure 9.22B	*Promotes shrinkage in a manner to allow prosthetic fitting; promotes tissue integrity*

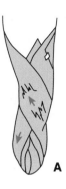

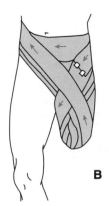

A   **B**

FIGURE 9.22

Action	Rationale
8. Instruct client on how to maintain dressings:	
• Client should remove shrinkage dressing daily to inspect residual limb.	*Allows early intervention if complications occur*
• Client should clean shrinkage dressings daily, allowing them to dry completely before reapplication.	*Reduces microorganisms; prevents skin irritation due to moisture*
• Client should air out any open areas of skin on residual limb for 1 hour four times a day.	*Promotes healing*
• Client should have at least two complete changes of shrinkage dressings.	*Avoids long periods of time without the device in place*
9. Demonstrate range-of-motion and isometric exercises of all extremities, including the residual limb.	*Promotes understanding; maintains strength and function*
10. Inform client that the prosthesis is usually fit by a specialist, called a prosthetist, 6 to 8 weeks after surgery.	*Allows client to anticipate timeline of continued treatment*

Evaluation

Were desired outcomes achieved? Examples of evaluation include:
- Desired outcome met: Client demonstrated proper residual limb care.
- Desired outcome met: Client's residual limb healed in a timely manner without contracture formation.
- Desired outcome met: Client's residual limb shrunk and allows for fitting and application of a prosthesis.

Documentation

The following should be noted on the client's chart:
- Residual limb incision, skin, and dressing appearance
- Positioning of residual limb
- Range of motion of residual limb and other limbs
- Client instruction and return demonstration; additional learning needs of client

---

Sample Documentation
Date: 2/17/05
Time: 2100

Positioned prone for 20 minutes. Able to state rationale to prevent contracture formation in residual limb. Able to demonstrate active range of motion in all extremities. Right below-the-knee closed residual limb incision well approximated, 22 cm in length. Remains dry and intact without redness or swelling. 6-inch elastic bandages reapplied via figure-8 method. Client able to assist with application and state relevance of shrinking residual limb in anticipation of prosthesis.

● Nursing Procedure 9.11

Using a Hoyer Lift

Purpose

Helps move and transfer clients who cannot assist nurse; particularly useful with obese clients
Prevents injury to client and undue strain on nurse's body

Equipment

- Hoyer lift (should include base, canvas mat, and two pairs of canvas straps)
- Large chair with arm support for client to sit in

Assessment

Assessment should focus on the following:
- Medical diagnosis
- Doctor's activity orders (e.g., positions contraindicated, amount of time client may be up)
- Client's ability to keep head erect
- Client's previous tolerance of sitting position (e.g., orthostatic hypotension, amount of time client tolerated sitting up)
- Need for restraints while sitting up
- Room environment (e.g., adequate lighting, presence of clutter and furniture in pathway between chair and bed)
- Condition of Hoyer device, hooks, and canvas mats

Nursing Diagnoses

Nursing diagnoses may include the following:
- Impaired physical mobility related to intolerance to activity and neuromuscular impairment

Outcome Identification and Planning

Desired Outcome

Sample desired outcomes include the following:
- Client is moved from and returned to bed by Hoyer lift without injury.

Special Considerations in Planning and Implementation

General

The nurse must be familiar with the Hoyer lift in order to operate it correctly (parts of the lift are labeled in Fig. 9.23). Practice using the lift without a client on the mat if you are unfamiliar with this device. Organization is crucial when performing numerous moving procedures on heavy clients to avoid client exertion and physical injury to the nurse. Plan activities such as changing bed linens while the client is out of bed; encourage client to use bedside toilet once out of bed.

Pediatric

Using the Hoyer lift can be frightening to a child. Demonstrate the procedure using a puppet or game and allow the child to participate in some way.

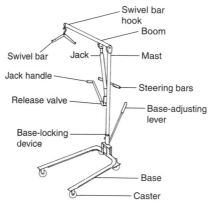

FIGURE 9.23

Geriatric

For elderly clients with chronic conditions, use extra caution when using the Hoyer lift. Clients with chronic cardiopulmonary conditions should be observed closely while sitting up and during transfer for exertion, respiratory difficulty, chest pain, and general discomfort.

End-of-Life Care

Care should be given to prevent complications of immobility that would compromise quality of life. If pain is a consideration, analgesia should be given.

Home Health

Help the family obtain the equipment, if needed. Educate the family on the use of the equipment and on proper body mechanics.

Delegation

Ascertain that assistive personnel have been trained in use of the Hoyer lift before using it. Reinforce the importance of monitoring cardiopulmonary status of clients likely to experience breathing difficulty, chest pain, or general discomfort.

Implementation

Action	Rationale
1. Perform hand hygiene.	*Reduces microorganism transfer*
2. Explain procedure and assure client that precautions will be taken to prevent falls.	*Decreases anxiety*

Action	Rationale
3. Provide privacy through-out procedure.	*Decreases embarrassment*
4. Place chair on side of bed client will be sitting on (lock wheels, if wheelchair).	*Places chair at close distance*
5. Adjust bed to comfortable working height; lock wheels.	*Prevents back and muscle strain in nurse; prevents bed movement*
6. Place client on mat as follows so that heaviest parts of body are centered on mat:	
• Roll client to one side and place half of mat under client from shoulder to midthigh, then roll client to other side and finish pulling mat under client.	*Positions client on mat with minimal movement*
• Be sure one or both side rails are up as you move from one side of the bed to the other.	*Prevents falls*
7. Roll base of Hoyer lift under side of bed nearest to chair with boom in cen-ter of client's trunk; lock wheels of lift.	*Moves mechanical part of lift to bedside; prevents lift from rolling*
8. Using base-adjustment lever, widen stance of base.	*Provides greater stability to lift*
9. Raise and then push jack handle toward mast, low-ering boom (this is accom-plished with appropriate button or control device in the electric Hoyer).	*Lowers booms close enough to attach hooks*
10. Place the strap or chain hooks through the holes of the mat (hooks of short straps go into holes behind back and hooks of long straps go into holes at other end), making certain that hooks are not putting exces-sive pressure on client's skin.	*Secures hook placement into mat holes; attaches rest of device to mat; prevents tissue injury*
11. Secure all equipment, lines, and drains attached to client and close off drains, if nec-essary (remember to reopen them after moving client).	*Prevents accidental dislodgment and client injury; prevents reflux of drainage*
12. Instruct client to fold arms across chest.	*Prevents injury*

Action	Rationale
13. Using jack handle, pump jack enough for mat to clear bed about 6 inches and tighten release valve.	*Assesses client stability and centering on mat*
14. Determine if client is fully supported and can maintain head support. Provide head support as needed throughout procedure.	*Assesses stability in relation to weight and placement*
15. Unlock wheels and pull Hoyer lift straight back and away from bed; instruct an assistant to provide support for equipment and client's legs throughout procedure.	*Promotes stability*
16. Move toward chair, with open end of lift's base straddling chair; continue until client's back is almost flush with back of chair.	*Moves and guides client into chair*
17. Lock wheels of lift.	*Provides stability*
18. Slowly lift jack handle and lower client into chair until hooks are slightly loosened from mat; guide client into chair with your hands as mat lowers. Avoid lowering client onto chair handles.	*Lowers client fully into chair*
19. Remove mat (unless difficult to replace or client's first time out of bed).	*Facilitates comfort*
20. Place tubes, drains, and support equipment for proper functioning, comfort, and safety:	*Prevents accidental dislodgment of tubes and drains and maintains necessary functions*
• Pillow behind head and shoulders	*Ensures client's stability in chair*
• Sheet over knees and thighs	*Facilitates warmth and privacy*
• Restraints where needed (e.g., Posey vest, sheet, arm restraints)	*Facilitates support of other body parts; reduces risk of falling*
• Phone and frequently used items within close range	*Places items desired or needed by client within reach*
• Catheter hooked to lower portion of chair	*Prevents reflux of drainage*
• IV pole close enough to avoid pulling	*Prevents shearing, mechanical phlebitis, or dislodging of cannula*
• Call light within reach	*Facilitates communication*

Action	Rationale
21. Assess client tolerance to sitting up.	*Reduces risk of falling*
22. Leave door to client's room open when leaving room unless someone else will be with client.	*Allows observation of unattended client*
23. Monitor client at 15- to 60-minute intervals.	*Reduces risk of falling*
24. Return client to bed.	
25. Perform hand hygiene and restore equipment.	*Reduces microorganism transfer; promotes clean environment*

Evaluation

Were desired outcomes achieved? Examples of evaluation include:
- Desired outcome met: Client was moved from and returned to bed by Hoyer lift without injury.

Documentation

The following should be noted on the client's chart:
- Status update, with indication for continued use of mobility-assist device
- Time of client transfer and type of lift used
- Client tolerance of procedure
- Duration of time in chair

Sample Documentation
Date: 2/17/05
Time: 2100

Client lifted out of bed using Hoyer lift. Placed in bedside chair. Tolerated procedure well, with respirations regular and nonlabored. Call light within reach. Door left partially open.

10

Rest and Comfort

OVERVIEW

- Each person's perception of pain is unique. Assessment of pain is considered the "fifth vital sign"; see Procedure 3.5, Appendix A.
- Cultural background may have a great impact on a client's pain threshold and pain tolerance, as well as on the client's expression of pain. The nurse must consider cultural impacts on the pain experience when planning care.
- Heat and cold may have special cultural significance for some clients (e.g., Asians or Hispanics), who classify conditions accordingly and expect corresponding treatments. Table 10.1 lists "hot" and "cold" conditions.
- Nurses must be sensitive to alternative pain relief measures used by clients and the cultural significance of those measures. Efforts should be made to reconcile religious rituals, herbal remedies, or other treatments with the established medical plan to facilitate culturally sensitive care.
- The assessment of pain should include its location, duration, intensity, and precipitating, alleviating, and associated factors.

● Table 10.1 Hot and Cold Conditions

Hot Conditions	Cold Conditions
Fever	Arthritis
Infections	Colds
Diarrhea	Indigestion
Constipation	Joint pain
Rashes	Menstrual period
Tenesmus	Earache
Ulcers	Cancer
Kidney problems	Tuberculosis
Skin ailments	Headache
Sore throat	Paralysis
Liver problems	Teething
	Rheumatism
	Pneumonia
	Malaria

The usual treatment for a hot or cold condition is thought to be the use of a food or substance of the opposite temperature.

- Appropriate duration of treatment is essential for the effective use of heat and cold.
- Cold therapy causes vasoconstriction; reduces local metabolism, edema, and inflammation; and induces local anesthetic effects.
- Heat therapy causes vasodilatation, relieves muscle tension, stimulates circulation, and promotes healing.
- Tissue damage can result if:
  - Excessive temperature is used (hot or cold)
  - Overexposure of site to treatment occurs
  - Electrical equipment is not checked for safety
- Some major nursing diagnostic labels related to rest and comfort are altered comfort, risk of altered comfort, and anxiety.

● Nursing Procedure 10.1

Administering Heat Therapy: Aquathermia Pad 🖐

Purpose

Stimulates circulation, thus providing nutrients to tissues
Reduces muscle tension

Equipment

- Aquathermia module (K-module) with pad (K-pad)
- Overbed or bedside table
- Disposable gloves
- Pillowcase
- Distilled water
- Tape
- Timer

Assessment

Assessment should focus on the following:
- Treatment order and response to previous treatment, if used
- Status of treatment area (redness, tenderness, cleanliness, dryness, sensation, integrity, and vascularity)
- Temperature, pulse rate and rhythm
- Degree of pain and position of comfort, if any
- Ability of client to maintain appropriate position without assistance
- Client's ability to perceive and report pain or burning sensation
- Presence of medical conditions that may impair sensation
- Proper functioning and safety of heating device
- Sensitivity of skin to heat treatment

Nursing Diagnoses

Nursing diagnoses may include the following:
- Acute pain related to joint pain
- Ineffective tissue perfusion related to vaso-occlusive process

Outcome Identification and Planning

Desired Outcomes

Sample desired outcomes include the following:
- Client verbalizes increased comfort after treatment.
- Client demonstrates increased mobility of affected extremity after treatment.
- Client does not experience any injury to skin integrity.

Special Considerations in Planning and Implementation

General

Schedule procedure for a time when the client can be assessed frequently. If the client is confused or cannot remain alone with a heating device, remain with the client or find someone to do so. Clients with decreased peripheral sensory perception, such as diabetics, must be monitored closely for heat overexposure.

Pediatric

Assess children more frequently because their epidermis is thin and fragile. Their ability to communicate discomfort associated with this procedure may be impaired.

Geriatric

Elderly clients may be extremely sensitive to heat therapy. Assess frequently.

Home Health

If a homebound client will be using a K-module when a nurse is not present, teach the client or family how to use the module safely. Ensure that the home environment is safe (e.g., electrical outlets are intact and not overloaded).

 Transcultural

Determine the client's cultural perspective regarding the use of heat to treat the condition. Discuss objections and incorporate hot/cold perception of illness and treatment into the plan of care. Omit treatment if client objects, and consult physician.

Delegation

Generally, this procedure may be delegated to unlicensed assistive personnel. Check agency policy. Emphasize importance of monitoring local skin area and maintaining time limits for therapy.

Implementation

Action	Rationale
1. Perform hand hygiene and organize equipment.	*Reduces microorganism transfer; promotes efficiency*
2. Explain procedure to client.	*Decreases anxiety; promotes cooperation*
3. Place heating module on bedside or overbed table at a level above the client's body level (Fig. 10.1).	*Facilitates flow of fluid*
4. Fill module two-thirds full with distilled water.	*Enables unit to function properly*
5. Turn module on low setting and allow water to begin circulating throughout the pad and tubing.	*Detects leakage of fluid or improper functioning before initiating therapy*
6. After water is fully circulating through the pad and tubing, check the pad with your hands to ascertain that it is warming and that there is no leakage of fluid.	*Checks for proper functioning and heating of unit*
7. Ensure that the water has reached the appropriate temperature (103°F to 110°F).	*Avoids thermal injury*

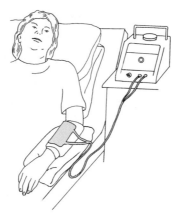

FIGURE 10.1

Action	Rationale
8. Put on disposable gloves, if indicated by risk for exposure.	*Decreases exposure to client secretions*
9. Position client appropriately to apply pad.	*Promotes comfort*
10. Place pillowcase over the heating pad and position pad on or around (if an extremity) treatment area.	*Prevents direct skin contact with pad, minimizing danger of burn injury*
• If pad needs to be secured, use tape. Do NOT use pins.	*Prevents puncture of pad and leakage of water*
11. After 60 seconds, assess for heat intolerance by: • Observing client's facial expression • Asking if heat is too high • Noting any dizziness, faintness, or palpitations • Removing pad and assessing for redness or tenderness; readjust temperature if necessary	*Prevents burn injury and complications of heat therapy*
12. Replace pad and secure with tape, if needed.	*Resumes treatment*
13. Instruct client NOT to alter placement of pad or heating module and to	*Promotes client cooperation and continued optimal functioning of unit; prevents burn injury*

Action	Rationale
call if heat becomes too intense.	
14. Leave call light within client's reach.	*Allows communication*
15. Recheck client every 5 minutes.	*Prevents burn injury*
16. After 20 minutes of treatment, turn module off, remove pad, and place pad on table with module.	*Terminates treatment; avoids reflex vasoconstriction*
17. Reposition client.	*Promotes comfort*
18. Return equipment.	*Maintains organized environment*
19. Remove gloves and perform hand hygiene.	*Reduces microorganism transfer*

Evaluation

Were desired outcomes achieved? Examples of evaluation include:
- Desired outcome met: Following treatment, client reports pain reduced from a 9 to a 5 on a scale of 1 to 10.
- Desired outcome met: Client demonstrates increased mobility of affected extremity after treatment.
- Desired outcome met: Skin remains intact with no evidence of injury.

Documentation

The following should be noted on the client's chart:
- Location and appearance of treatment area
- General response of client (weakness, faintness, palpitations, diaphoresis, extreme tenderness, if any)
- Duration of treatment
- Position of client during and after procedure
- Status of pain

Sample Documentation

Date: 2/3/05
Time: 1400

K-module applied to right calf for 20 minutes. No redness, warmth, or tenderness to touch at treatment area. Vital signs stable during and after treatment. Tolerated procedure well and indicates pain reduced from level 7 to level 2. Lying comfortably with left foot elevated on pillow.

Administering Heat Therapy: Commercial Heat Pack/Moist, Warm Compresses 🧤

Purpose

Promotes comfort and muscle relaxation
Stimulates circulation and promotes localization of purulent matter in tissues

Equipment

- Prepackaged heat pack
- Tape
- Two pairs of nonsterile gloves

If a prepackaged heat pack is unavailable or not preferred, substitute the following materials to make a warm, moist compress:

- Small towel or washcloth to place between heat and skin
- Warmed solution, per physician orders, 43°C (110°F)
- Heating pad or aquathermia pad (optional)
- Distilled water (for aquathermia pad)
- Petroleum jelly
- Plastic-lined underpad
- Clean basin
- Bath thermometer
- Pack of 4 × 4-inch gauze pads
- Bath blanket
- Two forceps (optional)

Assessment

Assessment should focus on the following:

- Treatment order, type of solution to be used, and response to previous treatments, if used
- Status of treatment area (edema, local bleeding, integrity)
- Temperature, pulse rate and rhythm
- Degree of pain and position of comfort, if any
- Ability of client to maintain appropriate position without assistance
- Client's ability to perceive and report pain or burning sensation
- Presence of medical conditions that may impair sensation
- Proper functioning and safety of heating device
- Sensitivity of skin to heat treatment

Nursing Diagnoses

Nursing diagnoses may include the following:
- Acute pain related to inflammation at IV infiltration site
- Impaired skin integrity related to wound infection
- Ineffective tissue perfusion related to impaired oxygen transport

Outcome Identification and Planning

Desired Outcomes

Sample desired outcomes include the following:
- Client verbalizes that pain is decreased within 1 hour after treatment.
- Client demonstrates increased mobility of affected extremity after treatment.

Special Considerations in Planning and Implementation

General

Schedule application of heat therapy when the client can be assessed at frequent intervals. Determine with client the best body position for comfort and alignment. If applying warm compresses, check heating device for safety and proper functioning. If using aquathermia pad for warm compress, set up heating device according to the guidelines in Nursing Procedure 10.1.

Home Health

Warn client that a clothing iron should never be used as a heat source for a warm compress. Use of a microwave oven for heating moist compresses can result in uneven heat distribution and may contribute to burns. Schedule the treatment when the client can be checked every 5 to 10 minutes by a caregiver or the home health nurse. Do not use heat therapy on clients with peripheral sensory deficits.

Pediatric

Children may require more frequent checks because skin may be more fragile and epidermis is thin. Their ability to communicate discomfort associated with this procedure may be impaired.

Geriatric

Duration of heat therapy in elderly clients may need to be reduced because their skin is often more fragile, with a thin epidermis.

 Transcultural

Determine cultural perspective regarding hot/cold perception of illness and appropriateness of treatment (see Table 10.1). Incorporate client preference when possible. Omit treatment if client objects, and consult physician.

Delegation

Generally, this procedure may be delegated to unlicensed assistive personnel. Check agency policy. Emphasize importance of monitoring local skin area.

Implementation

Action	Rationale
1. Explain procedure to client.	*Decreases anxiety; promotes cooperation*
2. Perform hand hygiene and organize equipment. Proceed to step 3 for Commercial Heat Pack or Warm, Moist compress, depending on equipment.	*Decreases microorganism transfer; promotes efficiency*

Preparing a Commercial Heat Pack

3. Remove heat pack from outer package, if present.	*Provides access to pack*
4. Break the inner seal: hold pack tightly in the center in upright position and squeeze. Do NOT use pack if leaking is noted (chemical burn may occur).	*Activates chemical ingredients to provide heat*
5. Lightly shake pack until the inner contents are lying in the lower portion of the pack. Proceed to step 6.	*Localizes activated chemicals*

Preparing a Warm, Moist Compress

3. Heat solution to desired temperature (43°C [110°F]) by placing the container in a bath basin filled with hot tap water. Check temperature of the solution with a bath thermometer. Discard hot tap water and pour warmed solution into bath basin. Place gauze into basin.	*Verifies safe and accurate temperature; promotes efficiency; saturates gauze with solution*
4. Prepare client: • Assist client into comfortable position for application.	*Facilitates compress placem*

Action	Rationale
• Place plastic pad under treatment area.	*Prevents soiling of linens*
• Drape client with loose bed linen.	*Provides privacy while allowing ease of access as needed*
5. Wring one layer of wet gauze until it is dripless.	*Removes excess solution*
6. Put on gloves.	*Reduces microorganism transfer*
7. Remove and discard old dressings, if present.	*Provides access to treatment site*
8. Remove and discard old gloves and put on new gloves.	*Reduces microorganism transfer*
9. If necessary, clean and dry treatment area. Proceed to step 10 for Commercial Heat Pack or step 10 for Warm, Moist Compress.	*Facilitates effectiveness of treatment*

Applying a Commercial Heat Pack

Action	Rationale
10. Place the heat pack lightly against treatment area.	*Allows for gradual initiation of dilatory effect*
11. After 30 seconds, remove heat pack and assess client for redness of skin or complaint of burning. Remove heat pack if not tolerated (problems noted) and notify physician.	*Prevents burn injury*
12. If no problems are noted, replace pack snugly against the area and secure with tape. Reassess treatment area every 5 minutes by lifting the corners of the pack. Proceed to step 13.	*Resumes treatment; stabilizes heat pack; monitors effects of treatment over time*

Applying a Warm, Moist Compress

Action	Rationale
If skin is intact, apply a thin layer of petroleum lly to the wound. Place mpress on the wound several seconds.	*Provides a protective barrier to client's skin; initiates vasodilation therapy*

Action	Rationale
11. Pick up edge of compress to observe initial skin response to therapy.	*Allows assessment of skin for adverse responses to therapy; promotes safety*
12. Replace compress gauze every 5 minutes, or as needed, to maintain warmth, assessing treatment area each time. Place towel over compress (a heating device, if available, may be placed over towel; instruct client not to alter settings of heating device).	*Provides for reassessment of treatment area; maintains heat of warm compress; promotes safety, as moist heat conducts heat more quickly and can cause burn injury*
13. Place call light within reach and raise side rails.	*Promotes communication and safety*
14. After 20 minutes, lower side rails, terminate treatment, and dry skin.	*Prevents local injury due to overexposure to treatment*
15. Apply new dressing over wound, if necessary.	*Promotes wound healing*
16. Reposition client and raise side rails.	*Facilitates comfort and safety*
17. Remove all equipment from bedside, remove gloves, and perform hand hygiene.	*Maintains clean environment; promotes asepsis*

Evaluation

Were desired outcomes achieved? An example of evaluation is:
- Desired outcome not met: After treatment, right foot remains cool to the touch and pale with +1 pedal pulse and sluggish capillary refill.

Documentation

The following should be noted on the client's chart:
- Size, location, and appearance of treatment area
- Status of pain and tissue perfusion
- Type of treatment
- Position of client
- Duration of treatment
- Client tolerance of treatment

Sample Documentation
Date: 2/3/05
Time: 140

Warm compress applied to right wrist for 20 minutes. Redness decreased from 2 to 1 cm. Site slightly warm to touch after treatment, capillary refill 3 seconds. Client reports pain reduced to level 1 from level 9. Tolerated treatment well; lying in bed with arm elevated on pillow.

● **Nursing Procedure 10.3**

Administering Heat Therapy: Heat Cradle and Heat Lamp 🖐

Purpose

Increases circulation
Promotes wound healing
Promotes general comfort
Assists with drying of wet cast

Equipment

- Heat lamp (with adjustable neck and 60-watt bulb) *OR* heat cradle (25-watt bulb)
- Disposable gloves
- Washcloth
- Towels
- Soap
- Warm water

Assessment

Assessment should focus on the following:
- Treatment order and response of client to previous treatment, if used
- Status of treatment area (presence of edema, redness, heat, drainage)
- Temperature, pulse rate and rhythm
- Degree of pain and position of comfort, if any

- Ability of client to maintain appropriate position without assistance
- Client's ability to perceive and report pain or burning sensation
- Presence of medical conditions that may impair sensation
- Proper functioning and safety of heating device
- Sensitivity of skin to heat treatment

Nursing Diagnoses

Nursing diagnoses may include the following:
- Altered skin integrity related to episiotomy
- Acute pain related to disruption of skin integrity
- Ineffective tissue perfusion related to edema

Outcome Identification and Planning

Desired Outcomes

Sample desired outcomes include the following:
- Site is clean, with no redness, edema, or drainage within 48 hours after beginning treatment.
- Client verbalizes that pain is relieved or decreased within 24 hours after beginning treatment.

Special Considerations in Planning and Implementation

General

Make sure lamp functions accurately and safely. Do NOT use if cord is frayed or cracks are noted. Schedule procedure at a time when client can be checked every 5 minutes. Be sure hands are thoroughly dry when handling electrical equipment.

Pediatric

Do not leave children unattended with heating apparatus. Assess frequently because of the fragile nature of their skin.

Geriatric

Duration of heat therapy may need to be reduced for elderly clients because their skin is often more fragile, with a thin epidermis.

Home Health

At home, a mechanic's trouble light with appropriate wattage bulb may be used as a heat lamp. Teach client/family safety precautions for using light. Ensure safety of home environment (e.g., electrical outlets are intact and not overloaded).

Transcultural

Determine cultural perspective regarding hot/cold perception of illness and appropriateness of treatment (see Table 10.1). Incorporate client preference when possible. Omit treatment if client objects, and consult physician.

Delegation

Generally, this procedure may be delegated to trained unlicensed assistive personnel. Check agency policy. Emphasize importance of monitoring local treatment area closely.

Implementation

Action	Rationale
1. Explain procedure to client.	*Reduces anxiety; promotes cooperation*
2. Perform hand hygiene and organize equipment.	*Reduces microorganism transfer; promotes efficiency*
3. Put on disposable gloves.	*Prevents contamination from secretions*
4. Position client for comfort and for optimal exposure of treatment area.	*Promotes optimal treatment results*
5. While it is turned off, place lamp 18 to 24 inches from wound to be treated.	*Prevents accidental burns from placing lamp too close*
6. Turn lamp on and observe client's response to the heat for 1 minute: • Observe facial and body gestures. • Observe wound area for redness. • Ask client if heat is too high.	*Determines initial response to treatment*
7. Cover client while keeping treatment area well exposed to the lamp; for heat cradle, place top sheet over cradle and client (Fig. 10.2). Be sure that neither clothing nor covers are touching the bulb of the lamp.	*Provides privacy; reduces electrical and fire hazard*
8. Remove disposable gloves and perform hand hygiene; put on gloves again, as needed (e.g., when direct	*Prevents microorganism transfer*

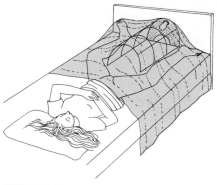

FIGURE 10.2

Action	Rationale
contact with body secretions is possible).	
9. Place call light within reach.	*Permits communication; promotes prompt response to client needs*
10. Assess client response to heat every 5 minutes.	*Prevents complications from treatment*
11. Remove covers and remove heat cradle after 10 minutes or heat lamp after 20 minutes.	*Terminates treatment; prevents local burn injury from overexposure to heat*
12. Reposition client and replace covers.	*Promotes comfort and safety*
13. Remove equipment from bedside and perform hand hygiene.	*Prevents hazards and microorganism transfer*

Evaluation

Were desired outcomes achieved? Examples of evaluation include:
- Desired outcome met: Site of treatment is clean with no redness, edema, or drainage 48 hours after beginning treatment.
- Desired outcome met: Client reports decreased discomfort following the heat lamp procedure.

Documentation

The following should be noted on the client's chart:
- Condition and appearance of wound or treatment area before and after treatment

- Pulse and temperature
- Duration and kind of treatment
- Position of client
- Status of pain
- Client tolerance of treatment

Sample Documentation
Date: 2/3/05
Time: 1400

Heat lamp applied to perineal area for 20 minutes. 3-cm moist red area noted around episiotomy site. After heat lamp treatment, episiotomy site intact and dry, with slight redness and 1-cm edema. Client reports no perineal pain. Tolerated procedure well, BP 130/76, pulse 80, temp 98.8. Lying in right lateral position in bed.

● **Nursing Procedure 10.4**

Administering Cold Therapy: Ice Bag/Collar/Glove/Commercial Cold Pack/Cold, Moist Compresses

Purpose

Reduces local edema, bleeding, and hematoma formation
Decreases local pain sensation

Equipment

- Ice bag/collar/glove/prepackaged cold pack
- Small towel or washcloth
- Tape
- Two pairs of disposable gloves

If an ice bag/collar/glove or prepackaged cold pack is unavailable or not preferred, substitute the following materials to make a cold, moist compress:
- Plastic-lined linen saver
  Clean basin
  Bath thermometer

- Pack of 4 × 4-inch gauze pads
- Solution cooled with ice, 15°C (59°F)
- Cotton swab stick
- Ice chips

Assessment

Assessment should focus on the following:
- Treatment order and response to previous treatment, if used
- Status of treatment area (edema, local bleeding, integrity)
- Temperature, pulse rate and rhythm
- Degree of pain and position of comfort, if any
- Ability of client to maintain appropriate position without assistance
- Client's ability to perceive and report pain or freezing sensation
- Presence of medical conditions that may impair sensation or circulation
- Proper functioning and safety of cooling device
- Sensitivity of skin to cold treatment

Nursing Diagnoses

Nursing diagnoses may include the following:
- Acute pain related to sprained right wrist

Outcome Identification and Planning

Desired Outcomes

Sample desired outcomes include the following:
- Client states that pain is reduced or relieved after treatment.
- No bleeding or hematoma is noted at treatment site.

Special Considerations in Planning and Implementation

General

Schedule the procedure at a time when the client can be checked frequently. Cold applications can cause further tissue damage in areas that have decreased circulation.

Pediatric

Children may require more frequent checks because their skin may be thinner and more sensitive to cold.

Geriatric

Elderly clients may require more frequent checks because their skin may be thinner and more sensitive to cold. Duration of cold therapy may need to be reduced because elderly clients are more likely to have diminished sensation and impaired circulation.

Home Health

In the home, a self-sealing plastic bag or a package of frozen small vegetables (e.g., peas) may be used as an ice bag, if necessary.

 Transcultural

Determine cultural perspective regarding hot/cold perception of illness and appropriateness of treatment (see Table 10.1). Incorporate client preference when possible. Omit treatment if client objects, and consult physician.

Delegation

Generally, this procedure may be delegated to unlicensed assistive personnel. Check agency policy. Monitor local treatment area closely.

Implementation

Action	Rationale
1. Explain procedure to client.	*Decreases anxiety*
2. Perform hand hygiene and organize equipment. Proceed to step 4 for Ice Bag/Collar/Glove, Commercial Cold Pack, or Cold, Moist Compress, depending on equipment.	*Reduces microorganism transfer; promotes efficiency*
Preparing Ice Bag/ Collar/Glove	
4. Fill bag/collar/glove about three-fourths full with ice chips.	*Provides cold surface area*
5. Remove excess air from bag/collar/glove by placing it on a flat surface and gently pressing on it until ice reaches the opening. Contain ice securely (fasten end of bag or collar or tie end of glove).	*Improves functioning of pack; prevents water seepage*
6. Cover bag/collar/glove with small towel or washcloth (if bag is made of a soft cloth exterior, this is not necessary). Proceed to step 7.	*Promotes comfort*

Action	Rationale
Preparing a Commercial Cold Pack	
4. Remove ice pack from outer package, if present.	*Promotes efficiency; provides access to pack*
5. Break the inner seal; hold pack tightly in the center in upright position and squeeze. Do NOT use pack if leaking is noted (chemical burn may occur).	*Activates chemical ingredients to provide cold*
6. Lightly shake pack until the inner contents are lying in the lower portion of the pack. Proceed to step 7.	*Localizes activated chemicals*
Preparing Cold, Moist Compresses	
4. Cool prescribed solution to desired temperature (15°C [59°F]) by running cold tap water over the container or by placing it in a basin of ice. Discard cold tap water or ice and pour cooled solution into bath basin. Place gauze into basin.	*Facilitates cooling of solution; saturates gauze with solution*
5. Prepare client:	
• Assist client into comfortable position for application.	*Facilitates compress placement*
• Place plastic pad under treatment area.	*Prevents soiling of linens*
• Drape client with loose bed linen.	*Provides privacy while allowing access to treatment site*
6. Wring one layer of wet gauze until it is dripless.	*Removes excess solution*
7. Put on gloves.	*Reduces microorganism transfer*
8. Remove and discard old dressings, if present.	*Provides access to treatment site*
9. Remove and discard old gloves and put on new gloves.	*Reduces microorganism transfer*
10. If necessary, clean and dry treatment area.	*Facilitates effectiveness of treatment*

Action	Rationale
11. Proceed to step 12 for Ice Bag/Collar/Glove and Commercial Cold Pack or Cold, Moist Compress.	

Applying Ice Bag/Collar/ Glove and Commercial Cold Pack

Action	Rationale
12. Place the pack lightly against treatment area.	*Allows for gradual initiation of vasoconstrictive effect*
13. Remove pack and assess client for redness of skin or complaint of freezing sensation after 30 seconds. Stop treatment if not tolerated (redness or complaint) and notify physician.	*Prevents cold injury*
14. Replace pack snugly against the area if no problems are noted, and secure with tape. Proceed to step 15.	*Resumes treatment; stabilizes cold pack*

Applying a Cold, Moist Compress

Action	Rationale
12. Place compress on the wound for several seconds.	*Initiates vasoconstrictive therapy*
13. Pick up edge of compress to observe initial skin response to therapy.	*Allows assessment of skin for adverse responses to therapy*
14. Replace compress gauze every 5 minutes or as needed to maintain coolness, assessing treatment area each time.	*Promotes safety; provides for reassessment of treatment area*
15. Place call light within reach and raise side rails.	*Promotes communication and safety*
16. Reassess treatment area every 5 minutes by lifting the corners of the gauze.	*Monitors effects of treatment over time*
17. After 20 minutes, terminate treatment and dry skin.	*Prevents local injury due to overexposure to treatment*
18. Apply new dressing over wound, if necessary.	*Promotes wound healing*
19. Reposition client and raise side rails.	*Facilitates comfort and safety*
20. Remove all equipment from bedside, remove gloves, and perform hand hygiene.	*Maintains clean environment; facilitates asepsis*

Evaluation

Were desired outcomes achieved? Examples of evaluation include:
- Desired outcome partially met: Site is clean but area remains edematous with limited mobility 48 hours after beginning treatment.
- Desired outcome met: Client reports decreased discomfort 24 hours after beginning treatment.

Documentation

The following should be noted on the client's chart:
- Size, location, and appearance of treatment area
- Status of pain
- Type of treatment
- Position of client
- Duration of treatment
- Client tolerance of treatment

Sample Documentation
Date: 2/3/05
Time: 1400

Ice bag applied to right wrist for 20 minutes. Edema decreased from 2 to 1 cm. Site slightly cool to touch after treatment, capillary refill 3 seconds. Client reports relief of pain. Tolerated procedure well, sitting in chair with wrist elevated on pillow.

● Nursing Procedure 10.5

Administering a Sitz Bath 🖐

Purpose

Promotes perineal and anorectal healing
Reduces local inflammation and discomfort

Equipment

- Clean bathtub filled with enough warm water to cov
  buttocks (or portable sitz tub, if available)

- Peri-care equipment
- Bath towel
- Bath thermometer, if available
- Bathroom mat
- Gown
- Small footstool
- Nonsterile gloves

Assessment

Assessment should focus on the following:
- Baseline vital signs
- Appearance and condition of treatment area
- Client's knowledge of benefits of sitz bath
- Client's inability to remain unattended in bathtub (e.g., confusion, weakness)
- Status of pain

Nursing Diagnoses

Nursing diagnoses may include the following:
- Impaired skin integrity related to episiotomy
- Acute pain related to disruption of skin integrity
- Ineffective tissue perfusion related to edema

Outcome Identification and Planning

Desired Outcomes

Sample desired outcomes include the following:
- Site is clean, with no redness, edema, or drainage, within 48 hours.
- Client verbalizes that pain is relieved or decreased within 12 hours after beginning treatment.

Special Considerations in Planning and Implementation

General

Avoid sitz baths during the initial injury phase (first 12 to 24 hours), as they may contribute to post-trauma swelling. Inflatable rings or cushions are generally discouraged because they can cause stretching and tension on perineal or anorectal tissue, which impairs wound healing. Schedule the procedure for a time when the client can be checked frequently. If client cannot remain alone, plan to remain with client or find someone to do so.

diatric

not leave children unattended during this procedure.

tric

atation from exposure to warm water could cause severe in blood pressure and cardiac function in elderly clients promised cardiovascular status. The duration and temperature of the sitz bath might need to be decreased, and clients must be watched closely for adverse reactions.

Home Health

Instruct client and family regarding the procedure. Emphasize the importance of a family member's checking on the client frequently if a potential safety hazard (e.g., falling in tub or on floor) exists.

Transcultural

See overview regarding hot/cold conditions and Table 10.1. Discuss therapy with client and relay any objections to physician. Adhere to cultural preferences regarding same-sex or opposite-sex care providers; family member should be instructed on procedure for sitz bath if preferred by client.

Delegation

Generally, this procedure may be delegated to unlicensed assistive personnel. Stress the importance of monitoring water temperature before contact with client's skin.

Implementation

Action	Rationale
1. Explain procedure to client.	Promotes relaxation and compliance
2. Perform hand hygiene, organize equipment, and put on gloves.	Reduces microorganism transfer; promotes efficiency
3. Check temperature of water with thermometer; water should be 40.5°C to 43°C (105°F to 110°F). If thermometer is unavailable, test water with your wrist (water should be warm).	Prevents skin damage from high water temperature
4. Assist client to bathroom and close door. Proceed to step 5 for a tub or toilet sitz bath.	Provides privacy

For Tub Sitz Bath

Action	Rationale
5. Place rubber ring at bottom of tub and place bathmat on floor.	Prevents accidental falls
6. Assist client into tub, using footstool if necessary.	Prevents accidental injury
7. Ascertain client's stability in the tub. Proceed to step 8.	Prevents complications from falling or unusual reaction to therapy

Action	Rationale
For Portable Sitz Bath Using Toilet Insert	
5. Prepare the equipment:	
• Raise the toilet seat and place the basin on the rim of the toilet bowl. Fill with warm water.	*Allows client to sit in the water*
• Fill water bag with warm water (40.5°C to 43°C [105°F to 110°F]). Prime tubing and close the clamp.	*Promotes comfort and vasodilation; prevents leakage*
• Hang the bag at approximately shoulder height.	*Higher heights may cause the water to leave the bag too quickly, creating a flow that is too forceful*
• Thread the tubing through the back of the basin and secure the tubing in the slot in the bottom of the basin (Fig. 10.3).	*Ensures that water is properly directed toward injured area and prevents spillage*

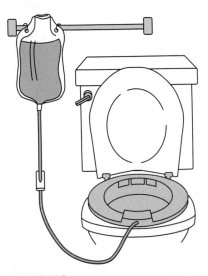

FIGURE 10.3

Action	Rationale
6. After the client is seated on the basin, demonstrate how to unclamp tubing to begin and adjust water flow.	*Allows client to adjust to comfort level*
7. Cover the client's lap with a towel or bath blanket.	*Promotes warmth and privacy*
8. Assess client's reaction to the treatment: • Observe facial expressions and body motions for signs of discomfort. • Ask if heat is too high. • Watch for dizziness, faintness, profuse diaphoresis. • Note any rapid increase or irregularity of pulse.	*Prevents complications from or unusual reaction to therapy*
9. Instruct client on use of call light, and place light within reach.	*Allows communication and immediate response to emergency*
10. Check client every 5 to 10 minutes.	*Allows assessment of unusual reactions*
11. After 15 to 20 minutes, help client out of the tub or up from the toilet.	*Terminates treatment*
12. Assist client with drying and dressing, then place linens in hamper.	*Prevents chilling*
13. Return client to room or bed.	*Promotes comfort*
14. Remove equipment and clean tub or sitz basin.	*Reduces microorganism transfer to others using tub or basin*
15. Remove gloves and perform hand hygiene.	*Reduces microorganism transfer*

Evaluation

Were desired outcomes achieved? Examples of evaluation include:
• Desired outcome met: Perineal tissue remains edematous, with episiotomy clean, dry, and intact 48 hours after beginning treatment.
• Desired outcome met: Client verbalizes that pain has decrea~ 12 hours after beginning treatment.

Documentation

The following should be noted on the client's chart:
• Appearance of treatment area before and after treat~
• Type of sitz bath used (tub or portable)

- Any unusual reactions to treatment, such as profuse diaphoresis, faintness, dizziness, palpitations, or pulse changes
- Duration of sitz bath
- Status of pain
- Client's reaction to treatment

Sample Documentation
Date: 2/3/05
Time: 1400

Tub sitz bath to perineal area for 20 minutes. Client states pain decreased from level 8 to level 1 after treatment. Redness decreased from pretreatment level. No drainage from open perineal wound. No complaints of dizziness.

● Nursing Procedure 10.6

Administering a Tepid Sponge Bath 🧤

Purpose

Provides controlled reduction of body temperature

Equipment

- Thermometer (oral or rectal)
- Basin of tepid water
- Gown
- Plastic-lined pads
- Bath blanket
- Six or seven washcloths
- Two towels
- Nonsterile gloves

Assessment

Assessment should focus on the following:
Doctor's order and client's response to previous treatment
Condition and appearance of skin
Pulse and temperature
Level of consciousness

Nursing Diagnoses

Diagnoses may include the following:

- Ineffective thermoregulation related to sepsis
- Risk for injury related to elevated temperature

Outcome Identification and Planning

Desired Outcomes

Sample desired outcomes include the following:
- Client maintains temperature within normal or acceptable limits (specified by physician).
- Client tolerates treatment with no adverse changes in status or vital signs.

Special Considerations in Planning and Implementation

General

Alcohol or Betadine baths are not recommended since they may be systemically absorbed. Discontinue bath if shivering occurs or if the client becomes agitated, as this may increase core temperature. An antipyretic should be given approximately 1 hour before the procedure (if ordered), as it reduces the hypothalmic set point. Otherwise, the body will superficially vasoconstrict and shiver during the procedure to maintain the set point.

Pediatric

The body temperature of children is less stable than that of adults and may require more frequent assessment. To lower a child's temperature, try placing the child in a tepid bath and splashing water over the body, and place the child on a wet towel and cover groin and axillary areas with wet washcloths for 20 minutes. This technique may reduce the temperature by 1F. Observe for rapid overcooling and discontinue if child begins to shiver or becomes agitated.

Geriatric

The body temperature of elderly clients can be unstable and may require more frequent assessment.

Home Health

Instruct client and family members on the procedure and precautions of the tepid sponge bath, and recommend that a thermometer be secured for the home.

Transcultural

Note overview regarding hot/cold conditions and Table 10.1. Adhere to cultural preferences regarding heat and cold, and same-sex or opposite-sex care providers; family member should be instructed on procedure for sponge bath if preferred by client.

Delegation

Generally, this procedure may be delegated to unlicensed assistive personnel.

Implementation

Action	Rationale
1. Explain procedure to client.	*Reduces anxiety; promotes compliance*
2. Close windows and doors.	*Eliminates drafts, thus preventing chilling; provides privacy*
3. Perform hand hygiene, organize equipment, and apply gloves.	*Reduces microorganism transfer; promotes efficiency*
4. Lower side rails and undress client, covering body with bath blanket and rolling topsheet to the bottom of bed. Position on back or for comfort.	*Prevents chilling; protects privacy*
5. Place plastic pads under client.	*Prevents linen soilage*
6. Fill basin with tepid water and place washcloths and one towel in basin of water.	*Cools cloths and towel*
7. Wring washcloths and place one in each of the following areas (loose towel can remain over private areas): • Over forehead • Under armpits • Over groin	*Promotes rapid cooling due to increased vascularity of these regions*
8. Rewet and replace washcloths as they become warm.	*Maintains coolness of cloths*
9. Wring the wet towel and place around one of client's arms (Fig. 10.4).	*Cools extremity*
10. Wring a washcloth and sponge the other arm for 3 or 4 minutes. Repeat steps 9 and 10 with the opposite arm.	*Gradually cools extremity*
11. Remove towel from arm and place in basin, dry both arms thoroughly, and replace light blanket over body.	*Prepares towel for future use; prevents chilling*

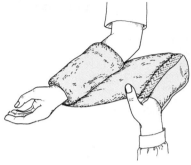

FIGURE 10.4

Action	Rationale
12. Observe for shivering, discomfort, or agitation. If present, terminate procedure and notify physician.	*Can cause increase in core temperature*
13. Check client's temperature and pulse. • If temperature is above 37.7°C (100°F), proceed with bath (continue with step 14). • If temperature is 37.7°C (100°F) or below, terminate the procedure (continue with step 15). • If pulse rate is significantly increased, terminate procedure for 5 minutes and recheck; if it remains significantly elevated, terminate procedure and notify physician.	*Prevents complications related to overcooling*
14. Continue by sponging and drying the following areas for 3 to 5 minutes each (you may use steps 9 to 11 when sponging legs): • Chest • Left leg	*Facilitates cooling by expanding the body surface area being treated*

Action	Rationale
• Back • Abdomen • Right leg • Buttocks *Note:* Stop every 10 minutes to reassess temperature and pulse in order to assess the effectiveness of treatment and prevent overcooling.	
15. Remove all cloths and towels and dry client thoroughly.	*Terminates treatment; promotes comfort*
16. Replace gown.	*Restores privacy*
17. Reposition client for comfort and raise side rails.	*Promotes comfort and safety*
18. Properly discard all washcloths, towels, plastic pads, and wet linens. (If necessary, obtain dry linens and remake bed.)	*Maintains cleanliness of environment*
19. Remove and discard gloves and perform hand hygiene.	*Reduces microorganism transfer*

Evaluation

Were desired outcomes achieved? Examples of evaluation include:
- Desired outcome met: Client's temperature reduced by 1.5°F and maintained within acceptable limits following tepid sponge bath.
- Desired outcome met: Client tolerated treatment with no adverse changes in status or vital signs.

Documentation

The following should be noted on the client's chart:
- Client's position before and after bath
- Pulse and temperature before, during, and after bath
- Client mentation and general tolerance of the bath
- Untoward reactions to the treatment
- Length of the treatment and percentage of body sponged

Sample Documentation
Date: 2/3/05
Time: 1400

Tepid sponge bath administered to trunk and extremities
for 20 minutes because client's temperature is 104.7°F.
Temperature after bath, 102.6°F; pulse, 118 and regular;
respirations, 28 and regular; BP, 110/62. Client tolerated
procedure well. Dozing quietly in bed in supine position.
Doctor notified of status.

● **Nursing Procedure 10.7**

Using a Transcutaneous Electrical Nerve Stimulation Unit

Purpose

Controls acute and chronic pain by delivering electrical impulse
    to nerve endings, which blocks pain message along pathway
    and prevents brain reception
Reduces amount of pain medication required to maintain comfort
Allows client to remain mentally alert, active, and pain-free

Equipment

- Transcutaneous electrical nerve stimulation (TENS) unit
- Lead wires
- Electrodes
- Fresh 9-volt battery
- Electrode gel (optional)
- Water (optional)

Assessment

Assessment should focus on the following:
- Status of pain (location and degree; alleviating and aggravating factors)
- Type and location of incision, if applicable
- Previous use of and knowledge level regarding TENS unit

- Presence of skin irritation, abrasions, or breakage
- Proper functioning of TENS unit
- Presence of medical conditions or equipment that may contraindicate the use of a TENS unit (e.g., pacemaker, defibrillator)

Nursing Diagnoses

Nursing diagnoses may include the following:
- Acute pain related to surgical incision
- Impaired physical mobility related to discomfort

Outcome Identification and Planning

Desired Outcomes

Sample desired outcomes include the following:
- Client ambulates in hallway with minimal complaint of pain.
- Client requests pain medication less frequently.
- Decreased dosages of medication are needed.

Special Considerations in Planning and Implementation

General

Apply electrodes to clean, unbroken skin only. If sensitivity to electrode adhesive is noted, notify doctor before application. If skin irritation is noted during TENS use, remove electrodes and notify doctor. Client should be informed that TENS unit may not totally relieve pain but should reduce discomfort.

Pediatric

Activities that may dislodge lead placement or accidentally change parameter settings may need to be limited.

Geriatric

Check skin frequently for tenderness and sensitivity. If client is confused and electrical stimulation increases irritation, decrease or stop stimulation and notify doctor.

Delegation

Specially trained personnel may apply TENS units in some agencies. Note agency policy.

Implementation

Action	Rationale
1. Perform hand hygiene and organize equipment.	*Reduces microorganism transfer; promotes efficiency*

Action	Rationale
2. Explain procedure to client.	*Promotes relaxation and compliance*
3. Wash, rinse, and dry client's skin thoroughly.	*Improves electrode adhesion*
4. Prepare electrodes as described in package insert.	*Promotes proper contact and energy conduction*
5. Place electrodes on body areas directed by doctor or physical therapist (often along incision site or spinal column or both, depending on location of pain).	*Places electrodes in position for optimal results*
6. Plug lead wires into TENS unit (Fig. 10.5).	
7. Ensure that unit is turned to the lowest setting before turning it on.	*Avoids client discomfort by having intensity level initially too high*
8. Regulate the TENS unit for client comfort:	
• Work with one lead (set) at a time.	*Ensures proper stimulation of each area addressed*
• Before beginning, ask client to indicate when stimulation is felt.	*Permits nurse to regulate stimulation within client tolerance*

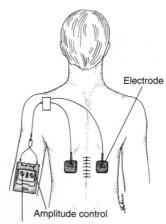

Electrode

Amplitude control

Pulse width control

FIGURE 10.5

Action	Rationale
• Beginning at 0, increase level of stimulation until client indicates feeling of discomfort (muscle contraction under electrode area).	*Achieves maximum stimulation to block pain sensation*
• When client indicates discomfort, reduce stimulation level slightly.	*Prevents continued contraction of muscles at pain site or around incision*
• Try to maintain highest tolerable level of stimulation. Repeat above steps with other lead (set).	*Promotes maximum blockage of pain sensations*
• Note color of blinking light on unit and change battery as needed.	*Indicates that unit is functional (red light may indicate low battery)*
9. Stabilize unit for client mobility, using one of the following methods:	
• Clamp unit to pajama bottom or gown (may place tape around unit and pin to gown with safety pin).	
• Place in pants pocket or clip to belt if client is ambulatory.	*Allows client mobility during treatment*
10. Monitor client for comfort level with vital signs assessment; check for increased respiratory rate, pulse, or blood pressure.	*Indicates effectiveness of unit; indicates need to adjust stimulation due to increased discomfort*
11. Be alert for malfunctions and correct them; the following guidelines should be used for general management of the TENS unit to prevent injury to client and damage to TENS unit:	
• Client should remove unit before a shower or bath.	*Prevents shock to client*
• If client complains of increased or sudden pain, check TENS connections and perform general assessment of incision, dressing, and client.	*Verifies function of unit and detects possible causes of increased discomfort*

Action	Rationale
• TENS unit should be off whenever removing or applying leads. If lead becomes disconnected, turn unit off, reconnect lead, then increase stimulation level from 0.	*Prevents shocking sensation*
• NEVER turn unit on when set at maximum stimulation: always start at 0 and gradually increase level.	*Prevents shocking sensation*
• If client complains of shocking sensation or muscle contraction, decrease stimulation level.	*Prevents excessive stimulation*
• Check battery status frequently.	*Prevents interruption of therapy due to loss of battery power*
12. Maintain therapy as ordered or as long as client desires, if on p.r.n. basis.	*Maximizes effectiveness of therapy through ongoing treatment*
13. Turn unit off and remove and discard electrodes to discontinue therapy.	*Stops stimulation to nerve endings*
14. Disinfect and store equipment according to facility policy.	*Decreases spread of microorganisms*
15. Perform hand hygiene.	*Reduces spread of microorganisms*

Evaluation

Were desired outcomes achieved? Examples of evaluation include:
• Desired outcome met: Client ambulating in the hall, reports pain decreased from a 7 to a 4 on a scale of 1 to 10 after TENS unit activated.
• Desired outcome met: Client requests pain medication less frequently.
• Desired outcome met: Decreased dosages of medication are needed.

Documentation

The following should be noted on the client's chart:
• Type and location of incision, if applicable
• Time, date, and duration of TENS application
• Level of stimulation of each lead (set)
• Area stimulated by each lead (set)

- Pain location, level, aggravating and alleviating factors
- Client's tolerance of treatment
- Client teaching done and accuracy with which client repeats instructions

---

Sample Documentation
Date: 2/3/05
Time: 1400

TENS unit applied for lumbar back pain reported at level 9. Electrodes applied to lumbar area with setting of 5.5 on lead 1 and 6.0 on lead 2. Client verbalized understanding of unit function and states that minimum pain (level 2) is felt at present. Tolerating treatment well, maintaining TENS therapy.

● **Nursing Procedure 10.8**

Using Patient-Controlled Analgesia

Purpose

Allows client to control delivery of pain medication in a safe, consistent, effective, and reliable manner using a programmable pump connected to a subcutaneous or intravenous catheter

Equipment

- Patient-controlled analgesia (PCA) infuser
- PCA administration set (pump tubing)
- Patent subcutaneous or intravenous line installed as the prescribed route of administration
- PCA infuser key
- PCA flow sheet or appropriate form
- Ordered narcotic analgesic vial bag or syringe (mixed by pharmacy)
- Vial injector (accompanies vial)
- Client information booklet
  IV start kit (unless venous access is already available)
  IV tubing and fluid as applicable
  Naloxone (Narcan) solution if giving opioid agonists
  i.e., morphine)

Assessment

Assessment should focus on the following:
- Doctor's orders for type of analgesic, loading dose, concentration of analgesic mixture, lock-out interval (minimum time allowed between doses), and supplemental medication or bolus for uncontrolled pain
- Type of illness or surgery
- Pain (type, location, character, intensity, aggravating and alleviating factors)
- Level of consciousness, orientation
- Catheter insertion site (patency, erythema, swelling, induration)
- Ability to learn and comprehend oral and written instructions
- Respiratory rate and depth (if less than 10/min, stop infusion and notify physician)

Nursing Diagnoses

The nursing diagnoses may include the following:
- Acute pain related to thoracic incision site
- Anxiety related to lack of pain control

Outcome Identification and Planning

Desired Outcomes

Sample desired outcomes include the following:
- Client states that pain is relieved within 2 hours of PCA initiation.
- Adequate relief from chronic pain is achieved.
- There is an increase in the client's activity that is currently limited due to constant pain.

Special Considerations in Planning and Implementation

General

Pain is very subjective; for pain management to be effective, it must meet the client's needs. Encourage clients to use nonpharmacologic measures to control pain (e.g., biofeedback, guided imagery). Often these techniques have synergistic effects with the medication that increase the client's activity tolerance and decrease the need for pain medication. Discourage family members from administering doses of analgesia for the client, as overdosage can occur.

Pediatric

PCA therapy is usually used in adolescents or adults. When it is used with a child, instruct the parents as well as the child.

Geriatric

The analgesic may have an adverse effect on some elderly clients (e.g., changes in level of orientation). Dosages may need to be titrated for those with impaired liver or kidney function.

Home Health

Teach family members how to recognize signs of overdosage in the homebound client. Naloxone must be readily available, and a plan for emergencies must be discussed with the client and caregiver. There are many types of pumps for home use. Discuss the specific pump applications with the client or caregiver.

💲 Cost-Cutting Tips

Portable infusion pumps are not necessarily trouble-free or less expensive for the client. The cost/benefit ratio must be considered with this method of controlling pain in the home setting. Refer client and family to home health agency for additional education and follow-up assessment of pain management effectiveness.

👥 Transcultural

Determine cultural perspectives regarding use of this procedure. Clients from various cultures may not feel comfortable with self-administration of medication.

Delegation

PCA pumps are managed by the RN and not delegated to others.

Implementation

Action	Rationale
1. Perform hand hygiene and organize equipment.	*Reduces microorganism transfer; promotes efficiency*
2. Explain use of system to client and provide written literature; assess accuracy of client's understanding with return demonstrations and client's verbal responses.	*Decreases anxiety; promotes compliance*
3. Prepare analgesic for administration after checking the five rights of drug administration (client, drug, dosage [concentration], route, time): • Connect injector to pre-filled vial or syringe (Fig. 10.6).	*Ensures delivery of appropriate medication and dosage*

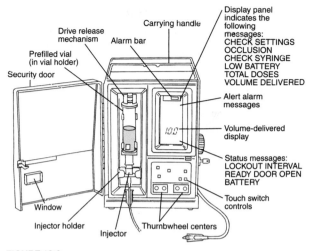

FIGURE 10.6

Action	Rationale
• Hold vial vertically and push injector to remove air.	
• Connect PCA administration set to vial, prime tubing, and close tubing clamp.	
• Plug machine into electrical outlet and use PCA infuser key to open pump door.	
• Load vial into machine according to equipment operation booklet.	
4. Prepare primary IV fluid and tubing (see Procedure 5.3).	*Provides access for connection of PCA tubing to client*
5. Attach primary IV tubing to Y-connector line of PCA tubing.	*Provides fluid to keep vein open between medication doses*
6. Open primary tubing clamp and prime lower portion of PCA tubing.	*Removes air from tubing*
7. Close clamp on primary IV.	

Action	Rationale
8. Put on gloves and prepare venous access: • Insert IV catheter (see Procedures 5.2 and 5.4); if venous access (IV lock or central line) is already present, verify patency and connect PCA tubing directly to IV catheter. • Release clamps on PCA and primary tubing. • Regulate primary IV to infuse at keep-vein-open (or ordered) rate (see Procedures 5.5 and 5.6).	*Maintains patency of vein between medication doses*
9. Administer loading dose if ordered: • Verify ordered dosage. • Set lock-out interval on pump at 00 minutes. • Set volume to be delivered, using dose-volume thumbwheel control. • Press and release loading-dose control switch.	*Delivers dose of analgesic to initiate pain relief*
10. Once loading dose is administered (if ordered), use the following steps to set parameters for dosage control: • Calculate volume of medication needed to deliver ordered dose (available dose per volume divided by ordered dose equals volume); often vials contain 200 mg Demerol per 20-mL vial or 30 mg morphine per 30-mL vial. • Set dose volume using thumbwheel control for desired volume for each dose.	*Determines volume that will deliver ordered dose* *Sets amount of fluid and medication to be delivered for each dose*

Action	Rationale
• If client is receiving a continuous infusion (basal rate), set the basal rate as ordered using the touchpad control.	*Delivers continuous rate of medication and allows patient-controlled supplement*
• Set lock-out interval using thumbwheel control to set the desired time interval.	*Sets minimum time between allotted doses; prevents medication overdose*
• To set 4-hour limit, push control switch to display current limit; if different limit is desired, depress again and hold switch until desired limit is reached, then release switch.	*Limits total volume to be infused over any consecutive 4-hour period*
• Close and lock security door using infuser key; "ready" message should appear indicating that PCA infuser is in client control mode and first dose can be administered. Place key with narcotic keys (or per agency policy).	*Secures narcotic and parameters set into machine*
11. Instruct client on administration of dose; inform client of the following information:	
• When pain is experienced, press and release control button.	*Delivers set dose of analgesic*
• Medication will be delivered and infuser will enter a lock-out period during which no additional medication can be delivered. A "ready" message will appear when next dose can be delivered.	*Prevents overmedication*
12. Ensure that the side rails are up and that the call bell and the PCA administration button are within reach before leaving the client.	*Provides a safe environment and allows for the client to administer analgesia*

Action	Rationale
13. Monitor the dosage received by client every 1 to 2 hours to maintain PCA therapy:	
• Press TOTAL DOSE switch and note number of client doses administered during past period.	
• Check pump function and notify physician of any need for changes in therapy.	*Assesses adequate control and physical response to medication level (high pain scores require reassessment)*
• Record temperature, pulse, respirations, pain relief, mobility, and sedation.	*Excessive sedation and any indication of respiratory depression require pump reprogramming.*
• At each assessment, monitor insertion site for erythema, inflammation, or drainage.	*Continuously assesses infection potential*
• Document doses delivered, volume remaining, and observations on flow sheet, and calculate total volume in appropriate column.	*Identifies total volume infused and remaining in vial*
• Check volume of medication delivered every 8 hours (or per policy); if agency policy, open pump door with infuser key and verify volume remaining in analgesic vial/bag (volume should equal initial volume minus total volume infused).	*Complies with federal narcotic administration laws*
14. If you are oncoming shift nurse, check drug infusing, dose volume, and lock-out interval with doctor's order.	*Verifies accuracy of infusion*
15. Change vial/bag and injector (when nearly empty or at end of 24-hour period, if agency policy) to provide fresh medication:	
• Assemble new vial/bag and injector.	
• Clear air from vial/bag and close tubing clamp.	

Action	Rationale
• Use infuser key to unlock and open PCA pump door. • Press on/off switch. • Close clamp to old vial and primary fluid tubing. • Remove empty vial (or old vial) and administration set from pump (see equipment operation booklet). • Attach new vial and injector to PCA administration set and prime to remove air. • Attach primary IV to Y-connector of new PCA administration set. • Insert administration set into pump (see equipment operation booklet). • Close and lock pump door. • Release tubing clamps. • Press on/off switch. • Record vial change on PCA flow sheet. • Send previous vial and tubing to pharmacy (per agency protocol).	*Identifies current volume of analgesic in PCA pump to comply with federal recording requirements*
16. To discontinue PCA therapy, follow step 15, omitting preparation of new vial; remove PCA tubing from IV catheter and replace with primary fluid tubing or infusion plug.	*Maintains IV site with fluid infusion or infusion lock*
17. Send vial and tubing to pharmacy (check agency policy).	*Adheres to federal regulations for narcotic control*
18. Discontinue epidural therapy per hospital policy. See Special Considerations in Planning and Implementation.	*Reduces risk of hematoma*
19. Discard or store equipment and perform hand hygiene.	*Restores client environment; prevents spread of microorganisms*

Evaluation

Were desired outcomes achieved? Examples of evaluation include:
- Desired outcome met: Client reports pain decreased from an 8 to a 2 within 2 hours of initiation of PCA therapy.
- Desired outcome met: Adequate relief from chronic pain was achieved.
- Desired outcome met: Client's activity has increased to level prior to pain.

Documentation

The following should be noted on the client's chart:
- Name and dosage of medication being infused
- PCA parameters (hourly dose, lock-out interval, and 4-hour limit)
- Level of consciousness (on scale of 1 to 5)
- Pain level (on scale of 1 to 10)
- Status of respirations
- Amount of medication (analgesic) used each hour
- Number of client attempts to obtain dose (if agency policy)
- Client response to and tolerance of treatment
- Condition of catheter insertion site
- Client or caregiver education activities

Sample Documentation
Date: 2/3/05
Time: 1400

Client received from recovery room after total hip replacement. Complains of pain at level 9. PCA therapy initiated, with 5 mg morphine given IV as loading dose. Dose volume set at 2 ml (2 mg), lock-out interval set at 60 minutes, and 4-hr limit set at 8 mg. Client alert and oriented (level 5). States pain measures 2 on a scale of 1 to 10, with 10 indicating severe pain. Respirations 14 and regular, used 4 mg over the past hour with one attempt for each dose. Return-demonstrated procedure for obtaining dose with 100% accuracy.

Using Epidural Pump Therapy

Purpose

Controls and reduces severe chronic and acute pain without
the more serious side effects of parenteral or oral narcotics

Epidural pump therapy may be ordered as continuous or
patient-controlled administration (PCA)

Equipment

- Patent epidural line installed as the prescribed route of
  administration
- Epidural pump setup
- Ordered narcotic analgesic vial bag or syringe (mixed by
  pharmacy; preservative-free bacteriostatic premixed
  solutions must be used)
- Vial injector (accompanies vial)
- Client information booklet
- Naloxone (Narcan) solution if giving opioid agonists
  (i.e., morphine)
- Povidone-iodine swabs

If PCA has been ordered, also include:
- PCA administration set (pump tubing)
- PCA infuser
- PCA infuser key
- PCA flow sheet or appropriate form

Assessment

Assessment should focus on the following:
- Physician's orders for type and dosage of analgesia and
  anesthesia
- Type of illness or surgery
- Pain (type, location, character, intensity, aggravating and
  alleviating factors)
- Level of consciousness, orientation, and sensation
- Catheter insertion site (patency, erythema, swelling, induration)
- Ability to learn and comprehend oral and written instructions
- Any contraindication for epidural analgesia, such as allergy
  to any proposed medication; any coagulopathy due to disease process or administration of systemic anticoagulants
  (administration of anticoagulants in combination with NSAI
  increases risk of epidural hematoma); localized infection
  inflammation of the area of the epidural catheter; diagno
  of meningitis or central nervous system infection; histo
  increased intracranial pressure

- Urinary retention (obtain an order for bladder scan or straight catheterization or to reinsert Foley catheter if indicated)
- Respiratory rate and depth (if less than 10/min, stop infusion and notify physician)

Nursing Diagnoses

Nursing diagnoses may include the following:
- Acute pain related to thoracic incision site
- Anxiety related to lack of pain control

Outcome Identification and Planning

Desired Outcomes

Sample desired outcomes include the following:
- Pain is relieved within 2 hours of initiation of epidural analgesia.
- Adequate relief from chronic pain is achieved.
- There is an increase in the client's activity that is currently limited due to constant pain.

Special Considerations in Planning and Implementation

General

Pain is very subjective; for pain management to be effective, it must meet the client's needs. See Procedure 3.5 and Appendix A for pain assessment procedures. Encourage clients to use non-pharmacologic measures to control pain, such as biofeedback, guided imagery, etc. Often these techniques have synergistic effects with the medication that increase the client's activity tolerance and decrease need for pain medication. Only preservative-free (nonbacteriostatic) opioid solutions or anesthetics are administered through an epidural catheter. Do not remove epidural catheter immediately after a dose of antithrombotic. Wait 12 hours after subcutaneous low-molecular-weight (LMW) heparin (enoxaparin [Lovenox], dalteparin [Fragmin]); remove within first 24 hours of initiating warfarin (Coumadin). You may resume anticoagulants/antithrombotics 2 hours after removal.

Pediatric

Epidural therapy is usually used in adolescents or adults. When it is used with a child, instruct the parents as well as the child.

Geriatric

Epidural therapy is usually well tolerated in elderly clients because the lack of systemic absorption of opioids via the epidural route.

Home Health

Teach family members how to recognize signs of overdosage in the rebound client. Naloxone must be readily available, and other emergencies must be discussed with the client and caregiver. There are many types of pumps for home use. Discuss the specific pump applications with the client or caregiver.

 Cost-Cutting Tips

Portable infusion pumps are not necessarily trouble-free or less expensive for the client. The cost/benefit ratio must be considered with this method in the home setting. Refer client and family to home health agency for additional education and follow-up assessment of pain management effectiveness.

 Transcultural

Determine cultural perspective regarding use of procedure.

Delegation

Epidural catheters are managed by the RN and not delegated. Other personnel should be instructed on management of the client in terms of positioning and moving.

Implementation

Action	Rationale
1. Perform hand hygiene and organize equipment.	*Reduces microorganism transfer; promotes efficiency*
2. Explain epidural therapy to client and provide written literature; assess accuracy of client's understanding with verbal client responses and return demonstration.	*Decreases anxiety; promotes compliance*
3. Prepare analgesic and anesthetic for administration by checking the five rights of drug administration (client, drug, dosage [concentration], route, time):	*Ensures delivery of appropriate medication and dosage*
4. Ensure that preservative-free nonbacteriostatic opioid solution has been prepared and placed in PCA or epidural pump according to manufacturer's directions.	*Preservatives are toxic to neural tissues.*
5. If epidural therapy will be administered using patient-controlled method, begin PCA setup: • Connect injector to pre-filled vial or syringe (see Fig. 10.6).	*Prepares machine to deliver medication as desired and triggered by client*

Action	Rationale
• Hold vial vertically and push injector to remove air.	
• Connect PCA administration set to vial, prime tubing, and close tubing clamp.	
• Plug machine into electrical outlet and use PCA infuser key to open pump door.	
• Load vial into machine according to equipment operation booklet.	
6. Attach PCA or epidural pump tubing to Luer-lok IV tubing that does not have Y-ports.	*Prevents inadvertent administration of other substances into the epidural catheter; minimizes the risk of separation of catheter and tubing*
7. Prime IV tubing.	*Eliminates air bubbles to prevent an air embolus*
8. Attach IV tubing to the distal end of the catheter and Luer-lok all connections.	*Prevents accidental leakage from separation of catheter and tubing; minimizes risk of infection*
9. Tape a tension loop of tubing to the client's body and securely tape to client's back.	*Minimizes risk of dislodging catheter by pulling on tubing*
10. Label tubing as epidural catheter with drug name, date, and time.	*Prevents inadvertent administration of other substances into epidural catheter*
11. Administer loading dose if ordered to initiate pain relief: Via PCA pump:	
• Verify ordered dosage.	*Initiates pain relief by providing effective medication dose to bloodstream*
• Set lock-out interval on pump at 00 minutes.	
• Set volume to be delivered, using dose-volume thumbwheel control.	
• Press and release loading-dose control switch.	
Via epidural catheter:	
• If loading dose (bolus) injection is to be given directly into an epidural catheter, ensure that a filtered needle is used and	*Alcohol is toxic to neural tissues.*

Action	Rationale
that the injection cap is cleansed with povidone-iodine. Alcohol should NEVER be used.	
12. Once loading dose is administered (if ordered), set parameters for dosage control:	
• Calculate volume of medication needed to deliver ordered dose.	*Determines volume that will deliver ordered dose*
• Set dose volume using thumbwheel control for desired volume for each dose.	*Sets amount of fluid and medication to be delivered for each dose*
• If client is receiving a continuous infusion (basal rate), set the basal rate as ordered using the touchpad control.	*Delivers continuous rate of medication*
If client is also receiving patient-controlled dosing:	
• Set lock-out interval using thumbwheel control to set the desired time interval.	*Sets minimum time between allotted doses; prevents medication overdose*
• To set 4-hour limit, push control switch to display current limit; if different limit is desired, depress again and hold switch until desired limit is reached, then release switch.	*Limits total volume to be infused over any consecutive 4-hour period*
• Close and lock security door using infuser key; "ready" message should appear indicating that PCA infuser is in client-control mode and first dose can be administered. Place key with narcotic keys (or per agency policy).	*Secures narcotic and parameters set into machine*
13. If client is receiving patient-controlled epidural therapy, instruct client on administration of dose and inform client of the following information:	

Action	Rationale
• When pain is experienced, press and release control button.	*Delivers set dose of analgesic*
• Medication will be delivered, and infuser will enter a lock-out period during which no additional medication can be delivered. A "ready" message will appear when next dose can be delivered.	*Prevents overmedication by client*
14. Ensure that the side rails are up and that the call bell and the PCA administration button are within reach before leaving the client.	*Provides a safe environment; allows client to administer analgesic*
15. For maintenance of epidural therapy:	
• Check pump function and notify physician of any need for changes in therapy.	*Assesses adequate control and physical response to medication level (high pain scores require reassessment)*
• Record temperature, pulse, respirations, pain relief level, mobility, sensation, and sedation.	*Excessive sedation and any indication of respiratory depression require pump reprogramming.*
• Assess for urinary retention.	*Determines if medication is impairing urinary elimination*
• At each assessment, monitor insertion site for erythema, inflammation, or drainage.	*Continuously assesses infection potential*
• At each assessment: Press "enter" button on the epidural pump and record volume remaining. Document volume and observations on flow sheet, and calculate total volume in appropriate column.	*Identifies total volume infused and remaining in vial*
• Check volume of medication delivered every 8 hours (or per policy); if agency policy, open pump door with infuser key and verify	*Complies with federal narcotic administration laws*

Action	Rationale
volume remaining in analgesic vial/bag (volume should equal initial volume minus total volume infused).	
16. If you are oncoming shift nurse, check drug infusing, dose volume, and lock-out interval with doctor's order.	*Verifies accuracy of infusion*
17. Change vial/bag and injector (when nearly empty or at end of 24-hour period, if agency policy) to provide fresh medication: • Assemble new vial/bag and injector. • Clear air from vial/bag and close tubing clamp. • Use infuser key to unlock and open PCA pump door. • Press on/off switch. • Close clamp to old vial and primary fluid tubing. • Remove empty vial (or old vial) and administration set from pump (see equipment operation booklet). • Attach new vial and injector to PCA administration set and prime to remove air. • Attach primary IV to Y-connector of new PCA administration set. • Insert administration set into pump (see equipment operation booklet). • Close and lock pump door. • Release tubing clamps. • Press on/off switch. • Record vial change on PCA flow sheet. • Send previous vial and tubing to pharmacy (per agency protocol).	*Initiates client-control mode* *Identifies current volume of analgesic in PCA pump*

Action	Rationale
18. To discontinue epidural or PCA therapy, follow step 17, omitting preparation of new vial; remove PCA tubing from IV catheter and replace with primary fluid tubing or infusion plug.	
19. Send vial and tubing to pharmacy (check agency policy).	*Adheres to federal regulations for narcotic control*
20. Discontinue epidural therapy per hospital policy.	*Reduces risk of hematoma*
21. Discard or store equipment and perform hand hygiene.	*Restores client environment; prevents spread of microorganisms*

Evaluation

Were desired outcomes achieved? Examples of evaluation include:
● Desired outcome met: Client reports pain decreased from an 8 to a 2 within 2 hours of initiation of epidural therapy.
● Desired outcome met: Adequate relief from chronic pain was achieved.
● Desired outcome met: Client's activity has increased.

Documentation

The following should be noted on the client's chart:
● Name and dosage of medication being infused
● Level of consciousness (on scale of 1 to 5)
● Pain level (on scale of 1 to 10)
● Status of respirations
● Amount of medication (analgesic) used each hour
● Condition of catheter insertion site
● Client response to and tolerance of treatment
● Client or caregiver education activities
● Physical mobility
● Level of sensation
● Elimination pattern
● For patient-controlled administration, the following should also be noted on the visit record:
   • PCA parameters (hourly dose, lock-out interval, and 4-hour limit)
   • Number of client attempts to obtain dose (if agency policy)

Sample Documentation
Date: 2/3/05
Time: 1400

Epidural therapy initiated while client was in active stage of labor complaining of pain at level 10 with contractions. 1 mg fentanyl and bupivicaine administered by anesthesiologist and maintained at 0.1 mg/hr. Client alert and oriented, with respirations even and unlabored at 12 per minute. Sensation level at umbilicus. Bladder non-palpable. States pain is at level 2 with contractions, using epidural in PCA mode with accurate return demonstration of procedure and one attempt per each obtained dose. Resting and tolerating therapy well. Side rails up and call bell within reach.

11

Perioperative Nursing and Wound Healing

OVERVIEW

- The aim of all barrier usage (i.e., gloves and gowns) is to decrease exposure to and spread of microorganisms and disease; all actions are aimed at breaking the chain of infection by eliminating the links.
- Gloves should be worn whenever exposure to body secretions is likely. ALWAYS WEAR GLOVES WHEN EMPTYING DRAINAGE CONTAINERS.
- If the sterility of materials, gloves, or gowns is in doubt, treat them as nonsterile.
- Some major nursing diagnostic labels related to biologic safety are risk for infection, impaired tissue integrity, acute pain, knowledge deficit, and anxiety.
- Unlicensed assistive personnel should be trained in safety protocols that prevent exposure to microorganisms, such as application of gowns and gloves. In general, procedures such as dressing changes are performed by the registered nurse or licensed practical nurse. For less complex dressings, some agencies train special personnel to assist with dressing changes. ALL ASSESSMENTS AND THE MANAGEMENT OF DRESSING CHANGES AND WOUND MANAGEMENT ARE THE RESPONSIBILITY OF THE LICENSED NURSE. See agency policy concerning delegation of specific procedures listed in this chapter to unlicensed assistive personnel.

Applying a Sterile Gown (11.1) 🧤
Applying Sterile Gloves (11.2) 🧤

Purpose

Preserves sterile field during sterile procedure

Equipment

- Sterile gown
- Sterile gloves
- Bedside table
- Sterile tongs (optional)

Assessment

Assessment should focus on the following:
- Client's ability to cooperate and not contaminate sterile gown or gloves

Nursing Diagnoses

Nursing diagnoses may include the following:
- Risk of infection related to incision site

Outcome Identification and Planning

Desired Outcomes

Sample desired outcomes include the following:
- Client exhibits no signs of infection after procedure.

Special Considerations in Planning and Implementation

Pediatric

If a child is restless or too young to understand the importance of maintaining a sterile field, restrain the child's arms and legs with linen or soft restraints during the sterile procedure. Encourage a parent to sit at child's bedside during the procedure, if possible.

Delegation

Procedures requiring maintenance of a sterile field generally require licensed personnel and should not be delegated. However, if agency policy and specialized training permits, sterile procedures may be delegated to an experienced, capable unlicensed person.

681

Implementation

Action	Rationale
Applying a Sterile Gown	
1. Perform hand hygiene and organize equipment; apply mask, if needed; enlist assistant to tie gown.	*Reduces microorganism transfer; promotes efficiency*
2. Remove sterile gown package from outer cover and open inner covering to expose sterile gown; place on bedside table, touching only outsides of covering. Spread covering over table; open outer glove package and slide inside glove cover onto sterile field.	*Maintains sterility of gown; provides sterile field; places gloves in convenient location and on sterile field*
3. Remove gown from field, grasping inside of gown and gently shaking to loosen folds; hold gown with inside facing you (Fig. 11.1).	*Prepares gown for application*
4. Place both arms inside gown at the same time and stretch outward until hands reach edge of	*Preserves sterility of gown*

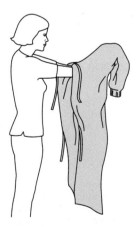

FIGURE 11.1

Action	Rationale
sleeves (i.e., keep hands inside the sleeves of the gown); don sterile gloves (see below).	
5. Have assistant tie the upper gown ties at the neck, then pull tie from back of gown and fasten to inside tie at the waist. Have assistant pull outside tie around with sterile tongs or sterile gloves. Nurse should grasp tie, pull around to front of gown, and secure to front tie.	*Secures gown without contaminating outer portion*
• IF GLOVE OR GOWN BECOMES CONTAMINATED, DISCARD AND REPLACE WITH STERILE GARB.	
Applying Sterile Gloves	
1. Perform hand hygiene. Don gown, if needed; otherwise, open glove package, place on bedside table, and remove inner glove covering; open inner package, using sterile technique, and expose gloves.	*Maintains sterile field*
2. Pick up one glove by cuff and slip fingers of other hand into glove (keep gown sleeve inside glove if applicable); pull glove over hand and sleeve.	*Applies glove while maintaining sterility*
3. Place gloved hand inside cuff of remaining glove and lift slightly; slide other hand into glove and pull cuff over hand, wrist, and sleeve of gown, if applicable (Fig. 11.2). DO NOT TOUCH SKIN WITH GLOVED HAND.	*Facilitates placing glove on hand without contaminating glove or gloved hand; stabilizes gown sleeve and creates continuous sterile hand-to-arm connection*
4. Pull gloves securely over fingers and adjust for fit, using one hand to fix the other.	*Places fingers deeply into gloves while maintaining sterility*

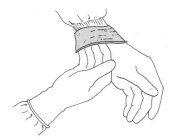

FIGURE 11.2

Action	Rationale
5. Proceed to sterile field, maintaining hands above waist; do not touch nonsterile items. IF GLOVE OR GOWN BECOMES CONTAMINATED, DISCARD AND REPLACE WITH STERILE GARB.	*Prevents contamination of gloves*

Evaluation

Were desired outcomes achieved? Examples of evaluation include:
- Desired outcome met: Procedure completed without contamination; wound appears clean with no signs of infection.

Documentation

The following should be noted on the client's chart:
- Sterile procedure performed
- Sterile garments used

Sample Documentation
Date: 2/17/05
Time: 2100

Temporary pacemaker inserted by Dr. Jones, with sterile technique used. Client tolerated procedure with no reports of unusual discomfort.

Changing Sterile and Nonsterile Dressings

Purpose

Removes accumulated secretions and dead tissue from wound
or incision site
Decreases microorganism growth on wound or incision site
Promotes wound healing

Equipment

- Nonsterile gloves
- 2-inch tape or Montgomery straps (paper tape, if allergic to
  others)
- Sterile dressing tray (forceps, scissors, gauze pads [optional])
- Additional sterile gauze dressing pads (2 × 2-inch, 4 × 4-inch,
  or surgical [ABD] pads, depending on drainage and size of
  area to be covered), or transparent dressing
- Sterile bowl
- Sterile gloves (for sterile dressing change)
- Towel or linen-saver pad
- Sterile cotton balls and cotton-tipped swabs (optional)
- Sterile irrigation saline or sterile water
- Cleaning solution as ordered
- Bacteriostatic ointment
- Overbed table or bedside stand
- Trash bag

Assessment

Assessment should focus on the following:
- Doctor's orders regarding type of dressing change,
  procedure, and frequency of change
- Type and location of wound or incision
- Time of last pain medication
- Client's level of pain
- Allergies to tape or solution used for cleaning

Nursing Diagnoses

Nursing diagnoses may include the following:
- Impaired tissue integrity related to pressure ulcer
- Risk for infection related to impaired skin integrity

Outcome Identification and Planning

Desired Outcomes

A sample desired outcome is:

- Client's wound is healing with no signs of infection.

Special Considerations in Planning and Implementation

General

Dressing changes are often painful. Assess pain needs and medicate client 30 minutes before beginning the procedure.

Pediatric

Children are often immunosuppressed and have decreased resistance; strict asepsis is needed to minimize exposure to microorganisms.

Geriatric

Elderly clients are often immunosuppressed and have decreased resistance; strict asepsis is needed to minimize exposure to microorganisms.

Home Health

Use newspaper to cover the table surface before arranging the work field. Pets should not be permitted in the area during the procedure.

Delegation

In general, procedures such as dressing changes are performed by the registered nurse or licensed practical nurse. For less complex dressings, some agencies train special personnel to assist with dressing changes. ALL ASSESSMENTS AND THE MANAGEMENT OF COMPLEX DRESSING CHANGES AND WOUND MANAGEMENT ARE THE RESPONSIBILITY OF THE LICENSED NURSE.

Implementation

Action	Rationale
1. Perform hand hygiene and organize equipment.	*Reduces microorganism transfer; promotes efficiency*
2. Explain procedure and assistance needed to client.	*Decreases anxiety; promotes cooperation*
3. Premedicate client for pain, if not previously medicated, and assess client's pain level and wait for medication to take	*Decreases discomfort*

Action	Rationale
effect before beginning dressing change.	
4. Place bedside table close to area being dressed.	*Facilitates management of sterile field and supplies*
5. Prepare supplies:	
• Place supplies on bedside table.	*Provides easy access to materials; promotes swift dressing change*
• Tape trash bag to side of table.	*Allows easy disposal of contaminated waste*
• Open sterile gloves and use inside of glove package as sterile field.	*Facilitates use of supplies without contamination*
• Open gauze-pad packages and drop several onto sterile field; leave some pads in open packages if in plastic container (if not, place some pads into sterile bowl).	*Maintains sterile field; prepares gauze for wetting*
• Open dressing tray and remove plastic from sterile bowl.	*Prepares tray and bowl for wetting solutions*
• Open liquids and pour saline on two gauze pads and pour ordered cleaning solution on four gauze pads (more if wet-to-dry dressing).	*Prevents transmission of organisms from table to supplies*
• Place several sterile cotton-tipped swabs and cotton balls on sterile field (use gauze instead if staples are present because cotton may catch on edges of staples).	*Prepares materials needed to clean wound*
6. Don nonsterile gloves.	*Prevents microorganism transfer*
7. Position client to allow access to wound and place towel or pad under wound area.	*Prevents soiling linens*
8. Remove old dressing: loosen the tape by pulling toward the wound and place soiled dressing in the trash bag (note appearance of dressing and wound). IF DRESSING ADHERES TO WOUND, SOAK IT WITH SALINE, THEN GENTLY PULL FREE.	*Permits observation of site and exposes site for cleaning*

Action	Rationale
9. Assess need for frequent (every 4 to 6 hours) dressing changes and effect of tape on skin. If indicated, apply Montgomery straps to hold dressings.	
10. If using Montgomery straps to hold dressing: • Place 8-inch strip of tape on table, sticky side up, and cover with 4-inch strip of tape, sticky side down. Apply safety pins or half-inch slits in spaces along the vertical nonsticky side of tape. • Place sticky side of tape on client, with nonsticky end reaching across half of wound area. • Repeat process on other side of wound; if wound is long, apply straps to upper and lower portions through the slits or using the safety pins.	*Holds dressing in place while preventing skin injury*
11. Discard gloves and perform hand hygiene.	*Reduces microorganism transfer*
12. Don sterile gloves (face mask optional) for sterile dressing change, or don nonsterile gloves for non-sterile dressing change.	*Prevents microorganism transfer*
13. Pick up saline-soaked dressing pad with forceps (forming a large swab) and remove debris and drainage from wound; move from center of wound outward, using a new pad for each area cleaned (Fig. 11.3). Discard old pads away from sterile supplies. Clean or replace forceps if soiled.	*Prevents contamination of wound from organisms on skin surface; maintains sterility of supplies*
14. Wipe wound with pads soaked with ordered cleansing solution, moving from	*Reduces microorganism transfer; avoids cross-contamination*

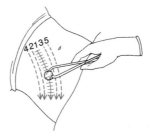

FIGURE 11.3

Action	Rationale
center of wound outward; discard pads and forceps.	
15. Apply antiseptic ointment, if ordered. Then place dressings over wound or incision in the following manner:	
• Pick up dressing pads by edge (saline-soaked, if wet-to-dry dressing) using sterile gloved hand or sterile forceps.	
• Place pads over wound or incision site until site is covered.	
• Cover with surgical pad (if wet-to-dry).	*Prevents contamination of dressing or wound*
16. Secure dressing by pinning, banding, or tying Montgomery straps together (the tying method may be used when frequent dressing changes are anticipated; Fig. 11.4).	*Keeps dressing in place*
17. Write the date and time of dressing change on a strip of tape and place tape across dressing.	*Indicates last dressing change and need for next change within 24 to 48 hours*
18. Dispose of gloves and materials, and store supplies appropriately.	*Decreases spread of microorganisms; maintains organized environment*
19. Position client for comfort with call light within reach.	*Facilitates comfort and communication*
20. Perform hand hygiene.	*Decreases spread of microorganisms*

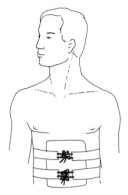

FIGURE 11.4

Evaluation

Were desired outcomes achieved? Examples of evaluation include:
- Desired outcome partially met: Delayed wound healing noted with poorly approximated wound borders, but no signs of infection noted.

Documentation

The following should be noted on the client's chart:
- Location and type of wound or incision
- Status of previous dressing
- Status of wound/incision
- Solution and medications applied to wound
- Type of dressing applied to wound or incision
- Client teaching done
- Client's tolerance of procedure

Sample Documentation
Date: 2/17/05
Time: 2100

Abdominal wound saturated with serous drainage. Wound bed is red with erythema around wound edges. Wound cleansed with normal saline, dressed with saline-moistened 4 × 4 gauze and covered with ABD pad secured with 2-inch paper tape. Client tolerated procedure well.

Removing Sutures

Purpose

Removing sutures in a timely manner avoids leaving marks and scars, since the need for wound support via suture closure decreases as wound healing occurs

Equipment

- Suture removal kit (scissors, forceps, gauze pads)
- Antiseptic solution or swabs (refer to physician orders or agency policy)
- Nonsterile gloves
- Waste disposal materials: trash can, bags (isolation bags optional)
- Steri-strips (optional)

Assessment

Assessment should focus on the following:
- Doctor's orders for suture removal and site of sutures (e.g., chest, scalp, knee)
- Client's knowledge of wound healing and signs of infection

Nursing Diagnoses

Nursing diagnoses may include the following:
- Risk for infection related to abdominal abscess
- Acute pain related to adhesions around suture site

Outcome Identification and Planning

Desired Outcomes

Sample desired outcomes include the following:
- Client shows no signs of infection or dehiscence after suture removal.
- Client reports no pain related to adhesions around suture site.

Special Considerations in Planning and Implementation

General

Sutures left in 14 days or longer may leave scars when removed. Clients with compromised healing (e.g., diabetes, nutritional deficiencies, immunosuppressive therapy) may have suture removal delayed. Clients with the potential for scar formation should be cautioned to minimize exposure to the sun to avoid an increase in scarring.

Pediatric

The child may need to be restrained with linen or soft restraints during the procedure. A parent may need to be available for comfort and reassurance, and a comfort object may be desired.

Geriatric

Sutures may need to remain in place in elderly clients for slightly longer periods due to delayed healing.

Home Health

If stitches come out too early, the wound edges may be re-aligned with butterfly-type bandages or tape. Call physician if area becomes red or swollen or drainage appears.

Delegation

In most facilities, suture removal is performed by physicians, nurses, physician assistants, or other licensed personnel.

Implementation

Action	Rationale
1. Perform hand hygiene.	*Reduces microorganism transfer*
2. Obtain and organize equipment: open suture removal tray, gauze package, and cleaning swabs/ solutions (if ordered).	*Promotes efficiency*
3. Explain procedure to client and position client for access to incision site.	*Decreases anxiety; facilitates cooperation and ease of suture removal*
4. Apply gloves.	*Prevents exposure to blood or exudate*
5. Remove and discard dressing, if any (see Procedure 11.3).	*Allows access to suture site*
6. Clean incision and assess status of healing.	*Removes blood or exudate; determines readiness for suture removal*
7. Use forceps to grasp suture.	*Supports suture for cutting*
8. Place tip (may be curved) of suture scissors under suture and cut (Fig. 11.5).	*Promotes removal of suture from skin*
9. Use forceps to slide suture out of skin in one piece.	*Ensures that all of suture is removed*
10. Discard suture onto gauze.	*Allows for examination of suture*
11. Remove remaining sutures as indicated (interrupted or continuous).	*Allows for observation of response to suture removal (e.g., no dehiscence)*

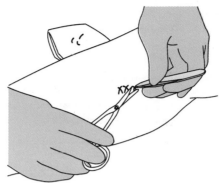

FIGURE 11.5

Action	Rationale
12. Swab suture site with anti-septic if ordered.	
13. Apply Steri-strips or dry gauze to incision, or leave open to air as ordered.	
14. Place all suture, gauze, and removal devices in plastic bag and discard appropriately.	
15. Remove gloves and per-form hand hygiene.	*Reduces microorganism transfer*

Evaluation

Were desired outcomes achieved? Examples of evaluation include:
- Desired outcome not met: 1-cm area of dehiscence noted after every other suture was removed.
- Desired outcome met: Client reports no pain related to adhesions around suture site.

Documentation

The following should be noted on the client's chart:
- Date and time of suture removal
- Number of sutures removed
- Location of sutures
- Any signs or symptoms of infection or dehiscence or excessive bleeding

Sample Documentation
Date: 2/17/05
Time: 2100

10 sutures removed from scalp wound. No redness, swelling,
or exudate noted. Skin edges continue to be approximated
without dehiscence. Client tolerated procedure well, stating,
"It wasn't bad, just a little uncomfortable."

● **Nursing Procedure 11.5**

Providing Preoperative Care

Purpose

Prepares client physically and emotionally for impending surgery

Equipment

- Assessment equipment (e.g., blood pressure cuff, stethoscope, pen light)
- Scale
- Teaching materials (films, booklet, sample equipment)
- Preoperative checklist
- Shave and preparation kit (razor, soap, sponge, tray for water) (optional; check agency policy)
- Procedure (hospital) gown
- Fingernail polish remover
- Denture cup (optional)
- Envelope for valuables (optional)
- Preoperative medications and administration equipment
- Nonsterile gloves
- Surgical scrub solution (e.g., povidone solution), if ordered
- Laxatives/enemas (if ordered)

Assessment

Assessment should focus on the following:
- Type of surgery
- Preparatory regimen for type of surgery (per doctor's order or agency policy)
- Signed consent form on chart before administering pre-operative sedation

- Client's perceptions of previous surgical experiences
- Admission history and physical examination for factors increasing risks of surgery (e.g., age, chronic or acute illness, depression, fluid and electrolyte imbalance)
- Learning or comprehension ability
- Reading ability
- Language barriers

Nursing Diagnoses

Nursing diagnoses may include the following:
- Deficient knowledge related to postoperative regimen
- Anxiety related to impending surgery

Outcome Identification and Planning

Desired Outcomes

Sample desired outcomes include the following:
- Client (and family if appropriate) verbalizes purpose of post-operative regimen.
- Client correctly demonstrates postoperative pulmonary and cardiovascular exercise regimens.

Special Considerations in Planning and Implementation

General

Assess the client's readiness to learn; if preoperative teaching time is limited, gear teaching toward essential items of concern. Prior exposure to the postoperative environment, staff, and regimen often decreases the client's anxiety and promotes cooperation.

Pediatric

Puppets may be used to explain the surgical procedure, pre-operative care, and the postoperative regimen. Some children may experience an intense fear of death. Provide emotional support and maintain presence of support systems for as long as possible before and after surgery. Answer children's questions simply, providing only necessary information and explanations. Ensure that legal guardian has signed consent form.

Geriatric

Fear of death may be particularly profound in some elderly clients, especially if this is a first hospitalization or first surgery. Supply clear and thorough explanations of all procedures. Encourage the client to participate in preoperative preparations.

Delegation

Preoperative teaching and physical/health assessment are performed by a licensed nurse and are not delegated to unlicensed assistive personnel.

Implementation

Action	Rationale
1. Perform hand hygiene and organize supplies.	*Reduces microorganism transfer; promotes efficiency*
2. Assess client's knowledge of impending surgery; reinforce information, and correct errors in understanding. It is the physician's responsibility initially to inform the client about surgery, options, and risks.	*Determines client's teaching needs; corrects misunderstandings*
3. Show films and provide booklets regarding surgery and postoperative care; encourage questions; answer questions clearly.	*Reduces anxiety; imparts knowledge*
4. Verify that operative permit is signed and on chart. It is the physician's responsibility to obtain proper informed consent.	*Avoids error in sending client to surgery without written consent*
5. Verify that ordered lab work and diagnostic studies (e.g., x-ray films, ECGs) have been done; check results of diagnostic studies, place copies on chart, and include results on preoperative checklist; alert doctor to abnormal values.	*Assesses client's preparation and readiness for surgery; determines if treatment of abnormalities is needed or if surgery must be postponed*
6. Make sure preoperative medications are available.	*Avoids delays on day of surgery*
7. Obtain client's height and weight; perform head-to-toe assessment, with in-depth assessment of areas related to surgery (see Nursing Procedure 3.7).	*Provides baseline data*
8. Instruct client about procedures or equipment that will be used to provide adequate oxygenation: • Demonstrate use of oxygen mask/cannula or of endotracheal tube and ventilator. • Explain related noises and sensations.	

Action	Rationale
• Arrange introduction to respiratory therapy personnel.	
• Demonstrate turning, coughing, and deep-breathing exercises, demonstrating use of pillow to splint incision site.	
• Explain techniques of chest physiotherapy, if applicable.	
• Stress the importance of pulmonary toilet in preventing secretion build-up.	*Prepares client for postoperative regimen; facilitates cooperation; decreases anxiety produced by postoperative regimen*
9. Discuss and demonstrate, if applicable, techniques for maintaining adequate circulation and pain control:	
• Demonstrate range-of-motion and leg exercises and check client's technique.	*Maintains circulation while client is bedridden*
• If transcutaneous electrical nerve stimulation (TENS) unit is to be used, explain procedure to client.	*Prepares client for use of TENS unit postoperatively*
• Arrange for physical therapist to visit client.	*Facilitates postoperative relationship and cooperation*
10. Discuss with client and family the postoperative unit or environment. Tour the unit and introduce client to staff. Inform family of special visiting hours, if applicable. Review tentative timetable of surgery and recovery room period. Inform family about agency's methods of communicating status updates during and after surgery.	*Reduces anxiety about unfamiliar setting and caregivers*
11. On the night before surgery:	
• Don gloves.	*Reduces microorganism transfer*
• Shave designated body areas.	*Prevents postoperative infection*
• Instruct client to shower with surgical scrub such as povidone	*Decreases microorganisms on skin surface*

Action	Rationale
solution, if ordered or if agency policy.	
• Administer laxative or other medications, if ordered.	*Helps flush bowel to prevent contamination of sterile field during procedure*
• Perform enema and check results.	*Evacuates bowel to prevent contamination of sterile field during procedure*
• Withhold foods and fluids after midnight the night before surgery (clear fluids may often be administered up to 3 to 4 hours before surgery, particularly if no IV fluids are infusing); consult agency policy.	*Prevents sterile field contamination secondary to incontinence; prevents bowel and bladder puncture because of distended organs*
• Check chart to determine which, if any, medications are to be given (permit sips of water) and at what time.	*Delivers drugs client needs to maintain therapeutic levels during surgery while eliminating those that may cause compatibility problems with drugs given during surgery*
• If applicable, mark the limb for which surgery is indicated.	*Prevents surgical error of operating on wrong limb*
• Remove gloves and perform hand hygiene.	*Reduces microorganism transfer*
12. On morning of surgery (or on the day before):	
• Verify presence of identification band (obtain duplicate band if needed).	*Ensure correct identification of client*
• Remove jewelry (may retain wedding ring, but wrap it with tape); ask client to send valuables and jewelry home with family or place in valuables envelope and store with security department or according to agency policy.	*Prevents loss of jewelry during surgery; secures valuables and belongings*
• Remove nail polish.	*Allows for good visualization of nail beds to monitor oxygenation status*
• Remove and label glasses, contact lenses, or other prostheses.	*Prevents loss*

Action	Rationale
• Remove full or partial dentures and label container (place with family or security department).	*Prevents loss*
• Assist client into hospital gown.	*Allows easy access to surgical site*
13. Thirty to 60 minutes before surgery (when operating room signals that client's preoperative medication is to be given):	
• Check client identification band.	*Verifies client's identity*
• Encourage client to void.	*Prevents contamination of sterile field and accidental bladder puncture*
• Obtain vital signs.	*Provides baseline data*
• Administer ordered medication.	*Induces mild sedation and achieves or maintains therapeutic levels*
• Raise side rails and instruct client to stay in bed.	*Prevents falls*
• Place call bell within reach and instruct client to call for assistance.	*Facilitates communication and safety*
• Encourage family to sit with client until stretcher arrives.	*Decreases anxiety*
14. When operating room personnel arrive to take client to surgery:	
• Compare client identification band with surgery call slip; note spelling of name and identification number.	*Confirms that correct client is being taken to surgery*
• Assist client onto stretcher.	*Prepares client for transport*
• Write final note in chart.	*Provides information on client's preoperative status*
• Place chart, stamp plate, and ordered medications on stretcher with client.	*Provides identifying information and preoperative meds for surgical staff*
15. Assist family to postoperative waiting room or instruct them to remain in client's room, if ordered by doctor.	*Ensures family members are nearby at conclusion of surgery*

Evaluation

Were desired outcomes achieved? Examples of evaluation include:
- Desired outcome met: Client and family verbalized purpose of postoperative regimen.
- Desired outcome met: Client correctly demonstrated pulmonary and cardiovascular exercises.

Documentation

The following should be noted on the client's chart:
- Presence of signed consent form
- Preoperative teaching done and client response
- Preparation procedures performed (e.g., enema, shave)
- Vital signs and other clinical data
- Preoperative medications given
- Disposition of valuables
- Completed preoperative checklist or areas pending completion
- Abnormal test results and time doctor was notified of these
- Further teaching or preparation needed

Sample Documentation
Date: 2/17/05
Time: 2100

Preoperative teaching done with instructions on
importance of pulmonary toilet and range-of-motion
and calf exercises. Client verbalizes understanding.
Preoperative checklist completed except for final vital
signs and medication.

● **Nursing Procedure 11.6**

Providing Postoperative Care

Purpose

Promotes return to state of physical and emotional well-being
Detects complications at early stage
Prevents postoperative complications
Facilitates wound healing

Equipment

- Assessment equipment (e.g., blood pressure cuff, stethoscope, pen light, scale)
- Respiratory therapy equipment (e.g., oxygen unit, incentive spirometer, nebulizer)
- Physical therapy equipment (e.g., transcutaneous electrical nerve stimulation [TENS] unit, mechanical percussor, vibrator)
- Emesis basin
- IV therapy equipment
- Nasogastric (NG) suction equipment
- Medications and medication administration record
- Teaching materials (e.g., films, booklets, sample equipment)
- Sterile gloves
- Personal hygiene/grooming supplies

Assessment

Assessment should focus on the following:
- Type of surgery
- Nature of supportive therapy (e.g., ventilator, feeding tube, IV therapy)
- Medication infusions
- Preoperative physiologic status
- History of chronic or concurrent illnesses that could delay recovery
- Monitoring equipment (e.g., telemetry unit, central venous pressure)
- Drainage systems (e.g., chest tube, wound, NG, or urine drainage systems)
- Communication barriers (e.g., language barrier, neurologic damage, presence of endotracheal tube)
- Level of consciousness and orientation
- Family support
- Emotional state

Nursing Diagnoses

Nursing diagnoses may include the following:
- Deficient knowledge related to postoperative regimen
- Anxiety related to postoperative situation
- Acute pain related to surgical incision
- Risk of infection related to disruption in skin integrity

Outcome Identification and Planning

Desired Outcomes

Sample desired outcomes include the following:
- Client verbalizes decreased anxiety regarding postoperative regimen.

- Client correctly demonstrates pulmonary and cardiovascular exercise regimen.
- Client verbalizes that pain is reduced to level 2 or less within 30 minutes of receiving pain medication.
- Client remains free of infection during the postoperative recovery period.

Special Considerations in Planning and Implementation

Pediatric

Puppets may be used to encourage cooperation with the postoperative regimen. Family members may be effective in persuading the child to participate.

Geriatric

Anesthesia may cause temporary disorientation and personality change. Reorient the client frequently; allow family members to remain with client as much as possible.

Home Health

If client has had outpatient surgery, arrange for follow-up by home health or public health nurse. Teach client and family information needed for safe and complete healing after surgery.

Delegation

Postoperative assessment, teaching, and dressing or wound management are the responsibility of a licensed nurse. Consult agency policy for assessments that can be performed by a registered nurse only.

Implementation

Action	Rationale
1. Perform hand hygiene, organize supplies, and apply gloves.	*Reduces microorganism transfer; promotes efficiency*
2. When client is admitted to unit:	
• Assist client from stretcher to bed; remove excess linens and cover client with sheet.	*Promotes warmth and privacy*
• Position client as ordered or with head of bed elevated 30 to 45 degrees; hook up oxygen, connect telemetry, begin drainage systems.	*Initiates support therapy; facilitates lung expansion*
• Assess respiratory, neurologic, and neuro-	*Provides baseline data on postoperative status*

Action	Rationale
vascular status; vital signs; apical pulse; bowel sounds; and ECG tracing from telemetry, as well as other parameters pertaining to specific body systems affected by surgery.	
• Assess incisional dressings and surgical wound drainage systems.	*Detects complications such as excessive bleeding or obstructed drains*
• Note urine output and output from drainage systems, as well as diaphoresis, emesis, and diarrhea.	*Enables early detection of fluid imbalances or systemic changes*
3. Orient client to staff and environment, especially location of call button.	*Decreases anxiety; promotes communication*
4. Allow family members at bedside as soon as possible.	*Reassures family; facilitates client comfort and orientation*
5. Review postoperative orders for therapy program:	
• Contact departments to schedule ordered lab work, x-ray films, ECGs, and other diagnostic tests.	*Facilitates early detection of complications*
• Note medications given after surgery and in recovery room, and arrange medication schedule at appropriate intervals.	*Returns client to routine medication regimen*
• Administer initial medication doses and treatments as soon as appropriate (if oral medication is needed, wait until client can tolerate fluids).	*Prevents GI upset from decreased peristalsis related to anesthesia*
• Monitor client for nausea or vomiting and return of bowel sounds.	*Indicates activity of bowel and possible development of ileus*
6. Monitor vital signs as indicated by client status or routine postoperative protocol (e.g., twice every half-hour, twice every hour, then every 2 to 4 hours if vital signs are stable).	*Allows early detection of postoperative complications*
7. Assess pain level and medicate as ordered; encourage client to request pain med-	*Promotes deep breathing and effective coughing; decreases the pain of turning*

Action	Rationale
ication before onset of severe pain; medicate client 30 minutes before exercises and pulmonary toilet.	
8. Begin pulmonary toilet immediately (if not contraindicated).	
• Reposition client regularly (every 2 hours); turn, deep breathe, and cough/suction client every 2 hours.	*Prevents buildup of secretions*
• Instruct client in use of incentive spirometry equipment and encourage use every hour.	*Facilitates lung expansion; mobilizes secretions*
9. Initiate range-of-motion and leg exercises, as well as chest physiotherapy, if applicable; if TENS unit is to be used, apply and turn on (see Nursing Procedure 10.7).	*Maintains circulation while client is bedridden; facilitates removal of accumulated secretions; promotes comfort by blocking pain reception of nerves*
10. Monitor surgical dressing and change or reinforce as needed and permitted. MANY DOCTORS PREFER TO REMOVE INITIAL DRESSING.	*Detects drainage and maintains secure wound coverage*
11. Help client to resume a normal state of personal grooming and hygiene:	*Promotes sense of well-being; increases self-esteem and sense of self-control*
• Obtain glasses, contact lenses, dentures, or other prostheses and apply, if appropriate and client desires.	
• Obtain valuables from security when client is fully awake and requests them.	
• Assist client in personal hygiene and grooming, when desired and not prohibited.	
12. Remove and discard gloves and perform hand hygiene.	*Decreases the spread of microorganisms*
13. Begin discharge teaching when client is fully awake	*Promotes self-care for client*

Action	Rationale
and family members are present.	
14. Reassess client's knowledge of and adherence to postoperative regimen and provide written instructions as indicated.	*Maximizes wound healing and postoperative recovery*

Evaluation

Were desired outcomes achieved? Examples of evaluation include:
- Desired outcome met: Client demonstrates minimal anxiety.
- Desired outcome met: Client states pain is level 2 with epidural.
- Desired outcome met: Client verbalized purpose of postoperative regimen and correctly demonstrated pulmonary and cardiovascular exercises.
- Desired outcome met: Client demonstrates no signs of infection during postoperative period.

Documentation

The following should be noted on the client's chart:
- Time client was admitted to room and area admitted from
- Complete assessment, with emphasis on abnormal findings
- Status of operative dressings, tubes, drains, and incisions
- Support equipment initiated
- Procedures performed
- Client's tolerance to therapy
- Abnormal test results noted and time doctor was notified
- Medications administered
- Client's and family's concerns
- Teaching needs noted

Sample Documentation
Date: 2/17/05
Time: 2100

Client admitted from recovery room after right thoracotomy. Alert and oriented. Vital signs obtained every 1 to 2 hours, with stable results. Skin warm and dry. Respirations deep and regular, rate of 16. Denies pain; epidural PCA functioning. Mediastinal tube to 20 cm H₂O suction. Serosanguineous drainage (50 mL) noted in Pleurevac. Chest dressing clean, dry, and intact.

Managing a Pressure Ulcer

Purpose

Removes accumulated secretions and dead tissue from wound
or incision
Decreases microorganism growth on wounds or incision site
Promotes wound healing

Equipment

- Dressing change materials as needed (forceps, scissors, transparent dressing, skin prep, tape [paper tape if allergic to other types of tape])
- Multipack gauze in plastic container or gauze pads and sterile bowl
- Nonsterile gloves and sterile gloves
- Towel or linen-saver pad
- Sterile irrigation saline (or non-cytotoxic cleanser)
- Irrigation kit (consider high-pressure irrigation system, if available)
- Topical-care agents (may vary from agency to agency, case to case)
- Moist wound barrier/transparent wound dressing or topical antibiotics, if ordered
- Overbed table or bedside stand
- Waterproof trash bag (adhering to specific guidelines for wound/drainage disposal materials)

Assessment

Assessment should focus on the following:
- Doctor's order regarding type of dressing change, procedure, and frequency of change
- Stage, size, appearance, and location of pressure ulcer (Fig. 11.6)
- Client factors contributing to development of pressure ulcer (e.g., prolonged immobility, poor circulation, nutritional status, incontinence, seepage of wound drainage onto skin)
- Risk assessment for development of pressure ulcer (using standardized tool, such as the Braden or Norton scale or agency-approved risk assessment tool)
- Time of last pain medication
- Allergies to tape or medication ordered
- Protective bed support (static or dynamic)
- Client's activity regimen (e.g., frequency of turning, getting out of bed)
- Client's knowledge regarding factors contributing to development of pressure ulcer
- Potential complications (e.g., sinus tract or abscess)

Sample pressure ulcer assessment guide

Patient Name: _____   Date: _____   Time: _____

Ulcer 1:				Ulcer 2:		
Site _____				Site _____		
Stage[a] _____				Stage[a] _____		
Size (cm)				Size (cm)		
Length _____				Length _____		
Width _____				Width _____		
Depth				Depth		
	No	Yes			No	Yes
Sinus tract	☐	☐		Sinus tract	☐	☐
Tunneling	☐	☐		Tunneling	☐	☐
Undermining	☐	☐		Undermining	☐	☐
Necrotic Tissue	☐	☐		Necrotic Tissue	☐	☐
Slough	☐	☐		Slough	☐	☐
Eschar	☐	☐		Eschar	☐	☐
Exudate	☐	☐		Exudate	☐	☐
Serous	☐	☐		Serous	☐	☐
Serosanguineous	☐	☐		Serosanguineous	☐	☐
Purulent	☐	☐		Purulent	☐	☐
Granulation	☐	☐		Granulation	☐	☐
Epithelialization	☐	☐		Epithelialization	☐	☐
Pain	☐	☐		Pain	☐	☐
Surrounding Skin:						
Erythema	☐	☐		Erythema	☐	☐
Maceration	☐	☐		Maceration	☐	☐
Induration	☐	☐		Induration	☐	☐
Description of Ulcers(s):						

Indicate Ulcer Sites:

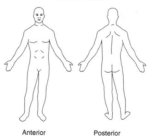

Anterior   Posterior

(Attach a color photo of the pressure ulcer(s) [Optional])

[a] Classification of pressure ulcers:

Stage I: Nonblanchable erythema of intact skin, the heralding lesion of skin ulceration. In individuals with darker skin, discoloration of the skin, warmth, edema, induration, or hardness may also be indicators.

Stage II;   Partial thickness skin loss involving epidermis, dermis, or both.

Stage II: Full thickness skin loss involving damage to or necrosis of subcutaneous tissue that may extend down to, but not through, underlying fascia. The ulcer presents clinically as a deep crater with or without undermining adjacent tissue.

Stage IV: Full thickness skin loss with extensive destruction, tissue necrosis, or damage to muscle, bone, or supporting structures (e.g., tendon or joint capsule).

FIGURE 11.6

Nursing Diagnoses

Nursing diagnoses may include the following:
- Impaired tissue integrity related to pressure ulcer
- Risk for infection related to decreased skin integrity

Outcome Identification and Planning

Desired Outcomes

Sample desired outcomes may include the following:
- Client regains skin integrity within 3 weeks.
- Client demonstrates no signs of infection or further infection during confinement.

Special Considerations in Planning and Implementation

General

Ulcer care may include débridement, wound cleansing, nutritional support, and other adjunctive care. The primary rule is to keep the ulcer tissue moist and the surrounding intact skin dry. Care of pressure ulcers is often very painful. Assess the client's pain needs and provide medication 30 minutes before beginning the procedure. A sterile, instead of clean, dressing change may be ordered. Consider using a high-pressure irrigation process to remove slough or necrotic tissue. You should NOT debride dry, black eschar on heels that are nontender, nonfluctuant, nonerythematous, and nonsuppurative. Pressure ulcer care tends to vary among agencies; consult the agency manual for guidelines.

Geriatric

Debilitation and decreased activity often accompany advanced age. Family members should be informed of the importance of preventing pressure to certain skin areas for extended periods of time.

Home Health

Use newspaper to cover the table surface during a dressing change. Do not allow pets in the area during the procedure.

Delegation

Pressure ulcer management is the responsibility of the nurse. Unlicensed assistive personnel should be instructed in prevention techniques such as turning and repositioning, use of positioning devices, and the importance of meticulous skin care.

Implementation

Action	Rationale
1. Perform hand hygiene and organize equipment.	*Reduces microorganism transfer; promotes efficiency*

Action	Rationale
2. Explain procedure and assistance needed from client.	*Promotes cooperation*
3. Assess pain level. Deliver medication, if needed, and wait for medication to take effect before beginning.	*Decreases discomfort*
4. Place bedside table close to area being dressed and prepare supplies:	
• Place supplies on bedside table.	*Organizes sterile field and supplies*
• Tape trash bag to side of table.	*Facilitates easy disposal of contaminated waste*
• Open sterile gloves and use inside of glove package as sterile field.	*Promotes use of supplies without contamination and prepares work field*
• Open gauze-pad packages and leave gauze pads in plastic container. If a plastic gauze container is not available, obtain a sterile bowl.	
• Open dressing tray.	
• Open liquids and pour saline on the gauze pads.	*Prepares gauze pads for wound cleansing*
• Lower side rails.	*Provides access to wound*
5. Don nonsterile gloves.	*Prevents exposure to drainage*
6. Position client to expose ulcer and place towel or linen-saver pad under wound area.	*Provides access to wound and prevents soiling linens*
7. Loosen tape by pulling toward the pressure ulcer and remove soiled dressing; note appearance of dressing and wound. MOISTEN DRESSING WITH NORMAL SALINE IF IT ADHERES TO WOUND, AND THEN GENTLY PULL FREE.	*Exposes site for cleaning; permits assessment of site*
8. Place soiled dressing in trash bag.	*Prevents spread of organisms*
9. Discard gloves in trash bag and perform hand hygiene. (Be sure to provide for client's safety when away from bed by raising the side rail.)	

Action	Rationale
10. Apply sterile gloves.	*Prevents introducing organisms into wound*
11. Pick up saline-soaked dressing pad with forceps and form a large swab.	*Provides means of cleaning wound*
12. Remove debris and drainage from the pressure ulcer, moving from center outward; use a new pad for each area cleaned, discarding the old pads.	*Prevents contamination of wound from organisms on skin surface; maintains sterility of supplies*
13. Use a dry gauze pad to dry the wound and surrounding skin and a skin prep on the surrounding skin; do not allow skin prep to touch broken skin areas. Discard forceps.	*Facilitates adherence of dressings/ pads; decreases microorganisms*
14. Place ordered topical agent into pressure ulcer or onto dressing, as appropriate for type of wound. DO NOT OVERPACK WOUND (Fig. 11.7).	*Provides necessary medication; minimizes exposure to infectious agents and promotes moisture. Overpacking may result in additional tissue damage from excessive pressure.*
15. Dress the pressure ulcer by covering it with a transparent wound dressing or other dressing as indicated by wound care protocol. Secure dressing with a window or frame of tape.	*Prevents additional exposure to microbes*
16. Write date and time of dressing change on a strip	*Indicates when dressing change was performed and need for next*

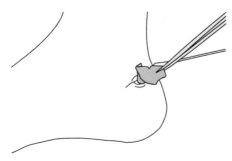

FIGURE 11.7

Action	Rationale
of tape and place tape across top of dressing.	*change*
17. Dispose of gloves and materials and store supplies appropriately.	*Decreases spread of microorganisms*
18. Position client for comfort using additional support devices as needed.	*Promotes comfort; support devices reduce pressure, friction, and shear*
19. Raise side rails and place call bell within reach.	*Promotes safety and communication*
20. Perform hand hygiene.	*Decreases spread of microorganisms*

Evaluation

Were desired outcomes achieved? Examples of evaluation include:
● Desired outcome met: Client regained skin integrity within 3 weeks.
● Desired outcome met: Client demonstrated no signs of infection or further infection during confinement.

Documentation

The following should be noted on the client's chart:
● Materials and procedure used for pressure ulcer management
● Location, size, and type of wound
● Solution and medications applied to wound
● Frequency of turning and repositioning client
● Support devices applied and to what areas
● Client teaching done and additional learning needs
● Client's tolerance of procedure

Sample Documentation
Date: 2/17/05
Time: 2100

Pressure ulcer site cleaned with saline. Sacral pressure ulcer approximately 3 cm in diameter, pink, with slightly granulated edges; no drainage or foul odor noted. Wound covered with saline-soaked pads and transparent dressing. Client turned to side with positioning pillow at back and is on Clinitron bed. Tolerated care with minimal discomfort.

Irrigating a Wound 🧤

Purpose

Removes secretions and microorganisms from wound

Equipment

- Irrigation solution
- Sterile irrigation set, including sterile syringe with sterile tubing (or catheter) attached
- Sterile basin
- Gauze pads
- Materials for dressing change, if applicable (see Nursing Procedure 10.2)
- Linen saver
- Large towel
- Waste receptacle
- Sterile and nonsterile gloves
- Overbed or bedside table

Assessment

Assessment should focus on the following:
- Doctor's order regarding irrigation
- Type and location of wound
- Irrigant (type of medication added, if applicable)
- Pain status and time of last pain medication

Nursing Diagnoses

Nursing diagnoses may include the following:
- Decreased tissue integrity related to poor circulation
- Risk for infection related to open abdominal incision

Outcome Identification and Planning

Desired Outcomes

Sample desired outcomes include the following:
- Client regains skin integrity within 1 month.
- Client demonstrates no signs of infection during confinement.

Special Considerations in Planning and Implementation

General

Wound irrigation can be painful; medicate client 30 minutes before beginning the procedure.

Pediatric

Children may contaminate the sterile field, gown, or gloves accidentally. Restrain child with linen or soft restraints during the procedure, if needed. Encourage a parent to sit with the child during the procedure, if possible, to provide reassurance and to help calm the child.

Home Health

Use newspaper to cover the table surface during wound irrigation. Do not allow pets in the area during the procedure.

Delegation

In general, this procedure is performed by the registered nurse or licensed practical nurse. See agency policy concerning delegation to unlicensed specially trained assistive personnel.

Implementation

Action	Rationale
1. Assess pain level. Give pain medication, if needed, and wait for it to take effect.	*Decreases discomfort*
2. Perform hand hygiene and organize supplies.	*Reduces microorganism transfer; promotes efficiency*
3. Explain procedure and assistance needed from client; provide privacy.	*Facilitates cooperation; decreases anxiety and embarrassment*
4. Place bedside table near wound area and open supplies (arrange for dressing change in addition to wound irrigation) (see Nursing Procedure 11.3).	*Permits dressing to be replaced after wound irrigation*
5. Don nonsterile gloves, lower side rails, position client, and remove old dressing (see Nursing Procedure 11.3).	*Provides access to wound*
6. Place linen saver and towel under wound.	*Catches overflow of irrigant and prevents soiling linens*
7. Discard nonsterile gloves, perform hand hygiene, and apply sterile gloves and goggles, if indicated.	*Maintains sterility*
8. Place basin beside wound and tilt client to side toward basin.	*Channels drainage of irrigation into basin*
9. Irrigate wound: • Insert irrigation tubing into upper portion of wound (or above cleanest portion of wound; Fig. 11.8).	*Allows fluid to flow from cleanest to dirtiest portion of wound*

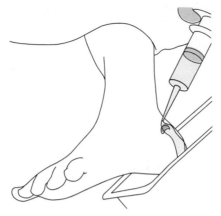

FIGURE 11.8

Action	Rationale
• Attach syringe to tubing or catheter and pour in irrigant; continue to pour irrigant until wound debris and drainage are washed into basin.	*Flushes debris and contaminants from wound*
• Move catheter to different part of wound and repeat irrigation until entire wound area has been irrigated and all irrigant has been used.	*Provides thorough irrigation of wound*
10. Use sterile gauze pads, if needed, to remove additional debris. Pack wound with gauze pads, if ordered. Apply sterile dressing.	*Protects wound*
11. Write the date and time of dressing change on a strip of tape and place tape across dressing.	*Indicates time of last dressing change and need for next change*
12. Dispose of gloves and materials and store supplies appropriately.	*Decreases spread of microorganisms*
13. Position client for comfort with call bell within reach.	*Promotes comfort and communication*
14. Perform hand hygiene.	*Decreases spread of microorganisms*

Evaluation

Were desired outcomes achieved? An example of evaluation is:
- Desired outcomes not met: Client still has altered skin integrity due to wound infection.

Documentation

The following should be noted on the client's chart:
- Location, appearance, and type of wound or incision
- Status of previous dressing
- Solution and medications applied to wound
- Client teaching done
- Client's tolerance of procedure

Sample Documentation
Date: 2/17/05
Time: 2100

Gaping abdominal incisional wound irrigated with sterile saline. Incision about 8 inches in length and gapes open at 2 cm crosswise along entire length of incision. No purulent drainage from wound. Open area pink, with whitish-yellow edges. Wound packed with moist saline gauze. Client turned to side with pillow at back. Tolerated procedure with minimal discomfort.

● Nursing Procedure 11.9

Managing a Wound Drain

Purpose

Removes accumulated secretions and dead tissue from wound or incision

Decreases microorganism growth on wounds or incision site

Promotes wound healing

Equipment

- Graduated container
- Sterile dressing tray (forceps, scissors, gauze pads [optional])

- Additional sterile gauze dressing pads (2 × 2-inch, 4 × 4-inch, or surgical [ABD] pads, depending on drainage and size of area to be covered), or transparent dressing
- Sterile bowl
- 2-inch tape or Montgomery straps (paper tape if allergic to others)
- Sterile and nonsterile gloves
- Towel or linen-saver pad
- Cotton balls and cotton-tipped swabs (optional)
- Sterile irrigation saline or sterile water
- Cleansing solution as ordered
- Bacteriostatic ointment
- Overbed table or bedside stand
- Trash bag (appropriate for type of disposal)

Assessment

Assessment should focus on the following:
- Type of drain
- Doctor's order or agency policy regarding frequency of drainage measurement
- Type, appearance, and location of wound or incision
- Time of last pain medication
- Client allergies to tape or solution used

Nursing Diagnoses

Nursing diagnoses may include the following:
- Impaired tissue integrity related to draining abscess
- Risk of infection related to decreased skin integrity

Outcome Identification and Planning

Desired Outcomes

Sample desired outcomes include the following:
- Client regains skin integrity within 3 weeks.
- Client demonstrates no signs of infection in wound.

Special Considerations in Planning and Implementation

General

Dressing changes and drain manipulation are often painful. Assess client's pain needs and medicate, if needed, 30 minutes before beginning procedure.

Pediatric

It may be necessary to have a parent assist while the procedure is being performed. Using dolls may be helpful in explaining to the child what drain management entails.

Home Health

Use newspaper to cover the table surface before arranging a sterile field. Do not allow pets in the area during the procedure.

Delegation

In general, this procedure is performed by the registered nurse or licensed practical nurse. See agency policy concerning delegation to unlicensed specially trained assistive personnel.

Implementation

Action	Rationale
1. Perform hand hygiene and organize equipment.	*Reduces microorganism transfer; promotes efficiency*
2. Explain procedure and assistance needed from client; provide privacy.	*Promotes cooperation; avoids embarrassment*
3. Assess pain level and administer pain medication 30 minutes before procedure, if needed; wait for medication to take effect before beginning.	*Decreases discomfort*
4. Place bedside table close to area being dressed.	*Facilitates management of sterile field and supplies*
5. Apply nonsterile gloves and goggles, if splashing is likely, and position client to expose wound.	*Eliminates drainage onto surrounding skin*
6. Place towel or pad under wound area and perform wound cleaning and dressing change (see Nursing Procedure 11.3). During wound cleaning, note condition of drain insertion site (intactness of sutures, presence of redness or purulent drainage).	*Avoids soiling linens; allows early detection of complications*
7. Clean wound with solution-soaked pads or swabs, moving from drain outward in a circular motion. Place gauze dressing around drain insertion site (Fig. 11.9).	*Prevents contamination of wound with microorganisms; decreases skin irritation from drainage*
8. Remove gloves, perform hand hygiene, and put on a clean pair of nonsterile gloves.	*Decreases microorganism transfer*

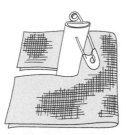

FIGURE 11.9

Action	Rationale
9. Check that drain tubings are not kinked, twisted, or dislodged. Proceed according to equipment used (Penrose drain, Hemovac, Jackson-Pratt [bulb drain], or T-tube).	*Promotes proper drainage*
Penrose Drain	
10. Place extra 4 × 4-inch pads over drain.	*Absorbs drainage*
11. Cover drain with one or two surgical pads.	*Provides for additional absorption of drainage*
12. Tape securely. Proceed to Step 13.	*Adheres pads to skin*
Hemovac	
10. Apply and secure dressing. Note drainage color and amount. Empty if half full or more by opening pouring spout, holding it inverted over graduated container, and squeezing Hemovac gently.	*Assesses drainage; empties drain to prevent overfilling and applying tension on suture areas; facilitates flow of clots and drainage*
11. Compress evacuator after emptying: • Place palm of hand on top of evacuator and press flat with top of spout open. • Replace stopper to spout while holding evacuator flat (Fig. 11.10). • Remove hand from evacuator and check that it remains flat.	*Activates suction needed to maintain drainage evacuation*

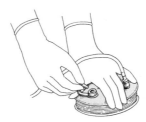

FIGURE 11.10

Action	Rationale
12. When assessing wound, drainage, and drain, make sure evacuator is still compressed; if not, empty drain and recompress. Proceed to Step 13.	*Maintains suction pressure*

Jackson-Pratt (Bulb Drain)

Action	Rationale
10. Apply and secure dressing. Note drainage color and amount. Empty if half full or more by opening pouring spout, inverting over graduated container, and squeezing bulb.	*Assesses drainage; prevents overfilling and tension pull on suture line; releases contents from bulb drain*
11. After emptying, recompress bulb by squeezing bulb in palm of hand with top of spout open, then closing spout and releasing bulb.	*Initiates suction needed for drainage evacuation*
12. When assessing wound, drainage, and drain, make sure evacuator is still compressed; if not, empty drain and recompress. Proceed to Step 13.	*Maintains suction pressure*

T-tube

Action	Rationale
10. Apply and secure dressing.	
11. Hang bag off trunk of body.	*Facilitates use of gravity for drainage*
12. To empty, open pouring spout, tilt to side with spout positioned over graduated container, pour, and recap spout.	*Prevents overfill of tube and tension on suture line*
13. Dispose of gloves and materials and store supplies appropriately.	*Decreases spread of microorganisms*

Action	Rationale
14. Position client for comfort with call bell within reach.	*Promotes comfort and communication*
15. Perform hand hygiene.	*Decreases spread of microorganisms*

Evaluation

Were desired outcomes achieved? Examples of evaluation include:
- Desired outcome met: Client regained skin integrity, as observed at 3-week check.
- Desired outcome met: Client demonstrates no signs of infection in wound.

Documentation

The following should be noted on the client's chart:
- Location and type of wound or incision
- Status of previous dressing
- Status of wound or incision site and drain
- Type and amount of drainage
- Solution and medications applied to wound
- Client teaching done
- Client's tolerance of procedure

Sample Documentation

Date: 2/17/05
Time: 2100

Abdominal wound dressing saturated with serous drainage. Dressing removed. Penrose drain intact, with moderate drainage. Area surrounding drain intact without redness. Site cleaned with saline solution. Dressing change performed. Client tolerated dressing change with minimal discomfort.

● **Nursing Procedure 11.10**

Collecting a Wound Specimen

Purpose

To identify causative agents/organisms in the chain of infection

Equipment

- Nonsterile gloves (latex-free if indicated)
- Sterile culture container appropriate for the organism to be collected
- Ancillary equipment (e.g., sterile swabs, forceps)
- Label identifying client, specimen, and date and time of collection
- Plastic, zip-closure biohazard bag
- Appropriate laboratory requisition
- Dressing/bandage for application after specimen collection when appropriate

Assessment

Assessment should focus on the following:
- Appearance of area of collection; color, odor, presence of exudates or other fluid
- Discomfort related to pain or pressure
- Adherence to proper sterile or clean technique

Nursing Diagnoses

Nursing diagnoses may include the following:
- Risk for infection related to poor wound healing

Outcome Identification and Planning

Desired Outcomes

A sample desired outcome is:
- Client shows no signs of infection.

Special Considerations in Planning and Implementation

Pediatric

A child may need to have a parent or other appropriate person nearby to provide support during specimen collection.

Geriatric

The skin of elderly clients may be fragile; avoid inadvertent tearing or bruising during specimen collection.

Home Health

Ice and a cooler may be needed to preserve the specimen until it can be transported to the laboratory.

Delegation

Ancillary staff may provide support and help transport specimen.

Implementation

Action	Rationale
1. Perform hand hygiene and put on gloves.	*Prevents microorganism transfer*
2. Arrange necessary equipment.	*Promotes efficiency*
3. Explain procedure to client, and position client to expose the wound.	*Decreases anxiety and increases cooperation*
4. Remove dressing if present (see Nursing Procedure 11.3).	*Provides access to wound*
5. Prepare culture material (open dish or remove sterile swab from culture tube kit).	*Provides access to culture medium*
6. Using swab from culture tube kit or sterile swab, saturate swab with material from site.	*Provides specimen of wound drainage*
7. Insert saturated swab into sterile culture tube, or smear culture plate with saturated swab. DO NOT BREAK SWAB STICK!	*Facilitates removal by lab personnel without contamination*
8. Apply top to the collection tube or culture plate.	*Protects sample from contamination*
9. Crush ampule of culture tube.	*Exposes medium to specimen*
10. Place specimen collection tube or plate into biohazard bag and zip closed.	*Promotes safe transfer of specimen*
11. Remove gloves and perform hand hygiene.	*Decreases microorganism transfer*
12. Label bag with date, time, and type of specimen.	*Ensures that information is recorded and reported properly*
13. Complete laboratory request slip.	*Identifies ordered test and source of specimen*
14. Apply new dressing, if needed.	*Protects wound*
15. Clean work area.	
16. Arrange for immediate transport of specimen, or deliver via delivery system if available.	*Provides a fresh specimen for increased accuracy of culture*
17. Document procedure in chart.	*Ensure prompt recording*

Evaluation

Were desired outcomes achieved? Examples of evaluation include:
● Desired outcomes met: Client shows no signs of infection.

Documentation

The following should be documented on the client's chart:
● Type of tissue collected
● Area of collection
● Time and date of collection

Sample Documentation
Date: 2/17/05
Time: 2100

Anterior nares cultured bilaterally. Culture material light green with no odor noted. Swab labeled, placed in Culturette and biohazard bag, and transported to laboratory.

12

Special Procedures

OVERVIEW

- The automatic implantable cardioverter defibrillator (AICD) is a life-saving device that can reverse a life-threatening dysrhythmia. However, it presents a risk of great physical and emotional injury to the client if it is improperly used or if the client is inadequately prepared for the sensation associated with it. The nurse, client, and family members or significant others need to be fully educated regarding its use and maintenance.
- Aggressive temperature-control therapy is crucial to regain the delicate balance necessary for vital organ function. If not closely monitored, temperature-control techniques can cause problems more serious than those originally being treated. Potential complications of hypothermia/hyperthermia include cardiac, vascular, pulmonary, and metabolic compromise.
- Improperly performed postmortem care could result in serious legal, ethnic/cultural, or ethical/moral dilemmas.
- When there is a threatened or actual death, caring for significant others also becomes a nursing concern.
- Caregivers should use gloves and gown while performing postmortem care because they may be exposed to body fluids.
- Some major nursing diagnostic labels related to special procedures are ineffective cardiopulmonary tissue perfusion, ineffective thermoregulation, ineffective coping, dysfunctional grieving, and risk for infection.

Managing and Providing Client Teaching for an Automatic Implantable Cardioverter Defibrillator (AICD) 🧤

Purpose

Ensures the client can care for the AICD properly. An AICD continuously monitors the client's heart rate and rhythm and delivers countershocks to the heart to terminate life-threatening recurrent ventricular dysrhythmias.

Equipment

- Gloves, if contact with body fluids is likely
- Basin of warm water
- Washcloth
- Soap

Assessment

Assessment should focus on the following:
- Level of knowledge of the client and family related to the AICD and follow-up care
- Cardiovascular and pulmonary status
- Signs of infection
- Effects of antiarrhythmia medications
- AICD activity diary
- Environmental safety
- Location of telephone
- Client's or significant other's reliability in carrying out home care instructions

Nursing Diagnoses

Nursing diagnoses may include the following:
- Knowledge deficit related to care of an AICD
- Ineffective tissue perfusion related to decreased cardiac output and dysrhythmia
- Anxiety related to life-threatening dysrhythmia

Outcome Identification and Planning

Desired Outcomes

Sample desired outcomes include the following:

- Client maintains stable vital signs within his normal parameters.
- Client's surgical incisions and abdominal pocket are healing without signs of infection.
- Client articulates feelings of acceptance and adaptation to the AICD.
- Client and/or caregiver demonstrate consistent ability to follow home care instructions.

Special Considerations in Planning and Implementation

General

Anxiety or residual neurologic impairment as a result of an episode of sudden cardiac death can interfere with integration and processing of information. Repeated teaching sessions may be necessary before the client and significant others can demonstrate an acceptable level of understanding about how to use the AICD. Touching the client when the AICD discharges will not cause harm. Local emergency medical services (EMS) should be informed in advance that the client has an AICD; encourage the client to wear a Medic-Alert bracelet.

∭ Transcultural

Ethnic and religious preferences vary regarding the use of life-preserving techniques. Individual and family communication is important in determining the client's preferences.

End-of-Life Care

Respect the client's wishes regarding the use of an AICD. A living will will help clarify the client's preferences.

Delegation

Nurses must be trained or certified in the use of AICD equipment. Training of other staff levels varies. Before delegating, make sure the person is trained or certified in use of AICD equipment.

Implementation

Action	Rationale
1. Perform hand hygiene and put on gloves if contact with body fluids is likely.	*Decreases microorganisms*

Action	Rationale
2. Instruct client to clean incisions daily with soap and water, taking care to clean the incision area in one direction and not reusing the same area of the washcloth.	*Decreases microorganisms*
3. Teach the client to inspect the insertion and generator site daily for redness, swelling, excessive warmth, or pain. The client may use a mirror to examine the lower aspects of the device pocket. Tell the client to report signs of infection to the physician immediately.	*Detects signs of infection early*
4. Instruct the client to avoid wearing tight clothing.	*Prevents chafing the skin over the protruding generator box*
5. Instruct the client to lie down when the AICD discharges.	*Decreases anxiety; prevent falls*
6. Reinforce and complete teaching begun in the hospital.	*Provides information; fear and anxiety may have interfered with earlier processing of information*
7. Review any activity restrictions (client should avoid any activity that involves rough contact).	*Avoids damaging the implant site or dislodging the device*
8. Instruct significant others to contact EMS and initiate cardiopulmonary resuscitation should cardiac arrest occur.	*Provides basic life support until EMS personnel arrive*
9. Examine the client's written diary of events resulting from each AICD discharge.	*Identifies malfunction of the AICD*
10. Assess for the effects of cardiac medications.	*Maximizes the chance of arrhythmia control*
11. Assess the home for environmental interference. Instruct the client to move away from any device that causes the AICD to emit a beeping tone, signaling AICD deactivation. Electromagnetic sources may cause inappropriate firing or deactivation of the AICD, but household	*Ensures continued correct functioning of the AICD*

Action	Rationale
appliances and microwave ovens will not interfere with the device.	
12. Assess client's adaptation to the AICD. Negative thoughts may create unpleasant emotions; ongoing support may be needed.	*Provides optimal client experience with AICD*

Evaluation

Were desired outcomes achieved? Examples of evaluation include:
● Desired outcome met: Client maintained stable vital signs within his normal parameters.
● Desired outcome met: Surgical incisions and abdominal pocket healing; no redness, drainage, or odor.
● Desired outcome met: Client verbalized feelings of comfort about AICD and ability to manage it.
● Desired outcome met: The client shows ability to follow home care instructions through return demonstration.

Documentation

The following should be noted on the client's chart:
● Teaching done and outcome of teaching
● Condition of surgical sites and generator pocket
● Current vital signs or trends, if applicable
● Responses to AICD shocks and whether they are appropriate
● Plans for future visits
● Discharge planning

Sample Documentation
Date: 2/17/05
Time: 2100

Left lateral thoracotomy and abdominal pulse generator pocket incisions without redness, drainage, swelling, or warmth. Temperature 99°F, pulse 84, BP 118/64. Denies dizziness or chest pain. Has Medic-Alert necklace on. Reviewed hospital discharge instructions with client and spouse.

Managing a Hyperthermia/ Hypothermia Unit

Purpose

Maintains client's body temperature within acceptable to normal range

Equipment

- Hyperthermia/hypothermia unit
- Hyperthermia/hypothermia blanket
- Appropriate solution for blanket (per manufacturer's recommendations)
- Disposable gloves
- Rectal probe
- Two sheets
- Linen blanket (optional)
- Linen savers (optional)
- Bathing supplies

Assessment

Assessment should focus on the following:
- Baseline data (vital signs, temperature, neurologic status, skin condition, circulation, ECG)
- Signs of shivering
- Proper functioning of hyperthermia/hypothermia unit and blanket
- Condition of electrical plugs (properly grounded) and wires (not frayed or exposed)

Nursing Diagnoses

Nursing diagnoses may include the following:
- Ineffective thermoregulation related to sepsis
- Hypothermia related to prolonged exposure to cold
- Risk for impaired skin integrity related to excess exposure to heating/cooling unit

Outcome Identification and Planning

Desired Outcomes

Sample desired outcomes include the following:
- Client's temperature is within acceptable or normal limits.

- No skin breakdown is noted.
- Nail beds and mucous membranes are pink; capillary refill time is 3 to 5 seconds.
- The client demonstrates minimal or no shivering.

Special Considerations in Planning and Implementation

General

Because there is a potential for skin damage with any electrical temperature-control device, treatment and temperature must be monitored closely.

Pediatric

Very young children are often highly sensitive to changes in heat and cold. Use blanket device to decrease or increase temperature gradually.

Geriatric

Chronically ill elderly clients are often very sensitive to changes in heat and cold. Use blanket device to decrease or increase temperature gradually.

End-of-Life Care

Respect the client and family's wishes regarding use of this treatment. Living wills help to clarify the client's preferences.

ᛜᛜᛜ Transcultural

Ethnic and religious preferences vary regarding use of heat and cold treatments. Individual and family communication is important in determining the client's preferences.

Delegation

Designated nursing staff who are trained to use hypo/hyperthermia units may set up the equipment and perform daily hygiene functions. The staff should be trained in observing for clinical signs of skin damage related to heat and cold treatments, but it is the registered nurse's responsibility to assess the client to determine the effectiveness of and continued need for treatment.

Implementation

Action	Rationale
1. Perform hand hygiene and organize equipment.	*Reduces microorganism transfer; promotes efficiency*
2. Prepare the hypothermia/ hyperthermia unit for use. When possible, prepare	

Action	Rationale
the unit away from the bedside.	
• Connect the blanket pad (cover with clear plastic cover to protect blanket from secretions, as needed) to the operating unit by inserting male tubing connector of blanket into inlet opening on unit (Fig. 12.1). Repeat same for outlet opening. Connect second blanket, if used, in same manner.	*Secures blanket tubing connection to unit*
• Check gauge for level of blanket solution. Solution should reach the fill line; add more recommended solution (usually mixture of alcohol and distilled water; see user's manual) into reservoir cap as needed. The solution is circulated through the coils in the blanket and warmed or cooled to maintain the blanket at the desired temperature.	*Facilitates proper functioning of unit*

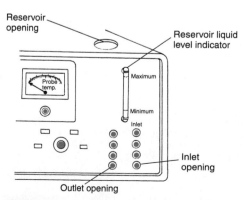

FIGURE 12.1

Action	Rationale
• Turn the unit on by moving the temperature control knob to the desired temperature (blanket coils will fill with solution automatically).	*Activates unit*
• Monitor blanket for adequate filling, watching gauge and adding solution to reservoir as needed to maintain fluid level.	*Prevents inadequate filling of blanket and improper functioning of system; ensures that unit is functioning properly before client use*
• Turn unit off.	*Allows safe transport of unit*
• Set master temperature control knob to either manual or automatic operation. When using automatic control, insert thermistor-probe plug into thermistor-probe jack on unit. When using manual control, set master temperature control knob to desired temperature.	*Adjusts unit to be controlled by temperature probe (automatic) or by nurse (manual)*
3. Transport equipment into client's room.	*Provides access to unit*
4. Explain procedure to client.	*Reduces anxiety; promotes cooperation*
5. Perform hand hygiene and don gloves.	*Prevents microorganism transfer*
6. Bathe client and apply cream, lotion, or oil to skin as directed. Replace gown. Remove gloves. Perform hand hygiene and don new gloves.	*Increases circulation; provides opportunity for skin assessment*
7. Place hypo/hyperthermia blanket on bed, place a sheet over the blanket, and apply linen saver, if needed.	*Protects skin from direct contact with blanket; avoids soiling of blanket*
8. Place client on blanket (may use side-to-side rolling, bed scales, or lifting apparatus).	*Positions client and blanket for treatment*
9. Remove gloves and perform hand hygiene.	*Reduces transfer of microorganisms*
10. Obtain baseline assessment data.	*Allows detection of change in status*

Action	Rationale
11. Don gloves, lubricate rectal probe, and insert probe into rectum.	*Ensures that temperature stays in desired range*
When using automatic control, check temperature control for accuracy of setting, check that automatic-mode light is on, and check pad temperature range for safe limits.	*Ensures that machine is functioning properly*
When using manual control, check that manual-mode light is on, check that temperature setting and safety limits are accurate, monitor client's temperature, and adjust blanket temperature to maintain body temperature.	*Allows nurse to monitor client's temperature continually and to adjust blanket temperature as needed to achieve desired body temperature*
12. Monitor client's response to treatment:	
• Measure temperature every 15 minutes until desired temperature is reached.	*Ensures that no excess change in body temperature occurs*
• Assess vital signs every 15 to 30 minutes, or as ordered initially, and every 1 to 2 hours until treatment is discontinued.	*Detects any adverse changes (e.g., arrhythmias, hyperventilation) caused by treatment*
• Watch for shivering (client's report, muscle twitching, ECG artifact). If present, obtain order for medication (tranquilizer).	*Shivering increases body metabolism and energy needs; tranquilizer will decrease shivering*
• Observe for edema.	*Edema is related to increased cell permeability*
13. Turn client every hour, and have client cough and deep breathe.	*Increases ventilation of airways and promotes secretion removal*
14. Every 2 hours, provide range-of-motion exercises, massage to bony prominences, and support stockings as ordered.	*Provides for exposure to maximum body surface area; decreases venous stasis*
15. Every 4 hours, remove rectal probe and clean according to manufacturer's instructions; use	*Allows monitoring for rectal irritation; checks probe accuracy*

Action	Rationale
glass thermometer to check temperature.	
16. Adjust master temperature control gradually until 98.6°F is reached over a period of 6 hours.	*Rapid changes in temperature could result in severe vital sign changes or arrhythmia.*
17. When machine is no longer needed, turn machine off, remove mat from bed, and return equipment to central supply for cleaning and reuse.	
18. Reposition client for comfort and raise side rails.	*Provides for comfort; prevents falls*
19. Perform hand hygiene.	*Reduces transfer of microorganisms*

Evaluation

Were desired outcomes achieved? Examples of evaluation include:
- Desired outcome met: Client's temperature returned to within acceptable limits (97.8°F).
- Desired outcome met: No skin breakdown noted.
- Desired outcome met: Nail beds and mucous membranes are pink; capillary refill time 3 to 5 seconds.
- Desired outcome met: Client demonstrated minimal shivering.

Documentation

The following should be noted on the client's chart:
- Baseline vital signs and client status
- Time treatment was initiated and initial temperature settings
- Initial and subsequent client response to treatment
- Client temperature and pulse
- Skin status

Sample Documentation
Date: 2/17/05
Time: 2100

Client placed on hypothermia blanket with master temperature set at 96.8°F and client temperature probe indicating 102.2°F, on automatic control. Vital signs stable, baseline BP 130/70, pulse 99. No shivering noted. Skin intact, with capillary refill less than 5 seconds.

Providing Postmortem Care

Purpose

Provides proper preparation of body of deceased client, with
minimum exposure of staff to body fluids and excrement, for
viewing by family members and for transport to funeral
home or morgue

Equipment

- Disposable gloves
- Clean linens
- Clean gown
- Wash basin with warm, soapy water
- Death certificate
- Isolation bags (optional)
- Cloth or disposable gown
- Two washcloths and towels
- 4 × 4-inch gauze or other dressing (optional)
- Moist cotton balls (optional)
- Identification bracelet or body tag
- Shroud (optional, unless agency policy)
- Dilute bleach mixture (optional)
- Tape
- Clamps
- Scissors
- Linen savers

Assessment

Assessment should focus on the following:
- Hospital policy regarding postmortem care and notification
  process
- Need for autopsy (if death occurs within 24 hours of hospitalization or is the result of suicide, homicide, or unknown
  causes; or if the family requests an autopsy)

Nursing Diagnoses

Nursing diagnoses may include the following:
- Ineffective coping by family with the death of loved one
- Dysfunctional grieving related to loss of loved one
- Risk for infection (caregiver), related to contact with
  contaminated body fluids

Outcome Identification and Planning

Desired Outcomes

Sample desired outcomes include the following:
- Body and environment are clean, with a natural appearance.
- Family views body with no signs of extreme distress at its physical appearance.
- There is no contact with body fluids.

Special Considerations in Planning and Implementation

General

The bodies of deceased clients with known infections requiring blood and body fluid precautions or isolation (e.g., tuberculosis, AIDS) should be tagged accordingly, and there should be appropriate disposal of soiled items and cleaning of nondisposable items. In some states, death may be pronounced by someone other than a physician (e.g., coroner, advanced practice nurse, home health nurse), particularly in out-of-hospital settings. Be familiar with agency and state policies and procedures related to pronouncement of death. Preferences regarding autopsy and organ harvesting vary widely among individuals, as well as cultures. Communication with the family on an individual basis is crucial, particularly if a living will is not in place. Current federal regulations mandate that for institutions receiving assistance through Medicare or Medicaid funding, permission must be sought to secure viable organs for harvesting in every case of death. Further, the Health Care Financing Administration (HCFA) mandates that a specially trained individual must seek permission from the family to do so.

 Transcultural

Staff should assist family members with emotional and spiritual needs before and at the time of death, such as summoning a spiritual advisor who shares the same faith or beliefs as the family members. Religious rites and practices differ with culture. Staff members should show respect for the deceased and should allow the family privacy. Before preparing the body, ask the family what postmortem practices are important; they may want to summon a priest, minister, rabbi, or other religious leader to the body.

Home Health

The client must be pronounced dead before the body can be removed from the home (unless being taken to a hospital or health facility). Follow agency policy for recording the pronouncement on the client's chart. When an autopsy is required or requested, the body must be left basically undisturbed until transported to the morgue.

Implementation

Action	Rationale
1. Record on the client's chart the time of death (cessation of heart function) and the time pronounced dead by a physician or other appropriate authority.	*Fulfills legal requirement for death certificate and all official records*
2. Notify family members that client's status has changed for the worse, and assist them to a private room until the physician is available.	*Provides privacy for family during initial grief; allows physician to notify family of client's death*
3. Return to client's room and close door.	*Prevents exposure of body to other clients and visitors; prevents family from seeing body before it is prepared*
4. Perform hand hygiene. Don gloves and isolation gown.	*Protects nurse from body secretions*
5. Hold eyelids closed until they remain closed. If they do not remain closed, place moist 4 × 4-inch gauze or cotton balls on lids until they remain closed on their own.	*Fixes eyelids in a natural, closed position before rigor mortis sets in*
6. Remove tubes, such as IV line, nasogastric (NG) catheter, or urinary catheter, if allowed and no autopsy is to be done.	*Provides a more natural appearance*
7. If unable to remove tubes: • Clamp IVs and tubes. • Coil NG and urinary tubes and tape them down. • Cut IV tubings as close to clamp as possible, cover with 4 × 4-inch gauze, and tape securely.	*Retains secretions while providing a clean and natural appearance*
8. Remove extra equipment from room to utility room.	*Allows mobility around bed; improves appearance of room*
9. Wash secretions from face and body.	*Improves appearance of body; decreases odor*
10. Replace soiled linens and gown with clean articles.	*Provides clean appearance; decreases odor*

Action	Rationale
11. Place linen savers under body and extremities, if needed.	*Absorbs secretions and excrement*
12. Put soiled linens and pads in bag (isolation bag, if appropriate) and remove from room.	*Decreases exposure to body fluids; removes odor; improves appearance of room*
13. Position client in a supine position with arms at side, palms down.	*Provides a natural appearance*
14. Place dentures (if present) in mouth, put a pillow under head, close mouth, and place rolled towel under chin.	*Gives face a natural appearance; sets mouth closed before onset of rigor mortis*
15. Remove all jewelry (except wedding band, unless band is requested by family members) and give to family with other personal belongings; record the name(s) of receiver(s).	*Prevents loss of property during transfer of body; ensures proper disposal of belongings*
16. Place clean top covering over body, leaving face exposed.	*Allows family to view client while covering remaining tubes and dressings*
17. Place chair at bedside.	*Provides seat for family member unable to stand or if momentary weakness occurs*
18. Dim lighting.	*Makes atmosphere more soothing and minimizes abnormal appearance of body*
19. After body has been viewed by family, tag client with appropriate identification. Some agencies require that body be placed in a covering or shroud and that an outer covering identification tag be applied.	*Ensures proper identification of body before transfer to funeral home or morgue*
20. Send completed death certificate with body to funeral home or complete paperwork as required by hospital and send body to morgue.	*Fulfills legal requirements for documentation of death*
21. Close doors of clients on hall through which body is transported, if hospital policy.	*Prevents distress to other clients and visitors*

Action	Rationale
22. Restore or dispose of equipment, supplies, and linens properly; remove gown and gloves and perform hand hygiene.	*Reduces microorganism transfer; maintains clean and orderly environment*
23. Have room cleaned: use special cleaning supplies if client had infection (e.g., 1:10 bleach dilution for AIDS clients, special germicides for isolation situations).	*Prevents transfer of microorganisms*

Evaluation

Were desired outcomes achieved? Examples of evaluation include:
- Desired outcome met: Body and environment are clean, with a natural appearance.
- Desired outcome met: Family viewed body with no signs of extreme distress at its physical appearance.
- Desired outcome met: There was no contact (staff or others) with body fluids.

Documentation

The following should be noted on the client's chart:
- Time of death and code information, if performed
- Notification of physician and family members
- Response of family members
- Disposal of valuables and belongings
- Time body was removed from room
- Location to which body was transferred

Sample Documentation
Date: 2/17/05
Time: 2100

Client pronounced dead by Dr. Brown; family members notified by doctor. Body viewed by family with no extreme reactions. Gold-colored wedding band taped to finger; gold-colored watch, clothing, and shoes given to Mr. Dale Smith (son). Body removed to James Funeral Home, accompanied by completed death certificate.

13

Community-Based Variations

OVERVIEW

- Time spent in planning and organizing visits allows the nurse to concentrate on care during visits and fosters more efficient use of resources.
- When entering the home, have all needed supplies and documentation materials available and well organized. Anticipate how to make appropriate substitutions for equipment or supplies in the home.
- A detailed initial assessment of the client, the environment, and the support system contributes to an effective, individualized plan of care.
- The nurse is a guest in the client's home and must be aware of cultural patterns and family dynamics and must make adjustments accordingly.
- Explain every action you take. If you are uncertain of the client's or family's reaction, ask permission before acting.
- Because home health care is delivered on an intermittent or part-time basis, support systems must be in place for each client so that consistent, adequate care is provided between visits.
- The safety of the nurse and the client must be carefully considered in the planning process. Be aware of the physical environment at all times.
- Password/passcode protection of electronic devices in the community setting is essential to avoid violating client privacy.

Preplanning and Organizing for Home Health Care

Purpose

Promotes efficiency and effective time management
Provides a plan for caring for clients scheduled to be seen the next day

Equipment

- Client case record (i.e., referral form, orders/treatment plan)
- Area map (manual or electronic)
- Medical supplies
- Scheduling notebook or personal digital assistant
- Cellular phone (or laptop computer for e-mail/fax)

Assessment

Assessment should focus on the following:
- Special needs of the client
- Problems detected at prior visits or before discharge

Nursing Diagnoses

Nursing diagnoses may include the following:
- Ineffective health maintenance related to knowledge deficit

Outcome Identification and Planning

Desired Outcomes

A sample desired outcome is:
- Client correctly demonstrates self-care measures and an appropriate plan for care management.

Special Considerations in Planning and Implementation

General

Always carry a list of local physicians' phone numbers and the name of a contact person in each office in case there are questions about care. Know where the laboratories are in the area, what requisitions and specimen containers are used by each lab, and how quickly specimens need to get to the lab. If using a Palm Pilot or laptop computer, secure all information with a security password or code to prevent unauthorized access to client data files and programs. Be aware of the nearest police or security stations in an area. Never risk your own physical safety.

Pediatric

Be alert for cues that may indicate a child is in an unsafe setting or is being neglected. Be familiar with agency policies and state or municipal legislation related to child safety and security within the home setting.

End-of-Life Care

Be familiar with hospice facilities and options within the community, as often clients must seek terminal-phase care outside of the home. Anticipate the family's needs as the client reaches the terminal phase.

Transcultural

If the client's culture is unfamiliar to you, check within the agency and community for people with specific knowledge of the culture. Obtain as much information as possible before making the visit.

Cost-Cutting Tips

Use less expensive home substitutions (see Appendix G).

Delegation

Ensure that a thorough assessment of the client's needs has been completed so that appropriate-level personnel can be assigned to visit the client, thus making efficient use of human resources. Plan periodic visits to coincide with the visits of home health aides so that you can evaluate the appropriateness and effectiveness of care provided. Review the plan of care with the home health aide and address any questions or concerns voiced by the client or aide.

Implementation

Action	Rationale
Planning	
1. Review chart of clients to be seen the next day.	*Allows an opportunity to obtain missing information; provides information about areas to focus on during visit and helps to prioritize care*
2. Determine special client needs (e.g., timed specimens to be obtained, IV medications to be administered at a certain time).	*Identifies priority concerns in the plan of care and orders*
3. Use an area map to determine the location of each client.	*Reduces travel time*

Action	Rationale
4. Determine the approximate time frame for each visit (i.e., 60 to 90 minutes for an initial visit, 30 to 60 minutes for a follow-up visit). If a specimen is to be obtained and taken to a lab, include the travel time to the lab in the total time for the visit.	*Allows for realistic scheduling of appointments; reduces chance of being late and keeping a client waiting*
5. Contact each client and set an approximate time for each visit. Remind each client that the time is approximate and is affected by travel conditions, emergencies, and so forth.	*Increases nurse flexibility; eliminates the need to rush through one visit to get to another by allowing a "time window" for each visit*
6. To the extent possible, take into account the client's preference for time of day, other appointments that the client may have, and the scheduling of other home health care providers.	*Promotes individualized care; increases compliance by considering client wishes; helps avoid the scheduling of multiple providers on the same day, which could exhaust the client*
7. List the day's scheduled visits, with client names and approximate times of visits, in the scheduling notebook. Follow agency policy regarding advising your supervisor about your visit schedule.	*Enables the supervisor to reach the nurse if new client information needs to be relayed*
8. For each client to be seen, assemble the needed documentation, including admission documentation, if applicable, appropriate lab requisitions, visit notes, and client education materials. Complete the demographic portion of each form as completely as possible before the visit. (If using a computerized system, be sure that all pertinent information is downloaded into the laptop or other device.)	*Promotes organization; allows efficient use of visit time; allows nurse to focus on the client during the visit*

Action	Rationale
9. Assemble any needed supplies and equipment for each client. Estimate and provide enough supplies for the client to use until the next scheduled visit, but do not overstock the home.	*Ensures that proper and adequate supplies are available for each client; reduces the need for extra visits to bring supplies*
10. If scheduling visits for a week or more for multiple clients, note the clients' physician appointments and the total number of visits scheduled for any one day of the week.	*Allows even distribution of caseload and grouping of clients for scheduling visits on specific days, thus decreasing travel time and enhancing efficiency*

Ensuring Personal Safety

Action	Rationale
1. Determine whether any client lives in an unsafe area. Check with agency supervisor to determine which areas are considered unsafe.	*Allows the nurse to schedule visits during the day, because some areas may be unsafe at night*
2. Determine if any clients are to be seen at specific times.	*Allows the nurse to prioritize the order of client visits*
3. Be aware of agency policy concerning the use of escorts or law enforcement officers when making visits in unsafe area.	*Permits time for advance notice and coordination if escorts are needed*
4. Before making any visits to clients in an unsafe area, be sure the supervisor knows where you are going and how long the visit is expected to take.	*Promotes safety by providing agency backup and support*
5. Inform the client of the approximate time of your arrival.	*Allows the client to watch for the nurse's arrival, allowing quick entry into the home*
6. Be sure your car is in good working order. If using public transportation, carry schedules with you.	*Reduces the risk of being stranded in an unsafe area*
7. Always lock the car. Avoid leaving anything in the car in plain sight.	*Reduces the risk of theft*
8. Be observant. Survey the area when approaching the client's home. Drive at	*Avoids drawing attention to the nurse; reduces risk of personal injury*

Action	Rationale
a normal rate of speed; if illegal or dangerous activity appears to be occurring, keep driving to a safe area and notify the agency and client.	
9. When entering a home, observe for exits; note any visible weapons or dangerous situations such as aggressive individuals or animals. Do not hesitate to terminate a visit if you believe your personal safety is at risk.	*Promotes awareness of risky situations*

Evaluation

Were desired outcomes achieved? An example of evaluation is:
- Desired outcome met: Client correctly demonstrated self-care measures and an appropriate plan for care management.

Documentation

The following should be noted on the client's chart:
- Schedule of visits
- Problems noted during visit
- Assistance required for next visit
- Findings from observation of home health aide (if applicable)

● Nursing Procedure 13.2

Maintaining Supplies and Equipment

Purpose

Ensures that an adequate stock of needed medical supplies is readily available for use
Promotes efficient client care

Equipment

- Nursing bag
- Paper towels
- Handwashing soap

- Waterless handwashing solution
- Gloves (sterile and nonsterile)
- Sterile dressing supplies
- Venipuncture supplies
- Blood pressure cuff
- Stethoscope
- Alcohol wipes
- Antiseptic solutions
- Tape
- Syringes
- Supplies specific to area of practice (e.g., tracheostomy care equipment, if applicable)

Assessment

Assessment should focus on the following:
- Types and amounts of items needed frequently for each client
- Specific supplies needed for area of practice
- Expiration dates, shelf life, and integrity of packaging of materials

Nursing Diagnoses

Nursing diagnoses may include the following:
- Impaired skin integrity related to surgical wound

Outcome Identification and Planning

Desired Outcomes

A sample desired outcome is:
- Client demonstrates intact skin integrity or adequate wound healing (wound approximation or granulation).

Special Considerations in Planning and Implementation

General

When stocking supplies, consider exactly which supplies are needed and how the cleanliness and integrity of each item can best be maintained. Supplies carried in the car are subject to extremes of temperature, which may cause deterioration (e.g., urinary catheters may become brittle, hydrocolloid dressings may dry out, vacuum tubes for blood collection may lose vacuum at high temperatures). Supplies in the car are also subject to dust and water contamination.

Carry a supply of plastic bags that may be used for disposal of used supplies that are not considered biohazardous waste.

When possible, adapt items commonly kept in the home to provide client care (see Appendix G).

✂ Cost-Cutting Tips

If appropriate, use less expensive home substitutions and re-usable supplies. When permitted, use clean technique instead of sterile technique.

Delegation

Perform a thorough assessment of the client's needs to ensure that appropriate-level personnel are assigned to visit the client, promoting efficient use of human resources. Periodically plan a visit to coincide with the home health aide's visit so that you can observe and evaluate the care that the aide provides.

Implementation

Action	Rationale
Maintaining Nursing Bag Supplies	
1. Keep paper towels, hand-washing soap, and water-less handwashing solution in the outside pocket of your nursing bag.	*Adheres to the principle that the outside of the bag is considered contaminated*
2. Carry items in the nursing bag, such as sterile gauze pads, venipuncture supplies, tape, syringes, blood pressure cuff, stethoscope, gloves, alcohol wipes, and antiseptic solutions, that may be needed unexpectedly or may be used frequently for a number of clients.	*Ensures easy access to frequently needed supplies*
3. Clean any item removed from the inside of the nursing bag before returning it to the bag.	*Keeps the inside of the nursing bag "clean"*
4. Check the bag and restock it at regular intervals. The specific items carried depend on your area of practice and typical client caseload.	*Ensure that items are available and in good condition*
5. For all supplies, make a written note of when the last item is used; restock the item as soon as possible.	*Eliminates extra trips to the agency office for supplies*
6. Avoid using stock supplies in the nursing bag to meet	*Ensures that necessary supplies are available*

Action	Rationale
a client's ongoing supply needs. Keep supplies provided for any particular client separate from the stock.	
7. When in the client's home, place your nursing bag on a clean, dry surface. If necessary, place a paper towel under the bag. If there is no suitable area in the home to place the bag, take into the home only those items needed for the visit.	*Prevents contamination of clean supplies*

Maintaining Car Supplies

Action	Rationale
1. Assign specific areas in your car for clean, sterile, and contaminated items.	*Adheres to the principles of medical asepsis*
2. Place supplies in washable plastic containers with lids. Do not place supplies directly on the trunk carpet. Label bins with type of supplies stored in each (Fig. 13.1).	*Maintains cleanliness; promotes organization; prevents water and dust contamination*
3. Carry the smallest amount possible of each supply.	*Ensures that supplies carried in the car will be used quickly,*

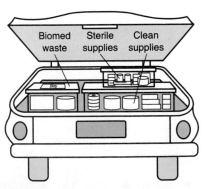

FIGURE 13.1

Action	Rationale
Supplies kept in the car may include Foley catheters, extra dressing supplies, drainage bags, paper towels, and antiseptic solutions.	*reducing the risk that they will deteriorate*
4. Regularly check all supplies kept in the car. Discard soiled or outdated supplies, and rotate all dated supplies.	*Maintains sterility, cleanliness, and proper condition of supplies*

Evaluation

Were desired outcomes achieved? An example of evaluation is:
● Desired outcome met: Client demonstrates intact skin integrity.

Documentation

The following should be noted on the client's chart:
● Skin status
● Treatment provided
● Supplies used and need for additional supplies for home
Agency policies vary as to how the use of supplies should be documented. Record the use of materials for client care so that the client can be charged for those items. Check agency policy and procedure for documentation.

● Nursing Procedure 13.3

Performing Environmental Assessment and Management

Purpose

Determines strengths and weaknesses of client's environment in relation to client's abilities, physical condition, and care required

Equipment

● Pen
● Comprehensive assessment form (agency-specific)

- Client history
- Completed physical assessment
- Client problem list or plan of care
- Physician's orders for care

Assessment

Assessment should focus on the following:
- Safety of the client in the current environment
- Status and adaptability of the environment to accommodate client's functional limitations
- Adequacy of environment for delivery of care ordered and indicated

Nursing Diagnoses

Nursing diagnoses may include the following:
- Risk for injury related to environmental clutter
- Toileting self-care deficit related to lack of wheelchair access to bathroom

Outcome identification and Planning

Desired Outcomes

Sample desired outcomes include the following:
- The client will function in a safe and supportive physical environment.
- The client will demonstrate toileting self-care measures within limitations imposed by wheelchair and physical environment.

Special Considerations in Planning and Implementation

General

Before performing an environmental assessment, make sure you are aware of the procedures and resources available to remove a client immediately from an unsafe environment.

If changes are needed in the home environment, enlist the help of the social worker, community resources, volunteer groups, and client family and friends as necessary to make the changes.

Pediatric

Is the house too hot or cold? Children are highly susceptible to physical illness during extremes of temperature.

Be alert to cues indicating that the child is in an unsafe setting or is being neglected. Be familiar with agency policies and state or municipal legislation related to child safety and security within the home setting.

Geriatric

Is the house too hot or cold? Elderly clients are highly susceptible to physical illness during extremes of temperature.

Look for poor lighting, scatter rugs, or clutter that might
cause the client to fall. Identify and inform the client of environmental modifications (e.g., grab bars, ramps and rails, nonskid
bath mats) that can be made to increase safety.

End-of-Life Care

Assess the emotional ability of the caregiver in supporting the
client and be prepared to offer emotional support. Be familiar
with hospice and other support facilities in the community that
can offer additional support services.

Transcultural

Assess the environment in the context of the client's culture. The
culture and belief system of the client is reflected in the home
environment. If you are unfamiliar with possible cultural implications, check within the agency for a resource person or consult
a text on cultural differences, particularly those related to the
primary contact person and customs (e.g., removing shoes
before entering the home).

Cost-Cutting Tips

Adaptations of the home environment may require structural
changes or additions. Items already in the home may be adapted
for client care (see Appendix G). Be knowledgeable about community or other resources that can provide low-cost help.
Certain items needed for care, such as oxygen concentrators that
operate on electricity, may increase the client's monthly electric
bill. Consider these factors when assessing the suitability of the
environment for care. Use social services and other resources to
help clients with financial needs.

Delegation

The environmental assessment is an ongoing assessment, and all
levels of personnel who visit the client in the home setting
should provide input.

Implementation

Action	Rationale
1. Review the client physical assessment, the care ordered, client history, and community assessment (Fig. 13.2).	*Helps determine whether the environment can support the client's needs*

Sample Assessment Form

NAME _____   DATE _____

ENVIRONMENTAL ASSESSMENT

NEIGHBORHOOD

Appears safe _____   Avoid after dark _____   Escort needed _____

Comments _____

PHYSICAL SETTING

Adequate space _____   Barriers to entry _____

Stairs inside home _____   Narrow doorways or halls _____

Inadequate floor, roof, or windows _____   Pets _____

Possible substance abuse by client/family _____

Comments _____

SAFETY

Inadequate lighting _____   Unsafe gas/electrical appliance _____

Inadequate heating _____   Inadequate cooling _____

Lack of fire safety devices _____   Unsafe floor covering _____

Inadequate stair railing _____   Lead-based paint _____

Unsafe wiring _____

Comments _____

SANITATION

No running water _____   No toilet facilities _____

Inadequate sewage disposal _____   Inadequate food storage _____

No cooking facilities _____   No refrigeration _____

Cluttered/soiled living area _____   No trash pickup _____

Insect infestation _____   Rodents present _____

Comments _____

SIGNATURE _____

FIGURE 13.2

Action	Rationale
2. Explain that a "walk-through" of the home is necessary to ensure that the client's needs can be met. Ask permission to look around the home,	*Increases client cooperation; enhances client control*

Action	Rationale
with emphasis on meeting the needs of the client/ family.	
3. Assess barriers to entrance and exit from the home, such as stairs. If needed, suggest ramps or alternative exits.	*Promotes client safety*
4. Assess internal barriers to mobility, such as stairs, narrow hallways, or uneven floors. If needed, work with client to find paths through the home that avoid or overcome these barriers (e.g., set up a temporary bedroom downstairs or obtain a narrow walker or wheelchair).	*Enhances client safety and mobility; includes client in making needed changes*
5. Find out how electricity is supplied (power company, generator, no electricity in the home). Assess electrical cords and outlets for fire hazards. Might the client trip over cords? Can the electrical system support the equipment needed for care, such as infusion or feeding pumps?	*Allows for adaptation of environment to promote safety; allows nurse and client to consider alternative methods of care delivery (e.g., if electricity is unreliable, consider using a manually controlled infusion without pump)*
6. Assess the adequacy of heating and cooling systems in the home. If needed, advise the client and family about safe heating units or fans. Assist client in using community resources to obtain needed equipment.	*Excessive heat or cold can have an adverse impact on the client's physical condition and medical progress.*
7. Assess the adequacy of the plumbing system. Is running water available?	*Identifies obstacles to good hygiene and infection control measures*
8. Assess fire safety, presence of smoke detectors, and client's plan for exit in case of fire.	*Reduces the risk of client injury from fire and smoke*
9. Assess the general cleanliness of the home and the adequacy of lighting for	*Evaluates setting for provision of care*

Action	Rationale
provision of care. Is there a refrigerator?	
10. Assess kitchen for safety, cleanliness, and safety hazards. Can the client function in the kitchen? Consider providing a home health aide to assist with kitchen upkeep and food preparation. If client has a new physical limitation, consider an occupational therapy referral to teach skills for independent and safe use of the kitchen.	*Promotes infection control and good nutrition; assists with promoting independence without risk for injury*
11. Considering the client's current functional limitations, assess the bathroom for safety and accessibility of tub, shower, and toilet. Obtain an order for adaptive equipment if needed, and consider physical therapy to instruct the client in safe techniques.	*Reduces risk of client injury from falls; maximizes client independence*
12. Look for signs of infestation by insects or rodents. Help arrange for treatment of environment, if needed.	*Reduces the risk of injury and infection; aids in adhering to principles of medical asepsis*
13. Assess the communication devices in the home (e.g., telephone, intercom, emergency call system).	*Allows the client to call for help in case of an emergency*
14. Ask whether there are any pets in the home. Evaluate their habits.	*Alerts home health care providers to presence of pets; evaluates possible impact of pets on client health*
15. With client assistance, assess the client's ability to move through the home, get in and out of chairs and bed, and so forth. Suggest using blocks to elevate furniture, using suitable chairs, and so forth. Consider a physical therapy referral for transfer training, and obtain order if indicated.	*Determines client's ability to safely perform activities of daily living; promotes client independence within functional limitations*

Action	Rationale
16. Ask the client if he or she feels comfortable and secure in the home.	*Determines client comfort level and desire to stay in home setting*
17. Review suggested alterations to the home setting, and set a timetable for completion.	*Assists client in setting goals; promotes client participation in care and enhances client control and independence*

Evaluation

Were desired outcomes achieved? Examples of evaluation include:
- The client functioned within his limitations in a safe and supportive physical environment.
- The client demonstrated toileting procedure with minimal assistance from care provider.

Documentation

The following should be noted on the client's chart:
- Safety hazards noted and actions taken to resolve them
- Adaptations that were needed to ensure safe and adequate care
- Client's ability to assist with environmental assessment
- Client's response to assessment, feelings about remaining in the home, and response to suggestions for adaptations
- Contact with other disciplines and resources regarding adaptations

Sample Documentation
Date: 2/17/05
Time: 1200

Environmental assessment completed with client cooperation. See assessment form. Suggestions made to client re: need for smoke alarms, removal of scatter rugs in hallway, and need for shower grab bars and elevated toilet seat. Client agreeable to adaptations but has concerns about financial factors; client will contact family in regard to assistance with finances. Client wishes to stay in the home. Will assess progress in making adaptations on next visit and will contact social worker if additional community resources are needed.

Assessing a Support System

Purpose

Determines extent of emotional support, physical assistance, and
assistance with care that can be provided to the client by others

Identifies the baseline for assistance that may be needed for
the client to receive care in the home

Equipment

- Pen
- Comprehensive assessment form (agency-specific)
- Client history
- Completed physical assessment
- Client problem list or plan of care
- Physician's orders for care

Assessment

Assessment should focus on the following:
- Client's relationship with family, friends, and others in the
  community
- Client's wishes regarding information given to others
- Client's financial status, ability to hire assistance or insurance
  coverage for assistant
- Availability, willingness, and ability of others to assist with
  client care

Nursing Diagnoses

Nursing diagnoses may include the following:
- Ineffective therapeutic regimen management related to
  extensive physical injury
- Bathing/hygiene self-care deficit related to pain and
  environmental barriers

Outcome Identification and Planning
Desired Outcomes

Sample desired outcomes include the following:
- Client demonstrates effective therapeutic regimen management with assistance from support person before discharge
  from agency care.
- Client maintains routine self-care hygiene with assistance
  from support persons, including home health care personnel
  as needed.

Special Considerations in Planning and Implementation

General

When assessing the client's support systems, provide the client with privacy to enable him or her to answer questions honestly. In some instances, the nurse will be unable to assess the client's support systems accurately until the client has developed trust in the nurse. Note any indications of abuse or neglect during an assessment of support systems. Elderly, pediatric, physically challenged, and emotionally challenged clients are particularly prone to abuse. Be knowledgeable in recognizing the signs of abuse and in determining which actions to take.

End-of-Life Care

Assess the caregiver's emotional ability to support the dying client. Be prepared to offer emotional support to the caregiver. Be familiar with hospice and other facilities in the community that can offer additional support services.

Transcultural

Cultures vary widely in their response to illness and to support of a person who is ill. In some cultures, offering assistance is considered insulting; in other cultures, everyone is involved with the client and is expected to know all details of care and the disease process. In some cultures certain diseases are considered shameful, and the client may be reluctant to risk any possibility of disclosure to another person. Be knowledgeable of the cultural factors that influence the client so that you can assess the support system in a nonjudgmental manner. Make every effort to provide resources that may support the client both emotionally and physically within the belief system of the client's culture.

Delegation

The nurse should perform the support system assessment but should receive input from all levels of personnel who visit the client. Include reports on support systems in information obtained from nursing care personnel.

Implementation

Action	Rationale
1. During all visits, observe the interaction between the client and others in the home.	*Provides insight into the client's relationships with others*
2. Initially, and on an ongoing basis, ask the client who is to be notified in an emergency and with whom information concerning the client may be discussed.	*Protects confidentiality and control of personal and medical information*

Action	Rationale
3. Explain to the client that you need to know who is available to assist with care, run errands, and so forth.	*Enhances client cooperation*
4. If the client lives with others, ask who can help with care, be responsible for decisions, provide emotional support, and so forth. Maintain a nonjudgmental attitude. Avoid asking about personal relationships, family matters, and so forth unless these have a direct impact on the client's care.	*Elicits information without violating the client's right to privacy*
5. Assess for indications of abuse, such as the client appears fearful, appears to be restricted to one room in home, has bruising or injuries that cannot be explained, family members will not allow the client to be alone with the nurse, or family members appear very hostile to the nurse's presence. Report suspicions of abuse to the appropriate authority; check agency policy and procedure.	*Enhances client safety*
6. If the client lives alone, inquire about friends, neighbors, or family members who could provide assistance. Note this information on the assessment form.	*Determines the existence of extended support*
7. Once support people have been identified, ask the client what information may be shared with them.	*Protects client confidentiality*
8. Ask support people what help they can provide, such as helping with care, errands, transportation, meals, and emotional sup-	*Determines the availability and willingness of support persons*

Action	Rationale
port. Approach support individuals in a nonjudgmental manner to elicit honest responses.	
9. If no support system is identified, refer the client to a social worker for assistance with use of community resources. Provide client with information on transportation services, grocery delivery, housekeeping services, and so forth. Assist client in using services, including use of computer and Internet services. Advise client of local groups that may provide help. Consider using home health aides to assist with care, if appropriate.	*Provides needed support services to client*
10. Review the results of the support system assessment only with other agency personnel involved in the client's care.	*Protects confidentiality while providing continuity of care*

Evaluation

Were desired outcomes achieved? Examples of evaluation include the following:
- Desired outcome met: Client demonstrates maintenance of therapeutic regimen with emotional and physical support from family members.
- Desired outcome met: Client maintains self-care and personal hygiene with support of significant others and supplemental care by home health aides.

Documentation

The following should be noted on the client's chart:
- Whom to notify in case of emergency
- Who has access to client information
- Availability, willingness, and ability of support people
- Name, address, phone number, and relationship of each support person to the client
- Any referrals made for supplemental or paid support

Sample Documentation
Date: 2/17/05
Time: 1200

Support system assessment completed. Client lives alone
but has several friends and neighbors willing to help with
care. Client has daughter who lives out of state but is to be
kept informed of care and condition. See assessment form
for specific names and information.

● **Nursing Procedure 13.5**

Preparing Solutions in the Home

Purpose

Provides a cost-effective method for obtaining necessary
solutions

Equipment

- Glass containers with tight-fitting lids (pint, quart, or larger
  for acetic acid or ordered solution)
- Large saucepan
- Tongs or oven mitts
- Salt
- White distilled vinegar
- Bleach

Assessment

Assessment should focus on the following:
- Economic need to prepare solutions at home instead of
  purchasing already prepared solutions
- Client/caregiver ability to learn and perform procedure
- Appropriateness of the environment for preparing and
  storing the solutions

Outcome Identification and Planning

Desired Outcomes

A sample desired outcome is:
- Client/caregiver will demonstrate correct technique in preparation and storage of solution.

Special Considerations in Planning and Implementation

General

If sterile saline, Dakins, or acetic acid solution is ordered for a client, check with the physician to determine if home preparation is acceptable. In some instances, it may be necessary to use purchased solutions, and the nurse should use community resources if cost is a factor. As applicable, treat the home preparation solutions as medication; see Box 5.1.

Delegation

As a basic standard, medication (solution) preparation, teaching, and administration are done by a licensed registered or vocational nurse, but some drugs may be given by RNs only. Policies vary by agency and state. NOTE SPECIFIC AGENCY POLICIES BEFORE DELEGATING ADMINISTRATION!

Implementation

Action	Rationale
1. Perform hand hygiene.	*Reduces microorganism transfer*
2. Organize equipment: glass jars with metal lids, clean saucepans large enough to hold jar, tongs or oven mitts, measuring spoons.	*Promotes efficiency*
3. Clean all equipment with warm soapy water and rinse thoroughly.	*Ensures that equipment is free of contamination*
4. Prepare container. Lay jar on its side in the saucepan. Fill saucepan with water; be sure jar is filled as well. Cover pan, bring water to a boil, and boil for 20 minutes. Remove from heat. Using tongs or oven mitt and handling only the outside of the jar and lid, re-	*Sterilizes container for use; prevents burns; maintains sterility of the inside of the container*

Action	Rationale
move the jar and stand it, empty, in a clean area. Remove the lid, handling only the outside. Place the lid loosely on the jar.	
5. To prepare a *sterile water solution:* Prepare jar as in Step 4. Boil 6 cups of water for 20 minutes in a clean saucepan. Slowly pour water into empty sterile jar until almost full. Place lid on jar. Allow to cool. Tighten lid and label with time and date of preparation. Prepare new solution every day.	*Prevents growth of microorganisms; indicates date of preparation and need for new solution*
6. To prepare *sterile saline 0.9% solution:* Prepare jar as in Step 4. Boil 6 cups of water as described above for sterile water solution. Pour 4 cups of sterile water into sterile jar. Using a teaspoon (sterilize with boiling water), add 2 teaspoons of table salt. Put lid on jar and shake well. Label with contents and date. Allow to cool before use. Prepare new solution every day.	*Creates proper percentage solution; prevents injury from using hot solution; prevents growth of microorganisms*
7. To prepare *acetic acid 0.25% solution:* Prepare jar as in Step 4. Boil 6 cups of water for 20 minutes as described for preparing a sterile water solution. Pour 5 cups of water into prepared jar. Let cool. Using a clean measuring spoon, add 4 tablespoons of white distilled vinegar. Close lid and shake to mix. Label with contents and date. Prepare new solution every day.	*Creates proper percentage solution; prevents growth of microorganisms*
8. To prepare a *Dakins solution:* Prepare pint jar as in Step 4. Boil water for 20 minutes as described for	*Creates proper percentage solution; prevents growth of microorganisms*

Action	Rationale
preparing sterile water solution and allow to cool. To create a *half-strength Dakins*, put 25 mL of bleach in the pint jar and fill to top with prepared, cooled, sterile water. To create a *full-strength Dakins solution*, put 50 mL of bleach in the jar and fill to top with prepared, cooled, sterile water. Place lid on jar. Label contents and date. Prepare new solution at least weekly.	

Evaluation

Were desired outcomes achieved? An example of evaluation is:
- Desired outcome met: Client and caregiver demonstrated correct technique in preparation and storage of solution.

Documentation

The following should be noted on the client's chart:
- Order from physician for home preparation
- Solution prepared, including amount, strength, and time and means of storage
- Client/caregiver ability to prepare solution

Sample Documentation
Date: 2/17/05
Time: 1200

Physician order received for instruction in home-prepared sterile saline solution. Observed client and caregiver preparing sterile container, sterile water, and proper measurement of salt to create 0.9% solution of sterile saline. Instructed in labeling and need to prepare daily. Caregiver demonstrated competence in procedure and proper storage of solution.

Pain Management

Basic Principles

- Pain is subjective and an individual experience; therefore, the client's report of pain characteristics must be considered accurate and valid.
- Pain tolerance is subjective and varies among individuals.
- Acute pain, by definition, generally lasts less than 6 months.
- Chronic pain, by definition, lasts more than 6 months.
- Successful assessment and management of pain depends, in part, on a good nurse–client relationship.
- Anticipatory pain management is best; intervene when pain is anticipated and before pain becomes significant.

Pain Assessment

- Self-report of the client's perceptions regarding pain must be considered valid.
- Assess factors/characteristics of client's pain:
  Location (Where is the pain? Can you point to it?)
  Intensity (On a scale of 1–10, how bad is it? Or use visual pain analog scale)
  Quality (Is it dull, sharp, nagging, burning?)
  Radiation (Does it radiate? Where does it radiate to?)
  Precipitating factors (What were you doing when it occurred?)
  Aggravating factors (What makes it worse?)
  Associating factors (Do you get nauseated or dizzy with the pain?)
  Alleviating factors (Do you know of anything that has made it better at times?)
- The following factors must be considered in assessing and managing the client's pain: medical diagnosis, age, weight, sociocultural affiliation (religion, race, gender).
- Self-management devices (such as patient-controlled analgesia pumps, PCA pumps) DO NOT exempt the nurse from performing frequent and careful client assessments.

- Assess clients receiving drug therapy for pain management every 1 to 2 hours (more often, if needed) to ensure adequate pain control and avoid complications of uncontrolled pain and complications of drug therapy.

General Pain Management Strategies

- Always assess pain first.
- Client/family teaching should be included as part of non-pharmacologic management to include factors such as what causes the pain, what the client can expect, what needs to be reported, instructions for reducing activity and treatment-related pain, and relaxation techniques.
- Consider general comfort measures such as client repositioning, back rub, pillows at lower back, bladder emptying, and cool or warm washcloth to area.
- Consider management of anxiety along with pain, using strategies of relaxation.
- Escalating and repetitive pain may be difficult to control. Early intervention is best.
- Around-the-clock (ATC) pain-therapy drug protocols are used to treat persistent pain, using the analgesia ladder standard as set forth by the World Health Organization. The use of oral medications, when possible, is recommended. Nonopioid or nonsteroidal anti-inflammatory drugs (NSAIDS) are used in the initial treatment, with progression to an ATC opioid and steroids, antidepressants, or anti-convulsants, as needed to control pain. Treatment proceeds to step 2 and step 3 of the analgesia ladder with increased potency of opioids and use of parenteral routes.
- Unrelieved pain has negative physical and psychological consequences.
- Take into consideration what the client believes will help relieve the pain and the client's ability to participate in treatment.
- If pain cannot be realistically relieved completely, educate client as to what would be considered a tolerable level of pain in consideration of the condition.
- Nonsteroidal anti-inflammatory drugs and drugs that inhibit platelet aggregation should be used with caution in clients with bleeding tendencies and conditions such as thrombocytopenia or gastrointestinal ulceration.

Postoperative Pain Management

- Always check the general surgical area for manifestations of postoperative complications when the client complains of pain. Watch for problems such as compromised circulation, excessive edema, bleeding, wound dehiscence and evisceration, and infection.

- Goals of postoperative pain management regimens include attaining a positive client outcome and reducing the length of stay.
- Administering nonsedative pain medications before ambulation should be considered to facilitate early and consistent ambulation postoperatively.
- The Agency for Health Care Policy and Research (AHCPR) and American Pain Society (APS) guidelines for management of acute pain indicate that surgical clients should receive nonsteroidal anti-inflammatory drugs or acetaminophen around the clock, unless contraindications prohibit use.
- Opioid analgesics are considered to be the cornerstone for management of moderate to severe acute pain. Effective use of opioid analgesics may facilitate postoperative cooperation in activities such as coughing and deep breathing exercises, physical therapy, and ambulation.
- Intravenous administration is the parenteral route of choice after major surgery.
- Oral drug administration is the primary choice of drug routes in the ambulatory surgical population.
- Oral administration of drugs should begin as soon as the client can tolerate oral intake.
- Acute or significant pain, not explained by surgical trauma, may warrant a surgical evaluation.

Complications of Drug Therapy

Watch for signs of narcotic overdose carefully—decreased respiratory rate and/or depth, decreased mentation, decreased blood pressure.

Administer naloxone as indicated by orders/agency policy immediately if signs of respiratory depression occur in clients receiving narcotics. Naloxone may increase rather than reverse the effects of meperidine.

A major sign of drug dependence is client need for increased dosages of medication (after other methodologic and drug alternatives have been attempted).

Check if narcotic administration produces consistent euphoria rather than just pain relief.

Pain Management in the Elderly

- Elderly clients often have complex pain because of multiple medical problems. Elderly clients are at a greater risk for drug–drug and drug–disease interactions.
- Elderly clients may experience a longer duration and higher peak effect of opioids. It is best to start with more conservative doses and increase as needed from that point. Meperidine (Demerol) should be given with caution, and monitor particularly for neurologic changes and seizures.

● Some elderly clients may experience more severe postsurgical pain than other age groups. In these cases, consider options such as oral morphine or hydromorphone, if ordered.

Special Considerations

● As a routine, pain medications are not given to clients with acute neurologic conditions, since assessment of the true neurologic status may be skewed with central or peripheral nervous system effects.
● The pain status of clients who have had recent vascular surgery should be monitored carefully. Excessive pain may result in increased blood pressure in response to stress, with subsequent rupture of newly grafted or anastamosed vessels.
● Note procedures on Patient-Controlled Analgesia (PCA) Management, Transelectrical Nerve Stimulation (TENS) Unit Management, Epidural Catheter Management, and Application of Heat/Cold Therapy in this procedure book.

Evaluation of Therapy

● Note verbal statement of pain decrease or increase.
● Note accompanying clinical indicators of pain increase or decrease.
● Note appearance of area of pain.
● Coping skills successfully used by client.
● Anxiety-reducing techniques successfully used.

Common Clinical Abbreviations

When multiple meanings are possible, consider the context.

abd	abdomen	exam	examination
ac	before meals	F	Fahrenheit
ADLs	activities of daily living	FBS	fasting/fingerstick blood sugar
ad. lib.	as desired	FHT	fetal heart tones
adm	admission	fl, fld	fluid
AKA	above-the-knee amputation	ft	feet
		fx	fracture/fractional
alb	albumin	g/gm	gram
amb	ambulate	gr	grain
ant	anterior	grav	gravida
AP	anterior-posterior	gt, gtt	drops
ATC	around-the-clock	h, hr	hour
ax	axillary	hg	mercury
approx	approximately	hct	hematocrit
b.i.d.	twice a day	hgb	hemoglobin
BKA	below-the-knee amputation	HOB	head of bed
		hx	history
BM	bowel movement	I & D	incision and drainage
BP	blood pressure		
BRP	bathroom privileges	I & O	intake and output
C	Centigrade, Celsius	ID	intradermal
c̄	with	IM	intramuscular
Ca	calcium	irriga	irrigation
CA	cancer	IV	intravenous
C & S	culture and sensitivity	K	potassium
		kg	kilogram
c/o	complains of	L	liter
CVP	central venous pressure	L, lt	left
		lat	lateral
cysto	cystoscopy	lb	pound
diab	diabetic	lymph	lymphatic
diag, DX	diagnosis	MAE	moves all extremities
DOA	dead on arrival	m	minims
dr	dram	mEq	milliequivalent
ECG	electrocardiogram	mg, mgm	milligrams
EENT	eye, ear, nose, throat	MI	myocardial infarction
et	and		

ml	milliliter	SOB	short of breath or side of bed
neg	negative		
NKA	no known allergies	sol	solution
noct	nocturnal	sp. gr.	specific gravity
NPO	nothing by mouth	S & S	signs/symptoms
N & V	nausea and vomiting	stat	immediately
OOB	out of bed	supp	suppository
oz	ounce	T, temp	temperature
p.c.	after meals	T & A	tonsillectomy and adenoidectomy
PO	by mouth, orally		
pr	per rectum	tab	tablet
PRN	when needed	tbsp	tablespoon
q	every	t.i.d.	three times a day
qAM	every morning	tinc	tincture
q.i.d.	four times a day	TKO	to keep open
qs	quantity sufficient	trach	tracheostomy
R	rectal	tsp	teaspoon
RBC	red blood cell	TUR	transurethral resection
rt, R	right		
resp	respirations	tx	treatment
RLQ	right lower quadrant	UA	urinalysis
RO or r/o	rule out	UGI	upper gastrointestinal
ROM	range of motion	vag	vaginal
Rx	prescription	vol	volume
sø	without	VS	vital signs
sub q	subcutaneous	WBC	white blood cell
sm	small	WNL	within normal limits
SL	sublingual	wt	weight

Selected Abbreviations Used for Specific Descriptions

ASCVD	arteriosclerotic cardiovascular disease	HCVD	hypertensive cardio-vascular disease
ASHD	arteriosclerotic heart disease	HEENT	head, ear, eye, nose, throat
BE	barium enema	HVD	hypertensive vascular disease
CMS	circulation move-ment sensation	ICU	intensive care unit
CNS	central nervous system or Clinical Nurse Specialist	LLE	left lower extremity
		LLQ	left lower quadrant
		LOC	level of conscious-ness; laxatives of choice
DJD	degenerative joint disease		
DOE	dyspnea on exertion	LMP	last menstrual period
DTs	delerium tremens	LUE	left upper extremity
D$_5$W	5% dextrose in water	LUQ	left upper quadrant
FUO	fever of unknown origin	Neuro	neurology; neurosurgery
		NS	normal saline
GB	gallbladder	NWB	non-weight bearing
GI	gastrointestinal	OPD	outpatient department
GYN	gynecology		
H$_2$O$_2$	hydrogen peroxide	ORIF	open reduction internal fixation
HA	hyperalimentation or headache		
		Ortho	orthopedics

OT	occupational therapy	RUE	right upper extremity
PAR	postanesthesia room		
PE	physical examination	RUQ	right upper quadrant
PERRLA	pupils equal, round, and react to light and accommodation	Rx	prescription
		STSG	split-thickness skin graft
PID	pelvic inflammatory disease	Surg	surgery, surgical
		THR; TJR	total hip replacement; total joint replacement
PI	present illness		
PM & R	physical medicine and rehabilitation	URI	upper respiratory infection
Psych	psychology; psychiatric	UTI	urinary tract infection
PT	physical therapy		
RL (or LR)	Ringer's lactate; lactated Ringer's	VD	venereal disease
		WNWD	well-nourished, well-developed
RLE	right lower extremity		
RR	recovery room		

Diagnostic Laboratory Tests: Normal Values

Test	Normal Values	(SI units)
Serum/Plasma Chemistries		
Arterial blood gases:		
pH	7.35–7.45	7.35–7.45 pH units
pCO_2	35–45 mm Hg	4.7–5.3 kPa
HCO_3	21–28 mEq/L	21–28 mmol/L
pO_2	80–100 mm Hg	10.6–13.3 kPa
	60–70 mm Hg (newborn)	8–10.33 kPa
O_2 saturation	95%–100%	Fraction saturated: > 0.95
	40%–90%	Fraction saturated: 0.4–0.9
Base excess	± 2 mEq/L	±2 mmol/L
AST (aspartate amino-transferase), formerly SGOT	8–35 U/L 16–72 U/L (newborn)	—same— —same—
Bilirubin:		
Direct (conjugated)	0.0–0.4 mg/dl	<5 umol/L
Indirect (unconjugated)	0.2–0.8 mg/dl	3.4–13.6 umol/L
Total	0.3–1 mg/dl	5–17 umol/L
Newborns	6–10 mg/dl	103–171 umol/L
Blood urea nitrogen (BUN)	5–20 mg/dl	1.8–7.1 mmol/L
	4–16 mg/dl (newborn)	1.4–5.7 mmol/L
Calcium (total)	8–10 mg/dl	2.05–2.54 mmol/L
Chloride	98–107 mEq/L	98–107 mmol/L
Cholesterol	120–200 mg/dl	—same—
Creatinine	0.7–1.3 mg/dl	62–115 umol/L
Creatinine phospho-kinase (CPK)	25–175 U/ml	—same—

(table continues on page 772)

Test	Normal Values	(SI units)
CPK isoenzymes	MM (skeletal) band 5–70 U/MB band (cardiac) < 5%	—same— —same—
Erythrocyte sedimentation rate (ESR)	Up to 20 mm/hr	—same—
Erythrocyte indices:		
Mean corpuscular volume 80–96 cu micron/micrometer (MCV)	80–96 fL	
Mean corpuscular hemoglobin (MCH)	27–31 picograms/ cell	27–31 pg
Mean corpuscular hemoglobin concentration (MCHC)	32%–36%	0.32–0.36 (mean concentration fraction)
Reticulocytes	0.5%–1.5% of red cells	0.005–0.15 fraction
Glucose	70–120 mg/dl	3.9–6.7 mmol/L
Hematocrit:		
Newborns	44%–64%	0.44–0.64 (volume fraction)
Infants	30%–40%	0.30–0.40 (volume fraction)
Children	31%–43%	0.31–0.43 (volume fraction)
Men	40%–54%	0.4–0.59 (volume fraction)
Women	38%–47%	0.38–0.47 (volume fraction)
Hemoglobin concentration:		
Newborns	14–24 g/dl	135–240 g/L
Infants	10–15 g/dl	100–150 g/L
Children	11–16 g/dl	110–160 g/L
Men	14–18 g/dl	135–180 g/L
Women	12–16 g/dl	120–160 g/L
Lactic dehydrogenase (LDH)	70–200 IU/L	—same—
Platelet count	150,000– 450,000 cell/ul	$150–450 \times 10^9$/L
Potassium	3.5–5.1 mEq/L	3.5–5.1 mmol/L
Partial thromboplastin time (PTT); (activated APTT)	20–45 seconds	—same—
Prothrombin time	10–13 seconds	—same—
Red blood cells (RBCs):		
Newborns	4.8–7.1 million/ cu mm	4.8–7.1 10^{12}/L

Test	Normal Values	(SI units)
Infants/children	3.8–5.5 million/ cu mm	3.8–5.5 10^{12}/L
Men	4.6–6.2 million/ cu mm	4.6–6.2 10^{12}/L
Women	4.2–5.4 million/ cu mm	4.2–5.4 10^{12}/L
Serum glutamic oxaloacetic transaminase (SGOT)	5–40 U/ml	
Sodium	136–145 mEq/L	136–145 mmol/L
White blood cells (leukocyte 5000– 10,000 cu mm count)		
Neutrophils	60%–70%	0.60–0.70 (mean number fraction)
Eosinophils	1%–4%	0.01–0.04 (mean number fraction)
Basophils	0%–0.5%	0.0–0.005 (mean number fraction)
Lymphocytes	20%–30%	0.20–0.30 (mean number fraction)
Monocytes	2%–6%	0.02–0.06 (mean number fraction)
Urine Chemistry		
Calcium	100–300 mg/24 h	2.5–7.5 mmol/24 h
Creatine	0–200 mg/24 h	< 5.0 mmol/24 h
Creatinine	0.8–2.0 g/24 h	7.1–17.7 mol/24 h
Creatinine clearance	100–150 ml of blood cleared of creatine per minute	
Osmolality	Males: 390– 1090 mM/kg Females: 300– 1090 mM/kg	
Potassium	25–125 mEq/24 h	25–125 mmol/24 h
Protein	40–150 mg/24 h	—same—
Sodium	40–220 mEq/24 h	40–220 mmol/24 h
Urea nitrogen	9–16 g/24 h	90–160 g/L
Uric acid	250–750 mg/24 h	1.48–4.43 mmol/ 24 h

Appendix D

Types of Isolation*

There are two tiers of transmission isolation precautions recommended by the Hospital Infection Control Practices Advisory Committee (HICPAC) and the Centers for Disease Control and Prevention (CDC). The tiers include Standard Precautions, for use with all clients, and Expanded Precautions (formerly Transmission-based Precautions) for clients with known or suspected infections with epidemiologically important pathogens requiring contact precautions, droplet precautions, and airborne infection isolation (AII). Expanded Precautions also includes creating a protective environment (PE) for severely immunocompromised clients.

Standard Precautions, the primary tier in the control of microorganism transmission, combines the major features of universal precautions and body substance isolation. HAND HYGIENE IS REQUIRED WITH ALL CLIENT CONTACT AND WITH ALL FORMS OF ISOLATION.

Standard precautions, in addition to hand hygiene, involves the use of protective equipment (PPE)—barriers and respirators used alone or in combination to protect mucous membranes, skin, and clothing from contact with infectious agents. Standard precautions are applied to blood; all body fluids, secretions, and excretions except sweat, regardless of the presence of visible blood; nonintact skin; and mucous membranes. Standard precautions are based on the principle that not all clients infected with blood-borne pathogens can be reliably identified before the possible exposure of health-care team members. Health-team members are instructed to use standard precautions with all clients and to add expanded precautions when indicated.

Expanded precautions include four types of precautions— airborne, droplet, contact, and, most recently added, protective environment (PE). Expanded precautions are employed if a client is known to have an infection involving highly transmissible pathogens, or the client is immunosuppressed, to interrupt transmission of infection or exposure to pathogens. Creating a PE dif-

*CDC Isolation Guidelines, AJIC, February 1996, pp. 32–52.

fers from the other types of precautions in that the goal of placing a high-risk client in a PE is to prevent the immunosuppressed client from acquiring infections from the environment. The goals of droplet, contact, and airborne precautions are to protect HCWs, visitors, and other clients from acquiring infectious agents from infected clients (see table for PPE required).

Pamphlets, fact sheets or other materials should be prepared to inform the client and significant others of the purpose of expanded precautions, when used. A notice is posted on the door of client's room requesting all visitors to see the nurse prior to entering the room. Expanded precautions involve the use of isolation procedures and appropriate protective equipment when caring for clients with diseases caused by specific microorganisms that are identified by the mode of disease transmission.

Gloves are used when handling any body part with broken skin, body secretion or secretion-soiled item. A gown is added when soiling of clothing is likely. A mask and goggles are worn whenever secretions are projectile or when an infection with a microorganism that is transmitted through air droplet transmission is suspected (an additional mask-precautions notice may be posted). All linens are handled with care to prevent contamination of the nurse's clothing. Reusable items used on clients known to be infected are tagged accordingly when sent for disinfecting.

Many facilities design isolation precaution signs that identify the necessary equipment (eg, the use of gloves, gown, masks, goggles, or special disposal of contaminated materials) in a yes/no format. The following table includes information found on most cards.

● Precautions Used by Health-Care Team Members

Isolation/Precaution Systems	Gloves	Gown	Mask	Goggles	Special Handling of Reusable Equipment
Standard precautions	Y	With possible soiling	If splashing likely	Y with projectile secretions	Y if contaminated with body substances
Expanded precautions	D	D	D	D	D
Contact	Y	Y	Y	Y with secretions	Y
Droplet	Y	Y	Y	Y if splashing	Y if soiled
Airborne	N	Y/D	Y	Y with secretions	Y if soiled

D = depends on disease; N = no, item is not generally required; Y = yes, item is needed in most circumstances (some listed). Some agencies require double-bagging of soiled materials before removal from the room; isolation card should identify these requirements.

Appendix **E**

Medication Interactions: Drug–Drug*

Some drugs (P 450 metabolism) may interact with other similarly metabolized drugs. Administer these medications with caution and explore possible need to avoid administering together. Choose times for drug administration that will place 2 to 4 hours between administering each drug (6 hours after taking extended-release dosage forms). Drugs with P450 metabolism include: amitriptyline, caffeine, haloperidol, theophylline, tacrine, carbamazepine, cyclophosphamide, diazepam, ibuprofen, naproxen, omeprezole, phenytoin, propranolol, tolbutamide, chlorpromazine, codeine, dextromethorphan, encainide, nortriptyline, timolol, verapamil, acetaminophen, ethanol, halothane, amiodarone, cisapride, cocaine, cortisol, cyclosporine, dapsone, dexamethasone, diltiazem, erythromycin, imipramine, lidocaine, lovastatin, nifedipine, progesterone, tacrolimus, tamoxifen, testosterone, valproate, vincristine, warfarin.

Type of Drug (examples)	Interacting Drug Type (examples)	Common Interaction
1. *Analgesics* Acetaminophen	Alcohol	Increased risk of liver damage
Ketoprofen (Orudis) Aspirin	Methotrexate (for cancer chemotherapy)	Increased risk of methotrexate toxicity: fever, mouth sores, low white blood cell production

(table continues on page 778)

*Most interactions included were those known to be severe, with some moderate interactions being noted. The degree of interaction for specific individuals may vary, however, thus this list is not all inclusive. Attempts were made to eliminate duplicate listings.

Type of Drug (examples)	Interacting Drug Type (examples)	Common Interaction
Aspirin Barbiturates amobarbital (Amytal) phenobarbital (Luminal) pentobarbital (Nembutal) and others . . .	Anticoagulants (oral) such as warfarin (Coumadin, Panwarfin)	Increases bleeding Decrease in anti-coagulation effect (Note: if dosage maintained and barbiturates are discontinued bleeding may occur.)
Ibuprofen Indocin	Lithium	Elevated levels of Lithium and risk of toxicity Sx: nausea, slurred speech, muscle twitching . . .
Meperidine (Demerol)	Chlorpromazine (Thorazine)	Increased sedation
2. *Antihyper-tensives* ACE inhibitors enalapril (Vasotec) lisinopril (Zestril) Atenolol (Tenorim) Thiazide drugs Bumex Lasix Hydralazine	Indomethacin (Indocin)	Inhibition of the anti-hypertensive drugs results in lack of control of hyper-tension
3. *Anticoagulants* Oral: dicumarol and warfarin (Coumadin, Panwarfin)	Amiodarone (Cordarone) Aspirin Ibuprofen Diflunisal (Dolobid) Naproxen and other NSAIDs	Increased risk of bleeding; enhanced anticoagulant effect Sx: hematemesis, blood in urine, stool, sputum . . .
4. *Anticonvulsives* Phenytoin (Dilantin)	Amiodarone (Cordarone) Disopyramide (Norpace)	Increased phenytoin levels and toxicity Sx: confusion, rapid eye movement, lack of muscle coordination Dysrhythmia and anti-cholinergic Sx: dry mouth, tachycardia . . .

ref E • Medication Interactions: Drug–Drug   779

Type of Drug (examples)	Interacting Drug Type (examples)	Common Interaction
5. *Antidepressants* Monoamine oxidase (MAO) Inhibitors such as: isocarbox-azid (Marplan) phenelzine (Nardil) tranylcypromine (Parnate) and others	Meperidine (Demerol)	Severe hypotension or hypertension, impaired breathing, convulsions, coma, and death
MAO Inhibitors	Pseudoephedrine Phenylpropanolamine Phenylephrine	(SEE RESP. DRUGS)
MAO Inhibitors Tricyclic drugs amitriptyline (Elavil) doxepin (Sinequan) and others . . .	Metaraminol (Aramine) Guanethidine (Ismelin)	Severe hypertension Hypertension due to the decreased anti-hypertensive effect of Ismelin
6. *Heart medications* Procainamide (Procan SR)	Pyridostigmine (Mestinon) for myasthenia gravis	Decreased effect Pyridostigmine with increased myasthenia gravis symptoms
Quinidine (Quinaglute)	Digoxin (Lanoxin) Digitoxin (Crystodigin)	Increased digoxin/ digitoxin effect Risk for toxicity Sx: poor appetite, visual abnormality, weakness, irregu-lar heart beat
7. *Gastrointestinal meds* Antacids	Anti-infection drugs: Ketoconazole (Nizoral), Tetracyclines. Ex: (Sumycin) (Doxycycline) (Vibramycin)	Reduced absorption with diminished effects of anti-infective drug
Acid Inhibitors Cimetidine (Tagamet)	Theophylline (Theo-Dur, Primatene)	Increased levels of theophylline with risk for toxicity: nausea, tremor, diarrhea, tachycar-dia, seizures

(table continues on page 780)

Type of Drug (examples)	Interacting Drug Type (examples)	Common Interaction
Cimetidine (Tagamet)	Warfarin (Coumadin)	Increased risk of bleeding Sx: blood in emesis, urine, stool
Famotidine (Pepcid) Omeprazole (Prilosec) Rantidine (Zantac)		
Sulcrafate (Carafate)	Varied oral anti-infection drugs: ciprofloxacin (Cipro) norfloxacin (Noroxin)	Decreased effectiveness of anti-infection drugs due to reduced absorption
8. *Antidiabetic drugs* Oral agents: chlorpropamide (Diabinese) glipizide (Glucotrol) glyburide (Micronase)	Sulfonamides Ex: sulfamethoxazole (Bactrim)	Increased effect of antidiabetic drugs, hypoglycemia Sx: tachycardia, tremors, diaphoresis, nausea, convulsions, coma and death
	Phenylbutazone (Butazolidin)	Risk for hypoglycemia
	Alcohol	Increased hypoglycemic effect from anti-diabetic agents with moderate to large intake of alcohol
	Nonselective beta blockers Ex: propranolol (Inderal), pindolol (Viskin), timolol (Blocadren), carteolol (Cartrol), nadolol (Corgard)	May decrease secretion of Insulin, thus reducing effectiveness of antidiabetic drugs resulting in continued or increased hyperglycemia
9. *Respiratory drugs* Theophylline (Primatene, Theo-Dur . . .)	Propranolol (Inderal)	Increased theophylline risk for toxicity Sx: nervousness, tachycardia
Asthma drugs:	Nonspecific beta blockers	Decreased effectiveness of epinephrine and isoproterenol

Type of Drug (examples)	Interacting Drug Type (examples)	Common Interaction
Epinephrine (Primatene, Epifrin) Isoproterenol (Isuprel)	Ex: propranolol (Inderal), pindolol (Viskin), timolol (Blocardren), carteolol (Cartrol), nadolol (Corgard)	Sx: continued respiratory distress or anaphylaxis Hypertension with systemic epinephrine treatment unrelated to allergy
Allergy or cold/ Cough Phenylephrine (Neo-Synephrine, Dristan, Night Relief . . . others)	Several Tricyclic Antidepressants Ex: amitriptyline (Elavil) doxepin (Sinequan)	Acute increase in blood pressure and cardiac contractility Sx: confusion, chest pain, palpitations, headache
Phenylpropanolamine (Allerest, Comtrex, Contac, Triaminic, Dimetapp, Sinarest and others); also diet aids Acutrim and Dexatrim	Antidepressants Monoamine oxidase (MAO) Inhibitors such as: isocarboxazid (Marplan), phenelzine (Nardil), tranylcypromine (Parnate) and others	Severe hypertensive reactions Sx: chest pain, flushing face, lightheadedness
Ephedrine (Primatene, broncholate and others) OR	MAO Inhibitors	Severe hypertension (as above)
Pseudoephedrine (Actifed, Benadryl, Tylenol cold med)	(See above)	(as above)
10. *Antimicrobials* Aminoglycosides Ex: gentamicin (Garamycin), amikacin (Amikin) tobramycin (Nebcin)	Ethacrynic acid (Edecrin)	Increased risk for hearing loss
Chloramphenicol	Oral antidiabetic drugs (Ex: Tobutamide)	Increased effect of antidiabetic drug and hypoglycemia

(table continues on page 782)

Type of Drug (examples)	Interacting Drug Type (examples)	Common Interaction
Ciprofloxacin (Cipro)	Theophylline (Theo-Dur, Primatene)	Increased levels of theophylline = toxicity: nausea, tremor, diarrhea, tachycardia . . .
Erythromycin (E-Mycin)	Cyclosporine (Sandimmune) Amioderone	Increased levels of each drug, and high risk of kidney or liver damage
Ketoconazole (Nizoral) or Troleandomycin (TAO)	Terfenadine (Seldane)	Increased levels of Terfenadine toxicity: dysrhythmia, dizziness . . .
Antituberculosis Drugs: Rifampin (Rifadin)	Immune suppressant cyclosporine (Sandimmune)	Decreased effect of cyclosporine
Rifampin (Rifadin)	Estrogen-containing oral contraceptives (Ex: Ortho Novum)	Decreased effect of contraceptive, high risk of pregnancy
Tetracyclines (Achromycin, Sumycin)	Calcium supplements or medications containing calcium	Reduced absorption and effect of tetracycline

Appendix **F**

Medication Interactions: Drug–Nutrient

Drug	Interaction With Food	Action
Acetaminophen	Ethanol increases hepatotoxicity	Avoid alcohol
Adenosine	Avoid food or drugs with caffeine Increase adenosine's effects	Avoid food or drugs with caffeine (Goody's®, Anacin®, Excedrin®)
Antibiotics		
Amoxicillin	No interaction with food	Take without regard to food
Ampicillin	Food decreases absorption	Take on empty stomach
Azithromycin	Better absorbed on empty stomach, do not give with antacids	Take on empty stomach
Cephalosporins	No interaction with food	Take without regard to food
Dicloxacillin	Food decreases absorption	Take on empty stomach
Erythromycin (take PCE dispertab without food**)	Possible gastric distress	Best if taken on empty stomach but may be taken with food
Fluoroquinolones	Complexes formed when given with iron or dairy products	Avoid iron and dairy products within 2 hours of dose
Nitrofurantoin	Possible gastric distress; improved absorption with food	Should be taken with food
Penicillin	Food decreases absorption (50%–80%)	Take on empty stomach

(table continues on page 784)

783

Drug	Interaction With Food	Action
Sulfonamides		Take with plenty of fluid and on an empty stomach if possible
Tetracycline	Decreased absorption due to chelation by milk, dairy, iron, antacids	Take with plenty of fluid and avoid interacting products
Antihypertensives Propranolol, metoprolol, HCTZ, and hydralazine	Food enhances bioavailability	Take consistently with food
Atovaquone	Absorption of tablets increased 3–4 times when given with fatty foods	Can take with food
Bisacodyl	Milk breaks down protective coating, which may lead to GI irritation	Avoid milk or antacids 1–2 hours before or after dose
Calcium acetate	Food increases absorption	Best if taken on an empty stomach, avoid antacids
Captopril	Food decreases absorption	Take at a constant time in relation to meals
Carbamazepine	Food-induced bile secretions improve drug dissolution	Take with food
Didanosine	Food decreases absorption due to acid secretion	Take on an empty stomach
Estrogens	Administration with food decreases nausea	Take with food
Etidronate	Forms complexes with polyvalent cations in food, decreasing absorption	Avoid food within 2 hours of dose
Griseofulvin	High-fat foods increase absorption	Take with high fat meal or nonskim milk
Hypoglycemics Chlorpropamide Glipizide Glyburide Tolbutamide	Drug takes 30 minutes to be absorbed and become effective	Take 30 minutes before meals

Drug	Interaction With Food	Action
Iron	Decreased absorption with antacids and certain foods (cheese, milk, ice cream)	Best if taken on empty stomach, but if taken with food, avoid interacting products
Isoniazid	Food decreases and delays absorption	Take on an empty stomach
Ketoconazole	Antacids decrease absorption	May be taken without regard to meals, but not with antacids
Levadopa	Decreased absorption with high protein diet	Take on an empty stomach
Lithium	Sodium is exchanged with lithium, which may lead to elevated lithium levels	Avoid abrupt changes in sodium intake or excretion
Lovastatin—excludes other HMGCoA drugs	Food maximizes absorption and increases bioavailability	Take with meals
Methoxsalen	Food impairs absorption	May take with food if nausea occurs, but better absorption on an empty stomach
Metroprolol	Food enhances absorption	Should be taken in a consistent manner with relationship to meals to avoid fluctuations in drugs levels
Mexiletine		Take with food for stomach irritation associated with administration
Monoamine Oxidase Inhibitors Isocarboxazid Tranylcypromine Phenelzine	Potentially life-threatening hypertensive episode due to tyramine interaction	Avoid cheeses, fermented meats, pickled herring, yeast, meat extracts, chianti wine
Moricizine	Food delays absorption	Best if taken on an empty stomach
Morphine	Food increases bioavailability	Take with food

(table continues on page 786)

Drug	Interaction With Food	Action
Nifedipine	Food alters release properties of drug	Take on an empty stomach
NSAIDs diflunisal, fenoprofen, ibuprofen, indomethacin, ketoprofen, meclofenamate, naproxen, piroxicam, salsalate, sulindac, tolmetin	Stomach irritation may occur	Take with food
Olsalazine	Increases residence of drug in body	Take with food
Omeprazole	Food delays absorption	Take on an empty stomach
Ondansetron	Food increases absorption by 17%	Take with food
Phenytoin	May decrease absorption with food	May be taken with or without food, but take consistently with or without food
Potassium (oral)	Stomach irritation and discomfort	Take with plenty of fluid and/or food
Pravastatin		May be taken with or without meals; avoid taking with high-fiber meals
Propafenone	Food increases absorption	Take with food
Quinidine	Possible stomach upset; increased absorption	May take with food if stomach upset occurs; avoid citrus fruit juices
Sotalol	Food decreases absorption	Take on an empty stomach
Sucralfate	Food inhibits therapeutic effects of drug (coats stomach)	Take on an empty stomach 1 hour before meals with plenty of water; avoid antacids 1–2 hours before or after dose

Drug	Interaction With Food	Action
Theophylline	Charcoaled meats cause decreased levels; high-fat foods increase absorption, raising levels	Avoid consumption of barbecued meats during therapy, avoid co-administration with high-fat food
Ticlopidine	High-fat meals in-crease absorption; antacids decrease absorption	Take with food to decrease GI upset
Warfarin	Vitamin K-containing foods (green leafy vegetables, lettuce, broccoli, brussels sprouts) decrease the PT	Avoid large amounts of, or changes in, consumption of vitamin K-containing foods; avoid alcohol
Zalcitibine	Food decreases bioavailability by 14%	Avoid administra-tion with food
Zidovudine	Food decreases con-centration of drug	Take on an empty stomach

Some drugs (P450 metabolism) may interact with grapefruit juice and cruciferous vegetables. Administer medications with water only and caution patient to avoid drinking grapefruit juice 2 hours before and 4 hours after taking these drugs (6 hours after taking extended-release dosage forms). Drugs with P450 metabolism include: amitriptyline, caffeine, haloperidol, theophylline, tacrine, carbamazepine, cyclophosphamide, diazepam, ibuprofen, naproxen, omeprezole, phenytoin, propranolol, tolbutamide, chlorpromazine, codeine, dextromethorphan, encainide, nortriptyline, timolol, verapamil, acetaminophen, ethanol, halothane, amiodarone, cisapride, cocaine, cortisol, cyclosporine, dapsone, dexamethasone, diltiazem, erythromycin, imipramine, lidocaine, lovastatin, nifedipine, progesterone, tacrolimus, tamoxifen, testosterone, valproate, vincristine, warfarin.

Equipment Substitution in the Home

Equipment	Substitution
Bed cradle, footboard	• Folding tray table, cardboard box
Bedrail	• Folding card table with legs under mattress
Male urinal	• Liter plastic soda bottle, cut to enlarge opening, cut edge taped
Electric adjustable bed	• Concrete block under corners of bed to elevate entire bed • Tightly rolled blankets under mattress to elevate head or foot of bed
Heel and elbow protectors	• Heavy-duty socks with padded heels, with the toe cut out
Hand mitts to prevent scratching	• Heavy-duty socks
Ice collar, bag	• Plastic bag of water frozen in desired shape
Linen protector	• Large plastic bag with towel taped on surface touching client
Device to prevent foot drop	• Well-fitted high-top sneakers
IV pole	• Cup hook • Wire hanger • Picture hanger
Trochanter roll	• Large towels rolled and taped
Weights	• Unopened food cans or bags of sugar/flour
Call bell	• Soda can filled with small stones
Medicine organizer and dispenser	• Egg carton, muffin tray

Potential Bioterrorism and Chemical Terrorism Agents Posing Greatest Public Health Threats

Bioterrorism Agents

CDC Category (Human)	Disease	Microorganism	Modes of Transmission	Respiratory	Ocular	GI Tract	Neurologic	Cutaneous	Septicemia	Incubation Period (Days)	Clinical Presentation	Clinical Management
				✓ = Potential Body Systems Affected								
A	**Anthrax**	*Bacillus anthracis*	Inhalation; contaminated foods; infected animals; soil	✓ ◆		✓		✓	✓	1–7	*Flu-like signs; respiratory distress; pustules; scabs; hematemesis; bloody diarrhea; abdominal pain; hypotension; sepsis; shock; death	Aggressive ventilatory support; IV fluids; pharmacological therapy = ciprofloxacin or doxycycline and 1 or 2 additional antimicrobials such as rifampin, vancomycin, penicillin, ampillin, and/or chloramphenicol.

A	**Botulism**	*Clostridium botulinum* toxin (Types A, B, and E)	Inhalation, contaminated foods	✓ ◆	✓	✓	✓	✓	✓	1–5	Muscle weakness; anticholinergic effects (dry mouth, constipation, urinary retention, ileus); descending paralysis; ptosis; diplopia; slurred speech; respiratory failure; death	Gastric decontamination and activated charcoal (if food borne); aggressive ventilatory support; IV fluids; pharmacological therapy = equine botulinum antitoxin (available from CDC and state/local health department)
A	**Plague (bubonic, pneumonic+, and septicimic)**	*Yersinia pestis*	Fleas; inhalation; infected animals	✓ ◆					✓	2–6	*Flu-like signs; enlarged painful lymph nodes; hypotension; pneumonia; respiratory failure; sepsis; shock; death	Isolate infected individual(s); aggressive ventilatory support; IV fluids; pharmacological therapy = streptomycin,

(table continues on page 792)

Bioterrorism Agents (continued)

CDC Category (Human)	Disease	Microorganism	Modes of Transmission	Respiratory	Ocular	GI Tract	Neurologic	Cutaneous	Septicemia	Incubation Period (Days)	Clinical Presentation	Clinical Management
				√ = Potential Body Systems Affected								
A	Smallpox	*Variola major*	Infected humans	√ ♦		√		√		7–17	*Flu-like signs; vomiting; macular rash developing into pustules in the mouth and throat and on the skin; hypotension; death	gentamicin, doxycycline, ciprofloxacin, or chloramphenicol Decontaminate intact skin, eyes, and mucous membranes with copious amounts of water (for skin add soap); IV fluids; there is no specific treatment for smallpox.

	Disease	Agent	Source/Transmission	Marks	Incubation (days)	Signs/Symptoms	Treatment
A	Tularemia	*Francisella tularensis*	Ticks, deer flies, mosquitoes; inhalation; infected animal tissues; contaminated foods: water	✓ ✓♦ ✓ ✓ ✓	1–14	*Flu-like signs; respiratory distress; pneumonia; chest pain; headache; delirium; enlarged painful lymph nodes; purulent conjunctivitis; sepsis; death	Isolate infected individual(s); ventilatory support as needed; decontaminate skin with soap and copious amounts of water; pharmacological therapy = streptomycin, gentamycin, or ciprofloxacin.
A	Viral hemorrhagic fevers	Ebola, Marburg, and Lassa	Infected humans; rodents	♦ ✓ ✓ ✓ ✓ ✓	2–21	*Flu-like signs; fever; headache; vomiting; diarrhea; petechiae; maculopapular rash; hemorrhagic rash; frank bleeding; hypotension; liver damage; renal failure; seizures; shock; coma; death	Isolate infected individual(s); decontaminate skin with soap and copious amounts of water; IV fluids; pharmacological therapy = ribavirin therapy; no antidote or vaccine is available.

*Flu-like signs include fever, body aches, malaise, anorexia, headache, weakness, chills, and sweats.

♦Has been weaponized in aerosolized form.

†Most likely to be used as a bioterrorism agent.

Sources: Centers for Disease Control: http://www.bt.cdc.gov/. PDR Guide to Biological and Chemical Warfare Response.

Chemical Terrorism Agents

Type	Examples of These Agents	Physiological Effects	Respiratory	Ocular	GI Tract	Neurologic	Cutaneous	Septicemia	Clinical Presentation	Latent Period
			✓ = Potential Body Systems Affected							
Nerve Agents (Vapor and Liquid forms)	GA (tabun) GB (sarin) GD (soman) GF VX	Disrupts normal transmission of signals between nerves and receiving organs by blocking acetyl-cholinesterase (responsible for destroying acetylcholine). Acetylcholine typically stimulates muscles and glands. Increased acetylcholine levels cause hyperactivity of muscles and glands.	✓	✓	✓	✓	✓		*Vapor:* (Dose dependent) Miosis; uncontrolled rhinor-rhea; salivation; tearing; sweating; airway constriction (causes SOB and coughing); uncontrolled se-cretions in the airways and GI tract; loss of conscious-ness; convulsions; paraly-sis; respiratory arrest	None (seconds to minutes)
									Liquid: (Dose dependent) skin contact causes sweat-ing and muscular twitching; nausea and vomiting; un-controlled secretions in the airways and GI tract; loss of consciousness; convul-sions; paralysis; respiratory arrest	30 minutes–18 hours

Pulmonary Agents	CG (phosgene) DP (diphosgene) PS (chloropicrin) CL (chlorine)	Damages the alveolar-capillary membranes on inhalation, allowing fluid to leak into the alveolar-capillary interstitial spaces, separating the alveolus from the capillary.	✓	Eye and throat irritation (leads to tearing, coughing, and chest tightness); anxiety; increasing dyspnea and tachypnea as pulmonary edema worsens; cyanosis; hypotension	2–24 hours
Cyanide Agents	AC (Hydrogen Cyanide) CK (cyanogens chloride)	Cyanide is distributed in the blood to the cells of organs and tissues and prevents intracellular oxygenation.	✓ ✓	*Low concentrations:* cause an increased RR and depth; dizziness; nausea; vomiting; and severe headaches *High concentrations:* increased RR and depth within 15 seconds of exposure; convulsions within 30–45 seconds; respiratory arrest within 2–4 minutes; cardiac arrest within 4–8 minutes	None (If dose is high, death can occur in 6 to 8 mins.)

(table continues on page 796)

Chemical Terrorism Agents (continued)

Type	Examples of These Agents	Physiological Effects	Potential Body Systems Affected — Respiratory	Ocular	GI Tract	Neurologic	Cutaneous	Septicemia	Clinical Presentation	Latent Period
Vesicant Agents (Vapor and Liquid forms)	H or HD (sulfur mustard) L (Lewisite) CX (phosgene oxime)*	Causes tissue damage upon contact.	✓	✓	✓	✓	✓	✓	Dose dependent: Skin erythema; vesicles (domed-shaped blisters); mild to severe conjunctivitis; photophobia; mild upper respiratory tract irritation to severe airway tissue damage leading to necrosis and hemorrhage; nausea and vomiting; CNS effects ranging from convulsions to sluggishness	2–48 hours

✓ = Potential Body Systems Affected

*CX does produces lesions, not vesicles.

Sources: Centers for Disease Control: http://www.bt.cdc.gov/. PDR Guide to Biological and Chemical Warfare Response.

NANDA-Approved Nursing Diagnoses

This list represents the NANDA-approved nursing diagnoses for critical use and testing.

Activity Intolerance
Activity Intolerance, Risk for
Adjustment, Impaired
Airway Clearance, Ineffective
Allergy Response, Latex
Allergy Response, Risk for Latex
Anxiety
Anxiety, Death
Aspiration, Risk for
Attachment, Risk for Impaired Parent/Infant/Child
Autonomic Dysreflexia
Autonomic Dysreflexia, Risk for
Body Image, Disturbed
Body Temperature, Risk for Imbalanced
Bowel Incontinence
Breastfeeding, Effective
Breastfeeding, Ineffective
Breastfeeding, Interrupted
Breathing Pattern, Ineffective
Cardiac Output, Decreased
Caregiver Role Strain
Caregiver Role Strain, Risk for
Comfort, Impaired
Communication, Impaired Verbal
Conflict, Decisional
Conflict, Parental Role
Confusion, Acute
Confusion, Chronic
Constipation
Constipation, Perceived
Constipation, Risk for
Coping, Ineffective

Coping, Ineffective Community
Coping, Readiness for Enhanced Community
Coping, Defensive
Coping, Compromised Family
Coping, Disabled Family
Coping, Readiness for Enhanced Family
Denial, Ineffective
Dentition, Impaired
Development, Risk for Delayed
Diarrhea
Disuse Syndrome, Risk for
Diversional Activity, Deficient
Energy Field, Disturbed
Environmental Interpretation Syndrome, Impaired
Failure to Thrive, Adult
Falls, Risk for
Family Processes: Alcoholism, Dysfunctional
Family Processes: Interrupted
Fatigue
Fear
Fluid Volume, Deficient
Fluid Volume, Excess
Fluid Volume, Risk for Deficient
Fluid Volume, Risk for Imbalanced
Gas Exchange, Impaired
Grieving
Grieving, Anticipatory
Grieving, Dysfunctional
Growth and Development, Delayed
Growth, Risk for Disproportionate
Health Maintenance, Risk for Ineffective
Health-Seeking Behaviors
Home Maintenance, Impaired
Hopelessness
Hyperthermia
Hypothermia
Identity, Disturbed Personal
Incontinence, Functional Urinary
Incontinence, Reflex Urinary
Incontinence, Risk for Urge Urinary
Incontinence, Stress Urinary
Incontinence, Total Urinary
Incontinence, Urge Urinary
Infant Behavior, Disorganized
Infant Behavior, Readiness for Enhanced Organized
Infant Behavior, Risk for Disorganized
Infant Feeding Pattern, Ineffective
Infection, Risk for
Injury, Risk for

Injury, Risk for Perioperative-Positioning
Intracranial, Adaptive Capacity, Decreased
Knowledge, Deficient
Loneliness, Risk for
Memory, Impaired
Mobility, Impaired Bed
Mobility, Impaired Physical
Mobility, Impaired Wheelchair
Nausea
Neglect, Unilateral
Noncompliance
Nutrition: Less Than Body Requirements, Imbalanced
Nutrition: More Than Body Requirements, Imbalanced
Oral Mucous Membrane, Impaired
Pain, Acute
Pain, Chronic
Parenting, Impaired
Parenting, Risk for Impaired
Peripheral Neurovascular Dysfunction, Risk for
Poisoning, Risk for
Post-Trauma Syndrome
Post-Trauma Syndrome, Risk for
Powerlessness
Powerlessness, Risk for
Protection, Ineffective
Rape-Trauma Syndrome
Rape-Trauma Syndrome: Compound Reaction
Rape-Trauma Syndrome: Silent Reaction
Relocation Stress Syndrome
Relocation Stress Syndrome, Risk for
Role Performance, Ineffective
Self-Care Deficit
Self-Care Deficit, Bathing/Hygiene
Self-Care Deficit, Feeding
Self-Care Deficit, Toileting
Self-Esteem, Chronic Low
Self-Esteem, Situational Low
Self-Esteem, Risk for Situational Low
Self-Mutilation
Self-Mutilation, Risk for
Sensory Perception, Disturbed
Sexual Dysfunction
Sexuality Patterns, Ineffective
Skin Integrity, Impaired
Skin Integrity, Risk for Impaired
Sleep Deprivation
Sleep Pattern, Disturbed
Social Interaction, Impaired

Social Isolation
Sorrow, Chronic
Spiritual Distress
Spiritual Distress, Risk for
Spiritual Well-Being, Readiness for Enhanced
Suffocation, Risk
Suicide, Risk for
Surgical Recovery, Delayed
Swallowing, Impaired
Therapeutic Regimen Management, Effective
Therapeutic Regimen Management, Ineffective
Therapeutic Regimen Management, Ineffective Community
Therapeutic Regimen Management, Ineffective Family
Thermoregulation, Ineffective
Thought Processes, Disturbed
Tissue Perfusion, Ineffective
Transfer Ability, Impaired
Trauma, Risk for
Urinary Elimination, Impaired
Urinary Retention
Ventilation, Impaired Spontaneous
Ventilatory Weaning Response, Dysfunctional (DVWR)
Violence, Risk for Other-Directed
Violence, Risk for Self-Directed
Walking, Impaired
Wandering

Bibliography

Adams, G., et al. (2000). Maximizing tolerance of enteral nutrition in severely injured trauma patients: A comparison of enteral feeding by means of percutaneous endoscopic gastrostomy versus percutaneous endoscopic gastrojejunostomy. *Journal of Trauma: Injury, Infection, and Critical Care, 48*(3), 459–465.

Altman, G. (2004). *Delmar's fundamental and advanced nursing skills* (2nd ed.). Clifton Park, NY: Delmar Thomson Learning.

American Nurses Association. (2002). *American Nurses Association's needlestick prevention guide.* Washington, D.C.: Author.

American Association for Respiratory Care (AARC). (1991). AARC clinical practice guideline: Incentive spirometry. *Respiratory Care, 36,* 1402–1405.

American Thoracic Society (1990). *Home mechanical ventilation of pediatric patients.* Retrieved December 17, 2003 from http://www.thoracic.org/adobe/statements/home1-2.pdf.

Amputee Resource Foundation of America, Inc. (2004). *Frequently asked questions.* Available at www.amputeeresource.org.

Anderson, D. J. & Webster, C. S. (2001). A systems approach to the reduction of medication error in the hospital. *Journal of Advanced Nursing, 35*(1), 34–41.

Armstrong, V. L. (2001). *Teaching pediatric tube feeding to care-givers.* Available at www.rosslearningcenter.com.

Atsuko, O. (2000). Intravenous line management and prevention of catheter-related infections in America: A cross-cultural seminar. *Journal of IV Nursing, 23*(3), 170–175.

Barber, P. (2003). Oh, my achin'. . . . at high risk for back injuries, nurses can prevent problems by practicing proper body mechanics and pushing for assistive technology, lift teams in their facilities. *Nurse Week (South Central), 8*(1), 16–17.

Barkley, T. W., & Myers, C. M. (2002). *Practice guidelines for acute care nurse practitioners.* Philadelphia: W. B. Saunders.

Bastin, R., Moraine, J., Bardocsky, G., Kahn, R., & Melot, C. (1997). Incentive spirometry performance: A reliable indicator of pulmonary function in the early postoperative period after lobectomy? *Chest, 111*(3), 559–563.

Beyerle, K. (2001). Focus on autotransfusion. *Nursing, 31*(12), 49–51.

Bjorvell, C., Wredling, R., & Thorell-Ekstrand, I. (2003). Prerequisites and consequences of nursing documentation in patient records as perceived by a group of Registered Nurses. *Journal of Clinical Nursing, 12,* 206–214.

Bick, D., & Stephens, F. (2003). Pressure ulcer risk: Audit findings. *Nursing Standard, 17*(44), 63–64, 66, 68, 70, 72.

Bonomini, J. (2003). Effective interventions for pressure ulcer prevention. *Nursing Standard, 17*(52), 45–50, 52, 54.

Callaghan, S., Copnell, B., & Johnston, L. (2002). Comparison of two methods of peripheral intravenous cannula securement in the pediatric setting. *Journal of Infusion Nursing, 25*(4), 256–264.

Camara, D. (2001). Minimizing risks associated with peripherally inserted central catheters in NICU. *American Journal of Maternal Child Nursing, 26*(1), 17–22.

Carpenito, L. (2003). *Nursing diagnosis: Application to clinical practice* (9th ed.). Philadelphia: Lippincott Williams & Wilkins.

Choate, K., Barbetti, J., & Sandford, M. (2003). Tracheostomy: Your questions answered. *Australian Nursing Journal, 10*(11), 1–4.

Clark, P. Rennie, I. & Rawlinson, S. (2001). Effect of a formal education programme on safety of transfusions. *British Medical Journal, 323*(7321), 1118–1120.

Conlan, A. A., & Kope, S. E. (2000). Tracheostomy in the ICU. *Journal of Intensive Care Medicine, 15*(1), 1–13.

Craven, R. F., & Hirnle, C. J. (2003). *Fundamentals of nursing: Human health and function* (4th ed.). Philadelphia: Lippincott Williams & Wilkins.

Cross, M. H. (2001). Autotransfusion in cardiac surgery. *Perfusion, 16,* 391–400.

Dobson, P. (2001). A model for home infusion therapy initiation and maintenance. *Journal of Infusion Nursing, 24*(6), 385–394.

Doenges, M. E., Moorhouse, M. F., & Geissler-Murr, A. C. (2002). *Nurse's pocket guide: Diagnoses, interventions, and rationales* (8th ed.). Philadelphia: F. A. Davis.

Dougherty, L. (2002). Delivery of intravenous therapy. *Nursing Standard, 16*(6), 45–52, 54, 56.

Dowding, D. (2001). Examining the effects that manipulating information given in the change of shift report has on nurses' care planning ability. *Journal of Advanced Nursing, 33*(6), 836–846.

Dreger, V., & Tremback, T. (1998). Blood and blood product use in perioperative patient care. *AORN Online, 67*(1), 154–190.

Fernandez, R. S., Griffiths, R. D., & Murie, P. (2003) Peripheral venous catheters: A review of current practices. *Journal of Infusion Nursing, 26*(6), 388–392.

Fish, J. (2003). *Tube feeding in the ICU: Overcoming the obstacles.* Available at www.rosslearningcenter.com.

Frey, A. M. (2003). Drawing blood samples from vascular access devices: Evidence-based practice. *Journal of Infusion Nursing, 26*(5), 285–293.

Gauthier, D. M (1999). The healing potential of back massage. *Online Journal of Knowledge Synthesis for Nursing, 6*(5).

Genesis Health System (2003). *How to use an incentive spirometer.* Retrieved December 1, 2003 from http://www.genesishealth.com/micromedex/quickdisease/nd0427.aspx?style=po.

Genzyme Biosurgery (2003). *Thoracic surgery: Pleur-evac chest drainage systems.* Retrieved December 1, 2003 from http://www.genzymebiosurgery.com/prod/cardio/gzbx_p_pt_cardio-thorac.asp.

Grant, M. J., & Martin, S. (2000). Delivery of enteral nutrition. *AACN Clinical Issues: Advanced Practice in Acute Critical Care, 11*(4), 507–516.

Hadaway, L. C. (2003). Skin flora and infection. *Journal of Infusion Nurses, 26*(1), 44–48.

Hammond, D. (1998). Home intravenous antibiotics: The safety factor. *Journal of IV Nursing, 21*(2), 81–95.

Hogan, M. A., & Wane, D. (2003). *Fluids, electrolytes, and acid-base balance: Reviews and rationales.* Upper Saddle River, NJ: Pearson Prentice Hall.

Intravenous Nurses Society. (2000). *Infusion nursing standards of practice.* Cambridge, MA: Intravenous Nurses Society.

Intravenous Nurses Society. (2000). Infusion nursing standards of practice. *Journal of Intravenous Nursing, 23*(6S).

JACE Systems. *JACE universal CPM–K100. Operating manual.* Cherry Hill, NJ: Author.

Jarvis, C. (2003). *Physical examination and health assessment* (4th ed.). St. Louis: Saunders.

Josephson, D. L. (2004). *Intravenous infusion therapy for nurses: Principles and practice* (2nd ed.). Clifton Park, NY: Thompson Delmar Learning

The Kendall Company. 15 Hampshire St. Mansfield, Massachusetts 02048 (SCD Response).

Klein, T. (2001). PICC's and midlines: Fine-tuning your care. *RN, 64*(8), 26–29.

Lewis, S. M., Heitkemper, M. M., & Dirksen, S. R. (2004). *Medical-surgical nursing: Assessment and management of clinical problems* (6th ed.). St. Louis: Mosby.

Lezon, K. (1999). Teaching incentive spirometry. *Nursing 99, 1,* 60–61.

Lynn-McHale, D. & Carlson, K. (Eds.) (2001). *American Association of Critical-Care Nurses: AACN procedure manual for critical care* (4th ed.). Philadelphia: W. B. Saunders.

Maher, A. B., Salmond, S. W., & Pellino, T. A. (2002). *Orthopaedic nursing* (3rd ed.). Philadelphia: W. B. Saunders.

Manias, E. (2003). Pain and anxiety management in postoperative gastro-surgical setting. *Journal of Advanced Nursing, 41*(6), 585–594.

Mason, D. J. (2003). Our aching backs: The rate of back injuries among nurses is soaring and inexcusable. *American Journal of Nursing, 103*(2), 11.

McConnell, E. A. (2002). Clinical do's and don'ts: Providing tracheostomy care. *Nursing 2002,* 17.

Metheny, N. A., & Titler, M. G. (2001). Assessing placement of feeding tubes. *American Journal of Nursing, 101*(5), 36–44.

Miller, L. (2002). Effective communication with older people. *Nursing Standard, 17*(9), 45–50, 53, 55.

Monarch, K. (2002). Legal aspects of infusion practice: Trends and issues. *Journal of Infusion Nursing, 25*(6 Supplement), S21–S30.

Murray, M. (1993). Principles of caring for residents with feeding tubes. *Nursing Homes, 42*(9), 37–39.

Myers, F., & Parini, S. (2003). Hand hygiene: understanding and implementing the CDC's new guideline. *Nursing Management, 34*(4), Suppl. 2, 3–16.

National Guideline Clearinghouse. (2002). *Prevention of thromboembolism in spinal cord injury.* Available at www.guideline.gov.

National Institute for Occupational Safety and Health. (2002). *Violence in the workplace: Occupational hazards in hospitals.* DHHS (NIOSH) Publication No. 2002-101. Retrieved July 16, 2003 from http://www.cdc.gov/niosh/2002-101.html.

National Institutes of Health. (2000). *Critical care therapy and respiratory therapy care section: Incentive spirometry.* Retrieved December 17, 2003 from http://www.cc.nih.gov/ccmd/pdf_doc/Bronchial%20hygiene/02-Incentive%20Spirometry.pdf.

Nettina, S. M. (Ed.). (2000). *The Lippincott manual of nursing practice* (7th ed.). Philadelphia: Lippincott.

North American Nursing Diagnosis Association (NANDA). (2003). *Nursing diagnoses: Definitions and classifications 2003–2004.* Philadelphia: NANDA International.

Oeltjen, A. M., & Santrach, P. (1997). Autologous transfusion techniques. *Journal of Intravenous Nursing, 20*(6), 305–310.

Overend, T. J., Anderson, C. M., Lucy, S. D., Bhatia, C., Jonsson, B. I., & Timmerman, C. (2001). The effect of incentive spirometry on postoperative pulmonary complications: A systematic review. *Chest, 120*(3), 971–978.

Ozawa, S., Shander, A., & Ochani, T. D. (2001). A practical approach to achieving bloodless surgery. *AORN Journal, 74*(1), 34–46.

Paice, J. A. (2002). Managing psychological conditions in palliative care. *American Journal of Nursing, 102*(11), 36–42.

Parker, L. (2002). Management of intravascular devices to prevent infection. *British Journal of Nursing, 11*(4), 240, 242–244, 246.

Passy-Muir. (2003). *Passy-Muir tracheostomy and ventilator speaking valves instruction booklet.* Retrieved December 2, 2003 from www.passy-muir.com/PDF%20Files/PMInternational Booklet.pdf.

Pennels, C. (2001). The art of recording patient care information. *Professional Nurse, 16*(9), 1359–1361.

Perry, A. & Potter, P. (2002). *Clinical nursing skills and techniques* (5th ed.). St. Louis: Mosby.

Pitorak, E. F. (2003). Care at the time of death: How nurses can make the last hours of life a richer, more comfortable experience. *American Journal of Nursing, 103*(7), 42–52.

Pomfret, I. (2000). Catheter care in the community. *Nursing Standard, 14*(27), 46–52.

Potter, P., Schallom, M., Davis, S., Sona, C., & McSweeney, M. (2003). Evaluation of chemical dot thermometers for measuring body temperature of orally intubated patients. *American Journal of Critical Care, 12*(5), 403–407.

Ralph, S., Craft-Rosenberg, M., Herdman, T., & Lavin, M. (2003–2004). *Nursing diagnoses: Definitions and classification.* Philadelphia: NANDA International.

Robinson, J. (2001). Urethral catheter selection. *Nursing Standard, 15*(25), 39–42.

Roe, S. (2003). *Delmar's clinical nursing skills and concepts.* Clifton Park, NY: Thompson Delmar Learning.

Scale-Tronix. 200 E. Post Road, White Plains, NY 10601 (Scale-Tronix Sling-Scale).

Seeman, S., & Reinhardt, A. (2000). Blood sample collection from a peripheral catheter system compared with phlebotomy. *Journal of Intravenous Nursing, 23*(5), 290–297.

Sheehan, D., & Schirm, V. (2003). End-of-life care of older adults: Debunking some common misconceptions about dying in old age. *American Journal of Nursing, 103*(11), 48–58.

Sheehan, J. (2001). Delegating to UAPs—A practical guide. *RN, 64*(11), 65–66.

Simpson, L. (2001). Indwelling urethral catheters. *Art & Science: Continuing Professional Development: Incontinence, 15*(46), 47–54, 56.

Smith, S. F., Duell, D. J., & Martin, B. C. (2004). *Clinical nursing skills: Basic to advanced skills* (6th ed.). Upper Saddle River, NJ: Pearson Prentice Hall.

Steinhauer, R. (2002). Bioterrorism. *RN, 65*(3), 48–55.

Stillwell, S. (2002). *Mosby's critical care nursing reference* (3rd ed.). St. Louis: Mosby.

Stone, J. T., Wyman, J. F., & Salisbury, S. A. (1999). *Clinical gerontological nursing: A guide to advance practice* (2nd ed.). Philadelphia: W. B. Saunders.

Stroud, M, Duncan, H., & Nightingale, J. (2003). Guidelines for enteral feeding in adult hospital patients. *Gut, 52*(Suppl. VII), vii1–vii2.

Teleflex Medical, Inc. (2003). *Fluid drainage with the Pleur-evac Sahara Chest Drainage System* (Media file). Fall River, MA: Author.

Truog, R. D., Cist, R., F., Brackett, S. E., et al. (2001). Recommendations for end-of-life care in the intensive care unit: The ethics committee of the Society of Critical Care Medicine. *Critical Care Medicine, 29*(12), 2332–2348.

U.S. Department of Health and Human Services, Centers for Disease Control and Prevention. (2002). Guideline for hand hygiene in health-care settings: Recommendations of the Healthcare Infection Control Practices Advisory Committee and the HICPAC/SHEA/APIC/IDSA Hand Hygiene Task Force. *Morbidity and Mortality Weekly Report, 51*(No. RR-16), 1–44.

U.S. Department of Health and Human Services, Centers for Disease Control and Prevention. (2003). Guidelines for environmental infection control in health-care facilities: Recommendations of CDC and Healthcare Infection Control Practices Advisory Committee (HICPAC). *Morbidity and Mortality Weekly Report, 52*(RR-10), 1–43.

U.S. Department of Health and Human Services, Centers for Disease Control and Prevention. (2003). *PDR guide to biological and chemical warfare response.* Available at http://www.bt.cdc.gov/.

U.S. Department of Health and Human Services, U.S. Food & Drug Administration, Center for Biologics Evaluation and Research. (2004). *Information sheet: Options for arm preparation.* Retrieved May 1, 2004 from http://www.fda.gov/CBER/blood/armpreprev.htm.

U.S. Department of Health & Human Services (Office of Civil Rights). (2003). *Protecting the privacy of patients' health information (fact sheet).* Available at http://www.hhs.gov/ocr/hipaa/; http://www.hhs.gov/news/facts/privacy.html.

Van Slyck, A., & Johnson, K. R. (2001). Using patient acuity data to manage patient care outcomes and patient care costs. *Outcomes Management for Nursing Practice, 5(1),* 36–40.

Virani, R., & Sofer, D. (2003). Improving the quality of end-of-life-care: Making changes at every level. *American Journal of Nursing, 103*(5), 52–60.

Wilkinson, J., & Wilkinson, C. (2001). Administration of blood transfusions to adults in general hospital settings: A review of the literature. *Journal of Clinical Nursing, 10*(2), 161–170.

Woodrow, P. (2002). Managing patients with a tracheostomy in acute care. *Nursing Standard, 16*(44), 39–48.

Woodruff, D. (2003). Protect your patient while he's receiving mechanical ventilation. *Nursing 2003, 33*(7), 32–34.

Zerwekh, J. V. (1997). Do dying patients really need IV fluids? *American Journal of Nursing, 97*(3), 26–30.

Index

Note: Page numbers followed by *f*, *t*, and *d* indicate figures, tables, and displays, respectively.